Historical Perspectives on the Role of the MRC

Essays in the history of the Medical Research Council
of the United Kingdom and its predecessor,
the Medical Research Committee, 1913–1953

Edited by

JOAN AUSTOKER
Cancer Research Campaign Science Policy Research Unit
Dept of Community Medicine and General Practice
University of Oxford

and

LINDA BRYDER
Dept of History, University of Auckland
Auckland, New Zealand

OXFORD   NEW YORK   TOKYO
OXFORD UNIVERSITY PRESS
1989

Oxford University Press, Walton Street, Oxford OX2 6DP
Oxford   New York   Toronto
Delhi   Bombay   Calcutta   Madras   Karachi
Petaling Jaya   Singapore   Hong Kong   Tokyo
Nairobi   Dar es Salaam   Cape Town
Melbourne   Auckland
and associated companies in
Berlin Ibadan

Oxford is a trade mark of Oxford University Press

Published in the United States
by Oxford University Press, New York

British Library Cataloguing in Publication Data
Historical perspectives on the role of the MRC.
1. Great Britain. Medicine. Research organisations:
Medical research council, to 1970
I. Austoker, Joan.   II. Bryder, Linda
610'.72041
ISBN 0-19-261651-X

Library of Congress Cataloging-in-Publication Data
Historical perspectives on the role of the MRC: essays in the history
of the Medical Research Council of the United Kingdom and its
predecessor, the Medical Research Committee, 1913–1953/edited by
Joan Austoker and Linda Bryder
1. Medical Research Council (Great Britain)—History.
I. Austoker, Joan.   II. Bryder, Linda.
R772.A6H57   1989   610'.72041—dc19   89-3122
ISBN 0-19-261651-X

Phototypeset by Dobbie Typesetting Limited, Plymouth, Devon
Printed in Great Britain
by Biddles Ltd,
Guildford & King's Lynn

Historical Perspectives
on the Role of the MRC

Preface

The Medical Research Committee was set up by the Government in 1913; in 1919 the Committee became the Medical Research Council (MRC). The aim of this book is to discuss the role of the MRC in shaping a national system of medical research in Britain. The lines of research adopted by the MRC are not self-evident but require explanation, and the essays in this volume explore why certain areas of research were favoured over others. It will be seen that resources were not divided equally in all possible areas of research. The influence exerted by administrators, particularly the MRC Secretaries, in the formulation of research policy is examined, as well as external influences such as the two world wars. The MRC's self-professed aim from the 1920s was primarily to promote basic biomedical research. However, its involvement extended over a wide range of medical problems and these essays examine the way in which through its medical research the MRC became involved with broader social problems. The essays explore the relationship and interaction between the MRC and the various other bodies concerned with medical research and its practical application, such as the Ministry of Health (also established in 1919), the universities, the Royal Colleges of Physicians and Surgeons, the Colonial Office, industry, and certain pharmaceutical companies.

The only general history of the MRC is that by A. Landsborough Thomson, who produced two volumes entitled *Half a Century of Medical Research. Vol. I. The Origins and Policy of the Medical Research Council (UK)* (London: HMSO, 1973) and *Half a Century of Medical Research. Vol. II. The Programme of the Medical Research Council (UK)* (1975, HMSO, London). Thomson joined the staff of the Committee in 1919 and was closely involved with the Council for the next forty years. This involvement gave him a unique knowledge of the inside workings of the MRC. However, it also made it difficult for him to distance himself from events when he came to writing its history. Moreover, Thomson is not, nor does he claim to be, a professional historian who has studied the history of medical research in its broader context.

The essays in this volume are selective; chosen to illustrate and highlight the directions of research and the role of the MRC in the first half of the twentieth century. We have drawn on the expertise of historians who are working on specific medical issues and who have made detailed studies of the part played by the MRC in their own particular field of interest. Having made a special study of a particular medical problem, they are able to place the work of the MRC in the context of national or international activities. It was felt that such a collective effort was essential if justice was to be done to the complex operations of research conducted by the MRC.

In the first chapter Linda Bryder discusses the origins of the Medical Research Committee, the original intentions to focus primarily on tuberculosis research, and the subsequent relative neglect of this area of research despite the persistence of tuberculosis as a medical problem. In chapter two Joan Austoker discusses the role of the first Secretary of the Medical Research Committee and Council (1913–33), Sir Walter Morley Fletcher, explaining his dominating influence over all aspects of MRC policy. It is clear that Fletcher set the parameters of future research by the Council. A third of the funds for medical research provided by the State were allocated to finance a central institute, and in chapter three Austoker and Bryder explore the lines of research undertaken at the National Institute for Medical Research, the central institute of the MRC. In the following chapter Bryder discusses the involvement of the MRC in bacteriology and public health research. She shows how such research advanced in relation to non-civilians during the First World War, but not until the late 1930s did the MRC evince an interest in public health research among the civilian population, and that it was the Second World War which provided the impetus for the setting up of the Emergency Public Health Laboratory Service from which the permanent Public Health Laboratory Service grew. In her contribution Celia Petty relates how the MRC moved rapidly to the forefront in nutritional research at an international level, but she also suggests how such scientific data were used to reinforce current prejudices regarding working-class ignorance and inefficiency and explains that where steps were taken to apply the 'newer knowledge of nutrition' the results were either irrelevant or counter-productive. A similar story is told by Jennifer Beinart in the colonial context, where researchers remained too preoccupied with laboratory research and showed themselves to be little aware of broader social ramifications of the medical problems that they were investigating. Helen Jones investigates the MRC's involvement in industrial health research, explaining how despite the sophisticated and elaborate research carried out by the MRC's Industrial Health Research Board, the research remained academic, little infuencing developments in industry. In its research into drugs the MRC interacted with pharmaceutical companies, and Jonathan Liebenau investigates an aspect of that interaction in his discussion of the MRC's involvement in the production of salvarsan and more especially insulin. One area in which the MRC became involved in clinical research was in radium therapy. David Cantor shows how the Council's involvement in this research brought it into conflict with the Royal Colleges of Physicians and Surgeons and how this conflict shaped experimental research in the biological effects of radiation. Sir Christopher Booth examines the wider involvement of the MRC in the field of clinical research, arguing that the MRC's contribution was valuable although at times the MRC was criticized for its lack of commitment to this vital area of medical research.

Many people assisted in the production of this volume. In particular, the editors would like to thank Sir Austin Bradford Hill, Dr Charles Fletcher, Dr Philip Mortimer, and Dr B. S. Lush, for their generous advice and assistance, and Mrs Mary Nicholas of the central MRC archives, Mr Robert Moore of the National Institute for Medical Research and the staff of the Rockefeller Archive Center, New York, for their archival guidance. Linda Bryder would also like to acknowledge with gratitude the financial support of the Queen's College, Oxford, and the British Academy for the British Academy Post-doctoral Fellowship which enabled her to work on this volume. Both editors would like to thank Dr Charles Webster and other members of the Wellcome Unit for the History of Medicine, Oxford, for general support and advice.

Oxford   J. A.
1988   L. B.

Contents

List of Contributors

Dr Joan Austoker
Cancer Research Campaign Science Policy Research Unit, Department of Community Medicine and General Practice, Oxford

Jennifer Beinart
Wellcome Unit for the History of Medicine, 45–47 Banbury Road, Oxford OX2 6PE

Sir Christopher Booth
Clinical Research Centre, Watford Road, Harrow HA1 3UJ

Dr Linda Bryder
Department of History, University of Auckland, New Zealand

Dr David Cantor
ARC Epidemiology Research Unit, Stopford Building (University of Manchester), Oxford Road, Manchester M13 9PT

Dr Helen Jones
Department of Sociology, Eleanor Rathbone Building, Myrtle Street, PO Box 147, Liverpool L69 3BX

Dr Jonathan Liebenau
Department of Information Systems, London School of Economics, Houghton Street, London WC2A 2AE

Dr Celia Petty
Centre for Human Nutrition, London School of Hygiene and Tropical Medicine, Keppel Street, London WC1E 7HT

Abbreviations

ASCC	American Society for the Control of Cancer
BDH	British Drug Houses
BECC	British Empire Cancer Campaign
BMA	British Medical Association
BMJ	*British Medical Journal*
CCHE	Central Council for Health Education
CCPR	Central Council for Physical Recreation
CIPD	Committee on Industrial Pulmonary Disease
CMAC	Contemporary Medical Archive Centre
CMO	Chief Medical Officer of the Ministry of Health
Colonial MRC	Colonial Medical Research Committee
DSIR	Department of Scientific and Industrial Research
EEF	Engineering Employers' Federation
EPHLS	Emergency Public Health Laboratory Service
HMWC	Ministry of Munitions' Health of Munitions Workers' Committee
HOSC	Chief Medical Officer of the Board of Education, *Annual Report, Health of the School Child*
ICRF	Imperial Cancer Research Fund
IFRB	Industrial Fatigue Research Board
IHRB	Industrial Health Research Board
ILM	Institute of Labour (now Personnel) Management
IWS	Industrial (Welfare) Society
LCC	London County Council
LGB	Local Government Board
LSHTM	London School of Hygiene and Tropical Medicine
MAB	Metropolitan Asylums Board
MOH	Medical Officer of Health
MRC	Medical Research Council
MRC PF	MRC Archives, Personal Files
MRC *SRS*	MRC *Special Report* Series
MRS	Medical Research Society
NAPT	National Association for the Prevention of Tuberculosis
NHS	National Health Service
NIIP	National Institute of Industrial Psychology
NIMR	National Institute for Medical Research
PHLS	Public Health Laboratory Service

PRO	Public Record Office, Kew
PRO CO	Public Record Office, Colonial Office Files
PRO MH	Public Record Office, Ministry of Health Files
PRU	Pneumokoniosis Research Unit
SAC	BECC's Scientific Advisory Committee
SRS	Special Report Series
TRC	Therapeutic Research Corporation
TTC	Therapeutic Trials Committee
TUC	Trades Union Congress
UCH	University College Hospital

1

Tuberculosis and the MRC

LINDA BRYDER

The Medical Research Committee was set up with a fund provided by the Government in Part I of the 1911 National Insurance Act. The money for medical research was included in the clauses in the Act relating to the control of tuberculosis. Landsborough Thomson argued in his history of the MRC that the inclusion in this section of the Act was merely a 'drafting convenience', that research was never meant to be confined to tuberculosis.[1] In this chapter it is argued that those formulating the 1911 National Insurance Act had tuberculosis specifically in mind when they set aside a fund for medical research. It was only subsequently that the opportunity was seized by medical scientists to broaden the scope of medical research. The process by which this occurred is discussed, and the subsequent research into tuberculosis is investigated, as an indication of the research priorities of this State-funded medical research organization.

The 1911 National Insurance Act and the Medical Research Committee

Part I of the 1911 National Insurance Act provided sickness and disability benefits and free medical treatment by general practitioners for all insured workers although not for their dependants. Two particular problem areas were isolated which received special attention under the Act. The first was maternity, and it was resolved to give insured workers a lump sum on the birth of each child (if both parents worked the amount was increased). The second was tuberculosis, and it was decided to provide free institutional treatment for this disease, for dependants of the insured as well as the insured themselves (called 'sanatorium benefit').

Introducing the 1911 National Insurance Act, David Lloyd George, Chancellor of the Exchequer, singled out tuberculosis as a problem warranting special consideration. He pointed out that, as a long drawn-out disease to which young people were susceptible and which was killing 75 000

---

[1] Landsborough Thomson, A. (1973). *Half a century of medical research*, Vol. I, *Origins and policy of the Medical Research Council (UK)*, p.12. HMSO, London.

people per annum in Great Britain and Ireland, tuberculosis could become a serious drain on the sickness and disability benefits which were to be introduced under the Act.[2] Friendly Societies, who had provided such benefits formerly, gave evidence of such a drain on their funds. Tuberculosis was responsible for one in three deaths among males aged 15–44, and for a half of deaths among females aged 15–24. Moreover, the medical profession was now arguing that tuberculosis could be cured through sanatorium treatment.[3] The experience of Germany was invoked; insurance committees in Germany had become involved in building tuberculosis institutions, with results that were 'amazing' with a large number of cures.[4] Tuberculosis was believed to be declining faster in Germany than in Britain. It was feared that if Britain did not follow the German example, it would fall behind in 'national efficiency', a consideration which had been at the forefront since the revelations of the poor physical standards of the recruits in the Boer War in South Africa, 1899–1902.

Tuberculosis thus became the only disease for which free institutional treatment was provided under the 1911 National Insurance Act, and was the only disease for which insurance commissioners were authorized to extend treatment to dependants of the insured. One and a half million pounds were allocated by the Treasury for the erection of tuberculosis institutions. One million pounds were to be expended annually on treatment, a rate of 1s. 4d. per insured person per annum. Of this amount 1d. was set aside for further research (amounting to approximately £56 000 per annum), on the argument that further research would ensure that State funds were expended to the fullest advantage. In an age in which the benefits of science and scientific research were increasingly considered self-evident, and possibly with an eye to Germany,[5] this clause, which in any case usurped only a small part of the total funds, was added at the last minute as a 'minor detail' and passed through Parliament relatively unchallenged.[6]

In an article published following his history of the MRC, Landsborough

[2] *Parliamentary debates (official report) House of Commons*, 5th series 1911, xxv (4 May 1911), 626.

[3] Latham, A. and Garland, C.H. (1910). *The conquest of consumption*, pp. 13, 173. Fisher Unwin, London.

[4] *Parliamentary debates (official report) House of Commons*, 5th series, 1911, xxv (4 May 1911), 627.

[5] On the possible influence of Germany on the research provision, see Kohler, R.E. (1982). *From medical chemistry to biochemistry. The making of a biomedical discipline*, p. 76. Cambridge University Press.

[6] Landsborough Thomson quoted W. J. Braithwaite's diary, the civil servant in charge of drafting the National Insurance Bill: 'Meeting in Chancellor's room, many persons, to finish up the bill. Many points decided of a smaller kind.... the Chancellor is setting aside a small sum for research': Landsborough Thomson, A. (1973). Origin of the British legislative provision for medical research. *Journal of Social Policy*, **2**, (1), 43; 'the Clause was very little discussed in either House': ibid. p. 49.

Thomson examined in detail the origins of the clause relating to research under the Act. Unlike his earlier assertion he now conceded,

> . . . it is conceivable that Lloyd George had envisaged research on tuberculosis alone; and it is at least probable that he had this disease chiefly in mind. . . . (The Clause may, on the other hand, have been merely the most convenient place for the insertion of a new item in the draft at the eleventh hour). The linkage is almost explicit in the Financial Resolution related to the Bill (6 July): '(1) To authorise payment out of moneys provided by Parliament . . . as respects sanatorium benefit, including research work in connection therewith, a sum not exceeding one penny a year for every insured person.'[7]

Landsborough Thomson devoted considerable time to discussing who was responsible for this 'farsighted measure', but did not come up with any definitive answer.[8] Indeed, ultimately it is of little significance who was responsible for suggesting the provision; what is important is that it was conceived as part of the 'sanatorium' clauses. The initiative could have come from any number of individuals, not least the members of the Royal Commission on Tuberculosis, who were involved in research into tuberculosis and subsequently showed themselves to be strongly in favour of a permanent research body into tuberculosis. This Commission had been set up following a statement by Robert Koch at the British Congress on Tuberculosis in London in 1901 that bovine tuberculosis was harmless to man. The Royal Commission had followed an unprecedented course of conducting its own laboratory research, not being satisfied with the evidence presented before it. The Commission had concluded that bovine tuberculosis was indeed responsible for causing tuberculosis among humans, and was spread mainly through infected milk supplies, a conclusion of vital importance to public health.[9] When consulted about the research fund by the Departmental Committee on Tuberculosis, which was set up in 1912 by the Treasury under the chairmanship of Waldorf Astor to advise on the 'sanatorium benefit' of the 1911 Act, the Commissioners claimed that there were many important questions still unanswered, that a Royal Commission could not sit in perpetuity, and that therefore they saw the fund as facilitating the continuation of the research which they had initiated.[10]

While it is of little consequence who was responsible for proposing the clause on research for the Act, the subsequent career of the clause in the hands of the Departmental Committee on Tuberculosis is of vital importance

---

[7] Ibid. p. 50.

[8] Ibid. pp. 44–9.

[9] *Final report of the Royal Commission appointed to inquire into the relations of human and animal tuberculosis*, Part I, Cd. 5761 (1911), pp. 37–40.

[10] Addison Papers Box 32: evidence before 1912–13 Departmental Committee on Tuberculosis —14 May 1912, Secretary of the Royal Commission, E. J. Steegman, pp. 7–18; 15 May 1912, G. Sims Woodhead, p. 4.

in the history of the Medical Research Committee. Composed of eminent medical scientists and practitioners, the Departmental Committee on Tuberculosis seized upon the research clause as an opportunity to expand medical research in general by the public purse. The extent to which research commanded its attention is seen by the disproportionate amount of time the Committee spent discussing how this fund should be expended, relative to time spent on discussing other aspects of the tuberculosis problem. The main point under discussion was whether the funds should be used on a central institution or distributed to existing research organizations, specifically the universities.

One early suggestion that the work of the new research organization might not be restricted to tuberculosis can be found in the evidence of Simon Flexner, Director of the Laboratories of the Rockefeller Institute for Medical Research in New York, whose opinion was sought on research organization. In his written evidence he confined his advice to the organization of tuberculosis research.[11] However, giving oral evidence before the Committee, he stated that he hoped that the research would not be confined to tuberculosis. He pointed out that at the Rockefeller Institute they believed in following leads and that at present there were no such leads in tuberculosis research.[12]

The Committee directly confronted the question of whether the research had to be restricted to tuberculosis, and decided to seek legal advice on the matter. Smith Whitaker, a member of the Committee and medical secretary to the British Medical Association, wrote to the Committee having asked the opinion of the legal Adviser of the Insurance Commission:

You asked me last week about the possibility of any of the money being applied to research respecting other diseases than tuberculosis . . . as we are at present advised, it would appear that the terms of the Act do not preclude the possibility of the money being applied to research in other diseases, but having regard to the context it would be proper that *the money should be applied solely for research in tuberculosis*, unless the Commissioners are satisfied in any year that all is being applied in that year that can usefully at that moment be so applied, and that a balance is available for other research. Even then the money could not be applied to research generally, but only to such research as bore some definite relation to improvement in the methods of prevention and treatment of disease; and perhaps there would have to be a further limitation that the diseases or the disease must be of a character which it was definitely contemplated would be brought within the scope of sanatorium benefit . . .[13]

Clearly not satisfied with this view, the Committee subsequently sought the opinion of the Law Officers' Department, which told them, 'We are of

---

[11] *Final report of the Departmental Committee on Tuberculosis* (Chair Lord Astor), Vol. II, Cd. 6654 (1913), pp. 47–8.

[12] Addison Papers Box 32: minutes of evidence, 5 November 1912, p. 31.

[13] Ibid. 5 November 1912, p. 4 (my emphasis).

opinion that the Insurance Commissioners may frame their regulations made under the proviso to section 16(2) of the National Insurance Act, 1911, so as to enable the monies therein referred to, to be applied for purposes of research in connection with any disease to which insured persons may be liable.'[14] Thus, in its final report, the Committee pointed out that legal opinion had advised that the funds need not be confined to tuberculosis, yet it anticipated 'that for the present, at any rate, the moneys will be applied mainly to research in connection with tuberculosis and its allied problems'.[15]

A memorandum was written by eminent medical authorities for the Departmental Committee, including among others T. Clifford Allbutt (Regius Professor of Physic, University of Cambridge), J. S. Haldane (Reader in Physiology, University of Oxford), G. Sims Woodhead (Professor of Pathology, University of Cambridge), James Ritchie (Superintendent of the Research Laboratory of the Royal College of Physicians, Edinburgh, and Secretary to the Pathological Society of Great Britain and Ireland, formerly Professor of Pathology, University of Oxford), and W. Bulloch (Professor of Bacteriology, University of London), as well as the Presidents of the Royal Colleges of Surgeons and Physicians. They approved the allocation of the funds to research into tuberculosis: 'presumably it is earmarked, at least for a few years, for research in connection with tuberculosis, and for the present it should be applied definitely and specifically to that purpose . . .'[16] The general belief indeed was at that time that the money would be devoted to a 'thorough study of tuberculosis', to quote the press, and that 'for every reason, it is desirable that it should be so.'[17] However, a writer in the *British Medical Journal* pointed out that tuberculosis itself was in many ways unsuitable for research, chiefly because when a question was addressed, the slow development of morbid lesions delayed the answer. It was held that, from the standpoint of pathology, tuberculosis should be regarded as one member of a group of infections, other members of which were more appropriate subjects for research. This opinion was, according to the author, supported by the fact that in institutions largely devoted to general investigations on infections, such as the Rockefeller or even the Pasteur Institute, comparatively little work had hitherto been done on tuberculosis.[18]

The Medical Research Committee, which was set up with this research fund, consisted of an executive committee comprising nine members, six of them professional and three of them lay. Lord Moulton of Bank, one of the lay members, was selected as chair of the committee. Other members were Christopher Addison (formerly Professor of Anatomy and Dean of St

---

[14] Ibid. 4 February 1913, p. 2.
[15] *Final Report Departmental Committee*, Vol. I, Cd. 6641 (1913), p. 14.
[16] Addison Papers Box 3: memorandum from Medical Schools, p. 4.
[17] Addison Papers, Box 79: *Pall Mall Gazette*, 23 June 1913.
[18] *British Medical Journal* (1913), **i**, 571.

Bartholomew's Hospital, and to be appointed the first Minister of Health in 1919), Waldorf Astor (who had chaired the Departmental Committee on Tuberculosis), Clifford Allbutt, Charles John Bond, William Bulloch, Matthew Hay, Frederick Gowland Hopkins, and William Boog Leishman. An advisory council was also set up, consisting of forty members appointed by the Minister of Insurance from names suggested by various government departments, by certain public medical and other scientific societies, and by the universities. There was a great deal of overlap in membership with the 1912 Departmental Committee on Tuberculosis, including David Davies, chair of the King Edward VII Welsh National Memorial Association (a voluntary anti-tuberculosis organization in Wales), and Sir Robert Philip (vice-chair and future chair of the National Association for the Prevention of Tuberculosis, NAPT). Thus, the tuberculosis connection was still in evidence. This council was to advise the Minister of Insurance on the research programme of the Committee annually before he gave his approval to the programme. However, the Advisory Council did not have much power. Sims Woodhead wrote to the newly appointed secretary to the Medical Research Committee, Walter Morley Fletcher, in June 1914 informing him that:

The members of the Advisory Committee (*sic*) complain that they had been called together on only a single occasion, and then after certain definite arrangements had been made. When they did meet, they were told, with a pistol at their head (for it practically came to that), that they must fall in with arrangements which had been made and concerning which they had not been consulted, or the whole work of the Executive would be wasted. From that time up to the present, they have heard not a word; and they resent this very much indeed. . . . The fact that the Advisory Committee know nothing of what is being done is creating among its members an intense feeling of dissatisfaction and an atmosphere of suspicion. . . . they do claim that their opinion is of some value, and that it is being ignored and wasted, while a few dominating minds are shaping a policy of which little is known, whilst even that little is, in their view, unsatisfactory. In short, the Advisory Committee feel that the Executive is magnifying its office and minimising that of the Advisory Committee.[19]

Four months later in another letter to Fletcher, Woodhead spoke of the 'functions, or perhaps I should say lack of functioning of the Advisory Council'.[20]

Some effort in the direction of tuberculosis research was made in 1914. A special committee on phthisis (pulmonary tuberculosis) in relation to occupations was set up in 1914 under the chairmanship of Christopher Addison, and included John Brownlee, E. L. Collis, Leonard Hill, Benjamin Moore, and Walter Fletcher. This committee was to ascertain whether

[19] MRC 1430: Woodhead to Fletcher, 25 June 1914, pp. 1-3.
[20] MRC 1430: Woodhead to Fletcher, 28 October 1914.

tuberculosis was unduly prevalent in the boot and shoe industry and, if so, what measures should be recommended for its prevention. In 1915 the committee issued a report upon the boot and shoe industry, and was also reported to be investigating the printing trade. J. Brownlee wrote a report in 1917 on tuberculosis among industrial workers, with special reference to female munition workers. There was also an investigation underway at Midhurst Sanatorium into the value of sanatorium treatment, and surgical treatment was being researched by L. S. T. Burrell and A. S. MacNalty (also in charge of tuberculosis services under the new Ministry of Health after 1919) on behalf of the Committee. Leonard Hill, Professor of Applied Physiology, included a discussion of the causes of tuberculosis in his two reports on ventilation, published in 1919 and 1920.[21]

However, as Fletcher later pointed out, the early programme of the Committee was almost immediately interrupted by urgent war work with the outbreak of the First World War in 1914. Woodhead stopped reproaching Fletcher for neglecting the Advisory Council, and C. Masterman, the Financial Secretary of the Treasury, gave his approval to any research work required in connection with the treatment of wounded.[22] The problem of tuberculosis itself intensified during the war; it was estimated after the war that almost 58 000 servicemen had contracted tuberculosis while on national service, and tuberculosis among young women increased by 35 per cent between 1914 and 1918.[23] Nevertheless, understandably little opposition was aroused when the Committee turned its attention away from tuberculosis to encompass the manifold health problems created by war, and the Committee's research programme during the war was far more successful in other areas. As a result of the war, Fletcher was able to point to the vital importance of not restricting the work of the Medical Research Committee to any one particular area. He outlined the many ways in which the work of the Committee had been crucial to the health of the nation during the war, medical research having yielded very practical results. Thus he claimed, 'In a

[21] MRC *SRS* 1: *First report of the Special Investigation Committee upon the incidence of phthisis in relation to occupations. The boot and shoe industry* (1915); MRC: *First annual report 1914–15* (1916), pp. 24, 25; MRC *SRS* 18: Brownlee, J. (1917). *An investigation into the epidemiology of phthisis in Great Britain and Ireland,* Parts I and II; MRC *SRS* 46: Brownlee (1920). *Epidemiology of phthisis,* Part III; MRC *SRS* 22: Greenwood, M. and Tebb, A. E. (1918). *An inquiry into the prevalence and aetiology of tuberculosis among industrial workers, with special reference to female munition workers*; MRC *SRS* 33: Bardswell, N. D. and Thompson, J. H. R. (1919). *Pulmonary tuberculosis mortality after sanatorium treatment, a report of the experience of the King Edward VII Sanatorium, Midhurst*; MRC *SRS* 67: Burrell, L. S. T. and MacNalty, A. S. (1922). *Report on artificial pneumothorax; MRC SRS* 32: Hill, L. E. (1919). *The science of ventilation and open-air treatment,* Part I; MRC *SRS* 52: Hill (1920). *Ventilation and open-air treatment,* Part II.
[22] MRC 1430: Fletcher to Woodhead, 31 October 1914.
[23] MacPherson, W. G., Leishman, W. B. and Cummins S. L. (ed.) (1923). *History of the Great War. Medical services. Pathology,* p. 477. HMSO, London; CMO: *Report 1939– 45* (1947), p. 59.

literal sense, the application of medical science has been one of the fundamental essentials of our victory.'[24] No one could deny the positive contributions of the Medical Research Committee (see Chapter 4). Fletcher's assessment certainly appeared to be accepted by the first Minister of Health in 1919, Christopher Addison, for one, who argued in favour of substantially increasing the grant for research and who also favoured placing the Medical Research Committee directly under the Privy Council rather than attaching it to the Ministry of Health, on the model of the Department of Scientific and Industrial Research founded in 1915.[25] In 1919 the Medical Research Committee was reconstituted to become the Medical Research Council directly responsible to the Privy Council and no longer responsible to the Insurance Commissioners.

Tuberculosis and the MRC, 1919 – 39

Once the financial basis for medical research was removed from the National Insurance Act, tuberculosis no longer enjoyed pride of place even nominally in the Council. The rate of decline of tuberculosis before the First World War was resumed after the war, but tuberculosis remained the major killer of young adults until after the Second World War, and yet little real interest was shown by the Medical Research Council in this disease. It seems clear that this was a reflection of the research interests of the administrators of the Council, particularly its secretary, Sir Walter Fletcher, whose interests lay elsewhere. Tuberculosis as a practical health problem could further legitimately be abandoned by the policy decisions following the war, which emphasized 'pure' research. It was explained in 1924, 'The best and earliest success can only come from their free and disinterested work in pursuit of clues that may lie here or there . . . The apparently academic and unpractical work of to-day may to-morrow give the key to a score of old problems and lead at once to new and unexpected powers. Faith must be put unreservedly in the scientific workers themselves.'[26] The MRC found work in areas other than tuberculosis to be, if not more interesting, then more rewarding in results.

Tuberculosis research was not entirely neglected by the MRC in the inter-war period, although MacNalty's summary of the tuberculosis research of the MRC in the *British Journal of Tuberculosis* in 1928 was necessarily brief.[27] The MRC set up a tuberculosis committee headed by C. F. Bond,

---

[24] Addison Papers Box 53: address by Fletcher to Research Defence Society, 1920, p. 2.

[25] Local Government Board: Addison, C. *Memorandum on the Provision of the Ministry of Health Bill, 1919, as to the work of the Medical Research Committee. (Clause 3 (1) proviso i)*, Cmd. 69 (1919): appendix: W. M. Fletcher.

[26] Addison Papers Box 67: notes for MRC annual report 1923–24, p. 19.

[27] MacNalty, A. S. (1928). *British Journal of Tuberculosis*, **22**, 16–18.

Fletcher, and MacNalty, to co-ordinate research into tuberculosis. The early interest in the epidemiology of tuberculosis, noted above, was not sustained. The committee on phthisis in relation to occupations did not meet after 1915. Despite the fact that the Registrar-General continued to report high tuberculosis death rates in the boot and shoe industry, no further investigations were undertaken by the Council until 1947. The only other report on tuberculosis in relation to occupation to appear before the Second World War was that by A. (later Sir Austin) Bradford Hill on the printing trade, which was published in 1929 in association with the Industrial Fatigue Board.[28]

The two committees of the MRC which dealt with tuberculosis research in the inter-war years were the tuberculin committee and the bacteriological committee, neither of which were prestigious committees within the MRC. Tuberculin had been developed as a diagnostic tool, a method of testing the presence of tuberculous infection. The tuberculin committee was set up in 1921 at the request of various stockowners who provided facilities for research into tuberculin testing of dairy cattle. As part of the attempt to regulate the milk supply, certain categories of milk had been devised after the First World War. Apart from the category 'pasteurized', there was a category of 'tuberculin-tested milk', which meant that cattle were periodically tested for tuberculous infection and reactors were removed. The MRC's tuberculin committee was asked to devise improved methods of testing dairy cattle by tuberculin in light of the anomalous and confusing results obtained by methods of tuberculin testing then in use. There was evidence given to the MRC of abuse of tuberculin, that cattle was sold under the guarantee of freedom from tuberculosis as shown by a tuberculin test when in fact the cows were suffering from tuberculosis.[29] By 1923 the MRC was spending £1 200 per annum on this research. Testing the efficacy of the tuberculin test was said to be an 'appropriate direction of effort for the Medical Research Council in view of the connected problems of the hygiene of milk and of bovine tuberculosis in man'.[30] While bovine tuberculosis was a serious problem, it was only responsible for approximately 6 per cent of the total deaths from tuberculosis. Nor did the Council extend its interest in the disease beyond the testing of cattle to encompass the related problems of the hygiene of milk and the disease in man, apart from issuing an authoritative statement in 1928 relating to a prevalent idea of drinking tuberculosis-infected milk to gain immunity: 'The Tuberculin Committee of the MRC

---

[28] MRC *SRS* 54: Hill, A. B. (1929). *An investigation into the sickness experience of printers (with special reference to the incidence experience of tuberculosis)*, MRC and Industrial Fatigue Board; see also Chapter 7.

[29] MRC 205/2: F. Knight (Secretary National Veterinary Medical Association of Great Britain and Ireland), 9 August 1927.

[30] MRC 205/2, Vol. I: Tuberculin Sub-committee, 9 June 1923.

strongly deprecate the suggestion which has been current in some quarters that children drinking milk containing bovine tubercle bacilli benefit in that way by obtaining some immunity against tuberculosis. Even if some degree of immunity be, in fact, thus obtained, . . . [a] method of such random and uncontrolled immunisation that carries with it grave risks of producing serious and even fatal disease is indefensible.'[31] The investment in research relating to tuberculin-testing of cattle was no doubt a result of the lobbying and financial support of cattle owners. In 1933, the tuberculin committee was replaced by a joint committee of the MRC and the Agricultural Research Council (set up in 1931) to continue to research tuberculin testing in cattle.

Research into the curative or preventive value of substances derived from cultures of the tubercle bacillus was the concern of the other subcommittee of the MRC for tuberculosis, the bacteriological committee. Public pressure to investigate the curative value of tuberculin as well as an anti-tuberculosis serum discovered by a Swiss bacteriologist, Henri Spahlinger, in the early 1920s was overridden in favour of sponsoring the work of Georges Dreyer, director of the Dunn School of Pathology, Oxford. A. S. MacNalty wrote a report in 1923 in which he pointed out that Dreyer's work was likely to revolutionize not only the treatment of tuberculosis but also that of other bacterial diseases.[32] However, by 1924 it was concluded that Dreyer's 'Diaplyte Vaccine', as it was known, was no more efficacious in the treatment of tuberculosis than other forms of tuberculin.[33]

Minimal attention was paid to a vaccine developed in France in 1921, Bacillus Calmette–Guérin (BCG). Investigations were carried out by A. Stanley Griffith, who continued to work in the laboratory set up under the Royal Commission on Tuberculosis. He reported unfavourably on the vaccine despite the enormous enthusiasm for it on the Continent.[34] Stanley Griffith himself might have contributed to the general lack of enthusiasm for BCG in Britain; he was described in 1929 as 'veering on the side of extreme scepticism and caution'.[35] In 1930, Dreyer, now also working on BCG, reported that, contrary to much research on the Continent, their own results supported their previous conclusion that vaccines of BCG were 'not necessarily safe for use in the preventive inoculation of man'.[36] A disaster in Lübeck, Germany, in 1930, in which at least 73 infants out of 249 inoculated with BCG died as a direct result of the inoculation, served to reinforce their reservations, despite the fact that the vaccine was later exonerated of all

[31] MRC 205/2, Vol. III: MacNalty to Ministry of Health, 9 November 1926.

[32] MRC 1220, Vol. I: Fletcher to Newman, 23 May 1923; ibid. report by MacNalty, 23 May 1923; ibid. Report for MRC members only, 11 June 1923; ibid. Fletcher to Cummins, 12 June 1923.

[33] MRC 205/2, Vol. II: *Final report on diaplyte vaccine*, 21 November 1924; MRC 1220, Vol. II: *Western Gazette*, 7 March 1924.

[34] MRC: *Annual report 1927–28* (1929), p. 100.

[35] MRC 1319, Vol. III: BCG, Fletcher to Middleton, 22 January 1929.

[36] MRC: *Annual report 1929–30* (1931), p. 84.

responsibility by a court of inquiry.[37] Calmette and Guérin were not particularly meticulous in their record-keeping, and thus the efficacy of BCG could be, and was, dismissed as based on unsound evidence.[38] Sir George Buchanan, chair of the Ministry of Health's Immunization Committee, asserted in 1933, 'One is not justified at the best in claiming more for the inoculation of BCG than that there is some prima-facie evidence to show that it is a useful temporary precaution to take.'[39] Major Greenwood, director of the MRC's Statistical Unit and professor of epidemiology and vital statistics at the London School of Hygiene and Tropical Medicine, expressed criticism of the figures quoted by Calmette and others in favour of the BCG results.[40] In the 1940s it was still argued that there had not been any properly controlled trials on BCG proving its worth, even though in Sweden, for example, thousands of people had been vaccinated with apparently successful results. Its worth in Sweden was not doubted, and A. J. Wallgren, a Swedish professor of paediatrics who had been largely responsible for introducing BCG into Sweden, urged Britain at least to undertake an 'unbiased trial' of the vaccine.[41]

Administrative objections were possibly more important than lack of scientific verification of its efficacy in the non-adoption of BCG in Britain in the inter-war period. Buchanan referred to administrative problems, such as the need for isolation of vaccinated children for about four weeks so as not to render the vaccination useless, and the need for revaccination. In his opinion, Britain had a well-developed anti-tuberculosis service in any case, which vaccination might interfere with.[42] Sir Wilson Jameson, Chief Medical Officer of the Ministry of Health, admitted during the Second World War that the official opposition rested on administrative grounds.[43]

In taking little interest in BCG, the MRC reflected the dominant opinion among tuberculosis specialists in Britain. L. S. T. Burrell, physician to the Brompton Hospital, was not alone in his remark, 'We shall not find salvation in inoculation.'[44] Tuberculosis specialists preferred to focus on curative measures and more traditional preventive measures, specifically education of the individual (see also Chapter 4). When a meeting was convened by the Health Committee of the League of Nations on BCG in 1928, it was decided

[37] Camille Guérin. In Rosenthal, S. R. (ed.)(1980). *BCG vaccine: tuberculosis-cancer* (2nd edn) pp. 35–8. PSG Publishing, Littleton, Massachusetts.

[38] Foster, W. D. (1970). *A history of medical bacteriology and immunology*, pp. 157–8. Heinemann, London.

[39] *Lancet* (1933), **i**, 654.

[40] *British Medical Journal* (1928), **i**, 793–5.

[41] *NAPT Bulletin* (1945), **7**, (3), 7, 8; ibid. (1948), **10**, (5), 155; *British Medical Journal* (1948), **i**, 1126–9.

[42] *Lancet* (1933), **i**, 654.

[43] MRC 1319/1: W. H. Tytler to Mellanby, 16 May 1944.

[44] *Transactions of 17th annual conference of the National Association for the Prevention of Tuberculosis (17 NAPT)* (1931), p. 149; *21 NAPT* (1935), p. 16.

by the MRC not to send any delegates, 'for it would not be satisfactory or particularly desirable for British scientific credit merely to send an officer who could not participate in the discussion and only acted as an observer'.[45] Here was an acknowledgement that Britain was not a world leader in tuberculosis research—and this possibly reinforced the tendency to develop other areas of research where Britain had some scientific standing internationally, such as vitamin studies (see also Chapter 5).

While there were no specific committees dealing with the surgery and chemotherapy of tuberculosis, these areas of research were not entirely neglected by the MRC. 'Artificial pneumothorax', a technique of temporarily collapsing the lung to rest it and in this way aid recovery, was discovered by an Italian doctor in 1892 and introduced into Britain in 1910. This technique was the subject of two MRC reports in 1922 and 1936.[46] However, the MRC showed little interest in thoracic surgery in general, although it was gaining widespread popularity in this period, particularly in Germany and USA.

Little work was done in research into chemotherapy, despite constant requests to investigate 'this or that wonderful cure for tuberculosis'.[47] In 1921 H. H. (later Sir Henry) Dale, director of the biochemistry department of the National Institute for Medical Research (and later director of the Institute), claimed that there appeared to be no real starting point for research into the chemotherapy of tuberculosis at that time. Nor did he discover much progress being made at the famous Henry Phipps Institute for tuberculosis research in Philadelphia, USA, which he visited that year.[48]

One treatment shortly to come to light was that discovered by Holger Moellgaard, professor of animal physiology at Copenhagen University, Denmark, in 1923, known as sanocrysin, with a gold content of 37 per cent. The MRC began a trial on sanocrysin in 1924, but the researchers found that the progress of the trial was hampered by the difficulty of distinguishing between actual effects of the treatment and the course the disease would have taken in any case, for the prognosis of tuberculosis was totally unpredictable. It was concluded in 1926 that sanocrysin was of benefit in a limited number of cases.[49] No further investigations were conducted by the Council into the

[45] PRO MH55/150: G. Buchanan, 11 October 1928.
[46] MRC *SRS* 67: Burrell, L. S. T. and MacNalty, A. S. (1922). *Report on artificial pneumothorax*; MRC *SRS* 215: Bentley, F. J. (1936). *Artificial pneumothorax: experience of the London County Council*.
[47] PRO MH55/148: Coutts, 14 August 1919; Landsborough Thomson, A. (1975) *Half a century of medical research* Vol. II, *The programme of the Medical Research Council (UK)*, p. 9. HMSO, London; see also Smith, F. B. (1985). Gullible's travails: tuberculosis and quackery 1890–1930. *Journal of Contemporary History*, **20**, 733–56.
[48] MRC 205/1: MacNalty, 'Conference on the future of tuberculosis work of the MRC', 5 March 1921, p. 9.
[49] MRC 1380/3: Sanocrysin Trials, 1924; ibid. MacLean to Fletcher, 8 February 1925; CMO: *Annual report 1927* (1928), p. 66.

treatment, but by the mid-1930s it was beginning to lose favour in general. It was later maintained that the results had not really been convincing and that some of the complications had been alarming, including kidney damage and severe skin rashes.[50]

The relative lack of interest in tuberculosis research within the MRC, as already noted, was related to the research priorities of the administrators, whose interests lay elsewhere. However, there was also little pressure from the medical profession to carry out research. As discussed above, BCG did not arouse much enthusiasm. The MRC claimed to have difficulty in finding candidates for carrying out tuberculosis research for which they offered a research fellowship, the Dorothy Cross Fellowship. Fletcher wrote 'My Council have been greatly disappointed at the field of candidates offering themselves for the valuable Cross Fellowships in tuberculosis . . . We have made these [Fellowships] known as widely as possible, but only a tiny group of third-rate candidates appeared, mostly Indians.'[51] This was despite the fact that the Dorothy Cross Fellowship was more valuable than a Rockefeller Fellowship. Yet that the MRC's own interests lay elsewhere was indicated in the attempt to broaden the scope of the Dorothy Cross Fellowship to include other diseases, as had been done for the initial medical research fund. Only the obstinacy of the donor, Mrs Cross, prevented this.[52]

Another reason for the dearth of tuberculosis research in Britain as opposed to Germany or the USA at this time may have been the absence of financial backing for such research outside the MRC. The type of tuberculosis research most highly developed was that associated with cattle which was backed by large cattle farm owners. Tuberculosis did not attract as much charity as did cancer for research purposes (possibly as a result of its differential class basis).[53] The structure of tuberculosis organizations in Britain also militated against research. In the USA, the National Tuberculosis Association sponsored a great deal of research.[54] The British counterpart, the National Association for the Prevention of Tuberculosis (NAPT), set up in 1898, primarily focused its attention on educating people in healthy, outdoor living as a preventive measure. Many tuberculosis specialists dissociated themselves from the NAPT, not considering it a professional organization, and focused their attention on the Tuberculosis

[50] *Tubercle* (1940), **21**, (2), 174; Houghton, L. E. and Sellors, T. H. (1949). *Aids to tuberculosis nursing. A complete textbook for the nurse* (3rd edn), pp. 68–9. Bailliere, Tindall and Cox, London.

[51] MRC 1615, II: Fletcher to Morriston Davies, 16 June 1931; ibid. Fletcher to Geoffrey Marshall, 18 June 1931.

[52] MRC 1615, III: Landsborough Thomson to Treasury Solicitor, 4 February 1935.

[53] Cole, G. D. H. and Cole, M. I. (1937). *The condition of Britain*, p. 105. Victor Gollancz, London.

[54] Shryock, R. H. (1947). *American medical research, past and present*, pp. 111–2. The Commonwealth Fund, New York.

Association (initially the Tuberculosis Society, set up in 1911).[55] However, the NAPT conducted the national fund-raising efforts related to tuberculosis, thus controlling the 'anti-tuberculosis funds', while the Tuberculosis Association had few resources at its disposal, conducting its research on a 'shoestring' budget.[56] Nor was there a close relationship between the NAPT and the tuberculosis committees of the MRC. Here personalities intervened. Sir Robert Philip, chair of the NAPT, claimed that he had been ignored by the MRC as an authority on tuberculosis, which did not inspire friendly co-operation.[57]

Tuberculosis and the Second World War

Thus, while the MRC did not totally neglect tuberculosis research in the inter-war period, nor could it be regarded as world leader in this area. Yet the situation of relative neglect of research into tuberculosis by the MRC was to alter with the onset of the Second World War in 1939, when pressure was placed on the Council to carry out research into tuberculosis as a result of a fear of the spread of the disease under wartime conditions.

P. D'Arcy Hart, director of the tuberculosis work of the MRC and a member of the Socialist Medical Association, argued in 1942: 'The present time, when production is of paramount importance, the demand for labour acute, makes it urgently necessary to arrive at a solution [to the tuberculosis problem]. We cannot afford to have unhealthy workers, nor can we permit the unnecessary spread of infection.' The experiences of the First World War were invoked as a warning of the potential dangers of warfare: 'If a repetition of the serious increase in tuberculosis during the last war is to be avoided in this—and some increase has already taken place—speedy action must be taken to minimise the effect of war stresses on industrial workers.'[58] The first two years of war did indeed see substantial increases in tuberculosis incidence and mortality. Moreover, the tuberculosis services had been disrupted at the start of the war, adding to fear of the spread of the disease. The evacuation of tuberculosis institutions involved the discharge of approximately 8 000

[55] P. D'Arcy Hart claimed that the NAPT was a 'society for ladies and gentlemen': interview, 20 May 1983. The Tuberculosis Society was set up in 1911, and this amalgamated with the Society of Medical Superintendents of Tuberculosis Institutions to form the Tuberculosis Association in 1928.

[56] *The British Thoracic Association (the first fifty years)* (1978), p. 74. British Thoracic Association, London.

[57] MRC 205/1, Vol. III: MacNalty to Fletcher (report of a visit to Sir Robert Philip in Edinburgh), 30 May 1931.

[58] D'Arcy Hart, P. and Daniels, M. *The war, tuberculosis and the workers, a report prepared by a Committee of the Socialist Medical Association of Great Britain* (2nd edn May 1942) Socialist Medical Association. Reprinted in *Medicine Today and Tomorrow* (June 1941), **3**, (2), 7.

tuberculous patients, some believed to be in a highly infectious state. One eminent surgeon contributed to the general scare of infection by his statement that 'every tuberculous person turned forth is like a bomb thrown among the public'.[59]

At the request of the Ministry of Health, the MRC set up the Committee on Tuberculosis in War-time in 1941 with Lord Dawson of Penn as chair and D'Arcy Hart as secretary 'to assist in promoting the investigation of the extent and causes of the war-time increase in the incidence of tuberculosis, particularly among young women, and also to advise the Council regarding possible preventive measures'.[60]

The Committee recommended the use of the newly discovered mass miniature radiography among selected groups of supposedly healthy persons to detect early cases of pulmonary tuberculosis. Miniature radiography, capable of taking one hundred 1.25 inch chest photos per hour, had been developed in the decade before the war, with Germany, the USA, the Netherlands, and Britain all contributing various inventions to the technique. It was first used in Britain by Hart and others at University College Hospital in 1940, from which it was estimated—together with other studies—that 1 to 2 per cent healthy adults would be shown to have tuberculous lesions.[61] The Committee also advocated the introduction of allowances for tuberculous patients and their families to ensure the voluntary co-operation of the workers in the radiography schemes. Some demands for allowances had been made before the war, and D'Arcy Hart and others would probably have pressed for the use of the newly developed mass radiography regardless of the Second World War, but war enabled him and others to present this as a solution to a national problem which was threatening the national effort.

The Ministry of Health introduced a scheme of mass radiography and allowances for curable cases of pulmonary tuberculosis in 1943 as a war emergency measure. The MRC then published another report guiding local authorities in the use of mass radiography, giving the results of some pilot studies undertaken in two factories, a large office, and a mental asylum in London. In these studies significant lesions had been discovered in 1 per cent of the apparently normal persons examined, four per thousand requiring treatment.[62]

The increased cases of tuberculosis discovered by miniature radiography and increases owing to war conditions contributed to a crisis in the

---

[59] *British Medical Journal* (1939), **ii**, 621; ibid. (1941), **ii**, 632.
[60] MRC *SRS* 246: *Report of the Committee on Tuberculosis in War-time* (1942).
[61] *Tubercle* (1940), **21**, (Suppl.), 20.
[62] MRC *SRS* 251: Clark, K. C., D'Arcy Hart, P., Kerley, P., and Thompson, B. C. (1945). *Mass miniature radiography of civilians for the detection of pulmonary tuberculosis (guide to administration and technique with a mobile apparatus using 35-mm film and results of a survey)*, Preface, and p. 88.

administration of tuberculosis institutions. Not only was there a shortage of beds, but more seriously there was a drastic shortage of staff. Staff shortage was at least partly a result of the growing fear of infection and it was in this context that BCG vaccination was given serious consideration for the first time in Britain. BCG was the subject of a Tuberculosis Association conference in 1943, at which the results of its use in Scandinavia and North America were discussed. J. Heimbeck's study of nurses in Norway had produced impressive results. He had found that 14 per cent of the nurses who had not been exposed to tuberculosis infection before they joined the hospital developed tuberculosis, while the rate among those previously infected was only 2 per cent. He therefore decided to inoculate nurses who had not been infected, and as a result the rate of this group contracting tuberculosis dropped to 2 per cent.[63] Other countries showed similarly impressive results from the use of BCG, although it was not favoured universally (for example, the USA continued to regard it with suspicion). At the close of the Tuberculosis Association meeting in 1943, it was resolved to ask the Minister of Health to facilitate a regular supply of BCG in this country and to instigate an extended investigation of its use. A deputation was sent to the Minister of Health, led by W. H. Tytler, Professor of Tuberculosis at the Welsh National School of Medicine, and including representatives of the NAPT and the Tuberculosis Association.[64]

There continued to be opposition to BCG vaccination in some quarters, among whom Sir Graham Wilson, the director of the MRC's Emergency Public Health Laboratory Service (EPHLS), figured. Nevertheless, in 1947 the Ministry of Health set up a committee to advise it on clinical trials of BCG. In 1948 a group of tuberculosis specialists visited Copenhagen to study the vaccine, and the first consignment of BCG arrived from Copenhagen in 1949. The Ministry issued a circular in 1949 instructing local authorities to offer BCG to persons who had known contact with tuberculous infection, with hospital nurses and medical students given a high priority.[65] They also requested the MRC to conduct a trial on BCG, which was begun in 1950. Vole bacillus vaccine, which had been discovered by A. Q. Wells at the Dunn School of Pathology in Oxford in 1937, was also included in the trial. By December 1952, over 56 000 children had been included in the trial, all in their final year at secondary modern schools in or near North London, Birmingham, and Manchester, and between the ages of 14 and 15.

A random process was used to allocate children with a negative reaction to

[63] Heimbeck, J. (1936). *Tubercle*, **18**, 97; *British Medical Journal* (1948), **i**, 1128.

[64] MRC 1319/1: W. H. Tytler to E. Mellanby, 16 May 1944; MRC 1319/1: G. S. Wilson to E. Mellanby, 1 June 1944.

[65] CMO: *Annual report 1949* (1950), p. 104; Ministry of Health Circular 72/49; Ministry of Health, Department of Health for Scotland: BCG vaccination, medical memorandum 322/ BCG, July 1949, p. 8.

tuberculin to three groups—those in one group were not vaccinated, those in another group received BCG vaccine, and those in a third group received vole bacillus vaccine. For the first nine years of the trial, the participants were followed by a repeated cycle of examinations by MRC teams, consisting of a postal enquiry, a home visit, and a chest radiograph and tuberculin test, each cycle lasting about fourteen months. Postal enquiries were continued for a further six years. Reports were published in 1956, 1959, and 1963. The reduction in the incidence of tuberculosis in the BCG vaccinated group compared with the tuberculin-negative unvaccinated group was approximately 80 per cent. BCG was found to be slightly more effective than vole bacillus vaccine.[66]

General vaccination in schools was introduced in 1953, before the MRC published their reports. By the end of 1954, 250 000 persons had been vaccinated in total, and 600 000 by 1956 (about half of these were schoolchildren). Vaccination in schools became much more general after the 1956 MRC report.[67]

The MRC Committee on Tuberculosis in War-time also recommended the pasteurization of milk throughout the country, and where this was not practicable, that all milk consumed by children should be boiled or else dried milk provided.[68] Further evidence in favour of pasteurization came from a study undertaken during the war by the MRC's EPHLS of the relationship between the wartime rise in the non-pulmonary tuberculosis death-rates and the quality of the milk supply. A preliminary report published in 1947 claimed that the nation's raw milk supply 'appears to be almost as heavily contaminated with tubercle bacilli now as it was twenty years ago'. In contrast to previous experience, the maximum incidence of infection with the bovine type of bacillus was the 5–9 age group instead of the 0–4 age group. The report suggested that the greater care in infant feeding resulted in partial protection of the pre-school child, while the introduction of the milk-in-schools scheme without adequate measures to safeguard the purity of the milk, might have led to the increase in the proportion of bovine infection in older children. The conclusion of the

[66] B.C.G. and Vole Bacillus vaccines in the prevention of tuberculosis in adolescents: First (Progress) Report to the Medical Research Council by their Tuberculosis Vaccines Clinical Trials Committee (1956). *British Medical Journal*, i, 413–27; 2nd report (1959). *British Medical Journal*, ii, 379–95; 3rd report (1963). *British Medical Journal*, i, 973–8. See also: Sutherland, I. (1959). *Tubercle*, **40**, 413–24; Heaf (1954). *Tubercle*, **35**, 154–63.

[67] A Vaccination Sub-committee of the Department of Health and Social Security in 1986 recommended that the BCG vaccination scheme in schools be abandoned by 1990 and replaced by a more selective scheme giving BCG vaccine to the 'neonates of Afro-Asian parents, Afro-Asian immigrants, and those who, because of their work or residence abroad, had a higher risk of infection': *British Medical Journal* (1986), i, 483–4.

[68] MRC *SRS* 246: *Report of Committee on Tuberculosis in War-time* (1942), p. 11; PRO MH55/1141: Tuberculosis Standing Advisory Committee of the Ministry of Health also passed a resolution on milk, 10 February 1942, p. 4.

report was that 'the value of this information for supporting the introduction of compulsory pasteurisation of all but T.T. milk needs no stressing'.[69]

The MRC thus played a major part in bringing about legislation that was to regulate the milk supply effectively, unlike the half-hearted attempts in that direction in the inter-war period.[70] By the Milk (Special Designations) Act of 1949, no milk was to be sold by retail in a given area except that which was designated under the categories 'Tuberculin Tested', 'Accredited' (for England and Wales) and 'Standard' (Scotland), and 'Pasteurized'. 'Accredited' and 'Standard', which were only applicable when the milk came from a single herd, were to be phased out as legal categories after five years. In 1969, the whole of Britain became an 'Attested Area'.

The 1940s saw a new era in tuberculosis treatment with the discovery of effective anti-tuberculosis drugs. In 1943 Selman A. Waksman discovered streptomycin at the Department of Microbiology of the New Jersey Agricultural Experiment Station, Rutgers University, USA. Laboratory and clinical experiments were immediately undertaken at the Mayo clinic, University of Minnesota, by W. H. Feldman and H. C. Hinshaw, who reported favourable results. In Britain the MRC set up a Streptomycin Committee in September 1946. However, at that time no supplies of the new drug were available for investigation. In December 1946, 50 kilograms were bought from America, enough to treat up to 200 cases. Domestic supplies were not fully established until 1949, by which time, over 350 kilograms had been bought from the USA at a cost of almost one million pounds.

Because of past difficulty in evaluating pulmonary tuberculosis treatment (for example, sanocrysin, as discussed above), the MRC decided to conduct a 'rigorously planned investigation with concurrent controls'. The type of patient to be investigated was carefully defined as 'acute progressive bilateral pulmonary tuberculosis of presumably recent origin, bacteriologically proved, unsuitable for collapse therapy, aged 15 to 25 [later extended to 30]'. The selection of this type of patient was justified as the parallel series of patients would be receiving the only other available treatment for that type of patient at that time—bed rest. It was also pointed out that there was not enough streptomycin to treat all patients in any case.

The first patients were admitted in January 1947 to the chosen centres— the Brompton and Colindale Hospitals in London, and Harefield Hospital, Middlesex. After three months when they still had not found enough patients

---

[69] MRC: *Report 1939–45* (1947), pp. 171–2; see also *Public Health* (1940), 105–8; Titmuss, R. M. (1950). *Problems of social policy.* In *History of the Second World War United Kingdom Civil Series* (ed. W. K. Hancock), p. 512, footnote 3. HMSO and Longmans, Green and Co., London.

[70] See Bryder, L. (1988) *Below the magic mountain: a social history of tuberculosis in twentieth-century Britain*, pp. 133–8, 245–7. Oxford University Press.

in the London and Middlesex areas, other authorities were approached—in Wales, Scotland, and Leeds. Another London hospital was also added. The trial included 107 patients, 55 were allocated to the streptomycin group and 52 to the control group.

Determination of whether a patient would be treated by streptomycin and bed rest or by bed rest alone was made by reference to a statistical series based on random sampling numbers drawn up for each sex at each centre by Sir Austin Bradford Hill; the details of the series were unknown to any of the investigators. Patients were not told before admission that they were to get special treatment. Control patients did not know throughout their stay in hospital that they were control patients in a special study. Clinicians were asked to adopt 'collapse therapy' (surgical collapse of the lung) only if the course of the disease so changed that some collapse therapy became indispensable and urgent—this happened in none of the streptomycin cases and in five of the control cases.

The trial lasted six months. The results were analysed by changes in the radiographic appearances. These were assessed by a panel of three, without knowledge of whether the films being viewed were those of streptomycin or control patients. The overall results left no doubt as to the beneficial effect of streptomycin. Seven per cent of the streptomycin patients and 27 per cent of the controls died before the end of the six months, a statistically significant difference. Considerable improvements were noted in 51 per cent of the streptomycin cases and 8 per cent of the controls. The results were published in the *British Medical Journal* in October 1948. The *British Medical Journal* noted that this was the first controlled investigation of its kind to be reported and quite apart from the results, would serve as a model for other such studies.[71]

Investigations were also being undertaken into tuberculous meningitis and miliary tuberculosis, organized by the MRC and the Ministry of Health, in London, Liverpool, and Glasgow. No controls were used in these investigations as no cure had previously been available. Initially only children up to the age of 7 were accepted for treatment. In September 1947 the MRC published preliminary results stating that, as available supplies of the drug permitted, patients suffering from tuberculous meningitis and miliary tuberculosis should be given the opportunity of receiving treatment with the drug. The number of beds for this treatment was, however, extremely limited, only 150 in 1947, rising to 200 in 1948.[72]

Early in the trials, the *British Medical Journal* published a particularly unfavourable appraisal of the new drug:

[71] *British Medical Journal* (1948), **ii**, 769–82.
[72] Ibid. (1948), **i**, 131.

The evidence of the trials already made in America leaves it at present quite uncertain whether streptomycin will prove, in the long run, to have greater therapeutic value in tuberculosis, and it may eventually be decided that the chief clinical uses of the drug lie in the treatment of certain other infections resistant to penicillin. The results of American and limited British tests of streptomycin in tuberculous meningitis have, in particular, been far less encouraging than originally hoped; there seems to be a very real risk that, even if the infection is controlled (as has only very rarely happened), the patient will usually be left mentally deficient, deaf, blind, or otherwise a hopeless invalid.[73]

This pessimism was possibly in part a response to the publicity the drug had previously been given leading to demands for the drug, sometimes desperate and far exceeding supplies.[74]

Subsequent reports assumed a quite different tone. For example, in 1950 a report from a hospital in Dublin, Ireland, claimed that prior to the introduction of streptomycin, almost 300 cases of tuberculous meningitis had been treated in the wards in thirteen years. All of these cases died in deepening coma within two or three weeks of admission. With streptomycin treatment one in every four or five cases recovered from the disease, provided that treatment was undertaken early and not abandoned too soon.[75]

However, scepticism of the new drug persisted among the medical profession. The Ministry of Health pointed out in 1950, 'There appears to be a belief prevalent among medical practitioners that streptomycin treatment does no more than prolong life or produce 'recovery' as a physical and mental wreck. This is not true . . .'. The Ministry reported that its investigation showed a 40 per cent recovery rate among cases treated early, as opposed to the previous 100 per cent mortality. Medical practitioners who doubted the efficacy of treatment were advised to visit some of the special units treating these patients.[76]

In the treatment of pulmonary tuberculosis with streptomycin, a new problem arose—was the appearance of streptomycin-resistant strains of bacilli. This caused a general fear that those who developed streptomycin-resistant strains could become a serious public health risk by passing on the resistant strain to others. However, this problem was solved by combining streptomycin with another recently discovered drug, para-aminosalicylic acid, PAS. PAS was first shown by J. Lehmann in Sweden in 1946 to have a pronounced action on tubercle bacilli. This discovery did not, however, at that time receive as much publicity as streptomycin. In 1948 the MRC undertook a second controlled trial to assess the new drug. The same type of

[73] Ibid. (1946), ii, 906; see also Mitchison, D. A. (1948). *NAPT Bulletin*, 10, (2), 52; *ibid.* 10, (3), 83.
[74] *British Medical Journal* (1946), ii, 906; ibid. (1947), ii, 138; ibid. (1948), ii, 276.
[75] *Tubercle* (1950), 31, 210.
[76] Ibid., 214; see also *Edinburgh Medical Journal* (1950), 57, 161.

case was used as in the first trial, and patients were grouped randomly for various treatments: streptomycin alone, PAS alone, or both drugs. Eleven hospitals were involved in the trials, which lasted three months. They demonstrated unequivocally that the combination of PAS and streptomycin prevented the development of streptomycin-resistant strains of tubercle bacilli.[77] Anti-tuberculosis chemotherapy continued to develop, although surgery and sanatorium treatment remained the dominant treatment for tuberculosis in Britain at least until 1960.

In conclusion, it has to be admitted that some qualification needs to be made to Landsborough Thomson's assessment of the MRC's work on tuberculosis that it played a vital role in the reduction of the disease and could be regarded as a world leader in that area.[78] The actual reduction of the disease appeared to occur independently of medical intervention and research in any case before 1945, but that is another story.[79] There is strong evidence to suggest that, although the MRC was initially set up with a fund provided for research into tuberculosis, tuberculosis quickly dropped in its order of priorities. It could not be described as a world leader in this area of research, for it did not initiate research so much as react to developments abroad, even in the late 1940s and 1950s when it did indeed carry out crucial research in chemotherapy and immunization.

[77] *British Medical Journal* (1949), **ii**, 1521.
[78] Landsborough Thomson, *Medical Research*, Vol. II, p. 5 (see note 47).
[79] See Bryder, *Below the magic mountain* (see note 70) and Smith, F. B. (1988). *The retreat of tuberculosis: 1850-1950*. Croom Helm, London.

2

Walter Morley Fletcher and the origins of a basic biomedical research policy

JOAN AUSTOKER

The development and expansion of the medical sciences in Britain was, to a considerable extent, dominated by a single individual. This was Walter Morley Fletcher, Secretary to the Medical Research Committee and then Council from 1914 until his death in 1933.[1] Medically qualified and a Cambridge graduate, Fletcher was a brilliant scientist working in Michael Foster's school of physiology. He collaborated with Gowland Hopkins in a series of notable experiments on the metabolism of muscle, for which he was elected a Fellow of the Royal Society in 1915. His broad interests in university life led him gradually away from the laboratory to an increasing involvement with his college, Trinity.[2] Here he combined his considerable intellectual gifts with an extraordinary flair for organization and administration. It was this ideal combination that prompted T. R. Elliot, another member of the Foster school, to advise Gowland Hopkins to propose Fletcher for Secretary of the Medical Research Committee. His acceptance of the post in 1913 ensured that biomedical science would be adequately represented in the development of a national science policy. It also secured the position of Cambridge as a leading centre of medical research. Fletcher was a Cambridge man 'first and foremost', and his devotion and loyalty to the University was reflected in the high position it occupied in his plans for the development of biomedical research.[3]

The mobilization of resources for war in August, 1914, served to reinforce rather than to halt Fletcher's activities. His position in organizing scientific resources for the war effort enabled him to establish co-operative relations with prominent groups in government, medical, academic, and scientific

---

[1] For an excellent account of Fletcher's contribution to biomedical research, and one on which many aspects of this chapter are based, see Kohler, R. E. (1978). Walter Fletcher, F. G. Hopkins, and the Dunn Institute of Biochemistry: a case study in the patronage of science. *Isis*, **69**, 331–55.

[2] Elliot, T. R. (1935). Sir Walter Morley Fletcher 1873–1933. *Obituary Notices of Fellows of the Royal Society*, **1**, 153–63.

[3] Ibid. p. 163.

circles.[4] He conceived his role to be the co-ordination and control of all aspects of medical research. He was a powerful and influential man whose wide-ranging experience and shrewd powers of analysis were highly respected. His opinion was frequently sought on the organization of the biomedical sciences. But, equally, he was outspoken in giving unsought advice and was sometimes 'too trenchant in his denouncement of others'.[5] His views on medical research differed radically from the opinions of those in the daily routine of clinical medicine and the care of patients, and his vigorous criticisms and intolerance of medical practice did not endear him to many in Harley Street.[6]

Fletcher believed that all medical research should be influenced by the MRC. His views on the needs of medical science became public policy in 1919. He visualized a national organization of biomedical sciences with himself as overseer of all policy within this system. He held the view that the MRC should not become a department within the proposed Ministry of Health. In this connection he received staunch support from both Robert Morant, the Permanent Secretary, and Christopher Addison, from 1917 the Minister of Reconstruction and later President of the Local Government Board for its closing days, and then the first Minister of Health. Addison felt that, while it was tempting and it would have been relatively easy to bring the Medical Research Committee wholly under the control of the Ministry of Health, it would have been 'a narrow and mistaken course'.[7] The recommendation of the Haldane Committee was that the MRC be incorporated under the direction of a Committee of the Privy Council, as was the case with the Department of Scientific and Industrial Research (DSIR) which was established during the war for the purpose of mobilizing the application of science to technology.[8] This would enable the MRC to provide a more general service, rather than being a body engaged upon research for the purpose of a single administrative department. It would thereby be freed from the restrictions imposed by bureaucratic departmental boundaries.

There is little doubt that, as Secretary of the MRC, Fletcher was in the appropriate strategic position to influence decisions relating to the reconstruction of medical sciences in post-war Britain. The provisions for an independent research body were achieved on 1 April 1920, providing the MRC with 'an unusual degree of freedom from Departmental

[4] Kohler, Walter Fletcher, F. G. Hopkins, and the Dunn Institute of Biochemistry, p. 334 (see note 1); Hopkins F. G. (1937). *Memorial to the late Sir Walter Morley Fletcher (1873–1933)*, pp. 13–26. Oxford University Press, London.

[5] Elliot, Sir Walter Morley Fletcher, p. 163 (see note 2).

[6] Ibid. p. 161.

[7] See MRC 1190 I and MRC 1331/A.

[8] Varcoe, I. (1970). Scientists, government and organized research: the early history of the DSIR, 1914–1916, *Minerva*, 8, 192–217.

intervention'.[9] The appointment of members of the Council was under the jurisdiction of a Committee of the Privy Council for Medical Research, but as this Committee met only once in all its years of existence, in practice the MRC had full executive powers and responsibilities to choose its own Secretary, to control its own administration, and to determine its own policy.[10] The constitutional position of the MRC therefore enabled it to promote a wide programme of research in medical science, free from territorial and administration limitations.

This suited Fletcher perfectly. From the outset he had strongly discouraged any attempts to organize medical research outside his sphere of influence. As early as 1915 he had warned the Board of Control and the Board of Education that their lines of research were impinging on what he regarded as his territory. He was displeased with the refusal of the Imperial Cancer Research Fund (ICRF) to comply with his request for some formal co-operation in the administration of funds for cancer research.[11] He was determined that *all* medical research in the future should come directly or indirectly under MRC control. As he had emphasized in 1918,

The Medical Research Committee . . . is able to organize and coordinate work at every centre of medical research in the Kingdom . . . If any fresh private endowment, given generally for medical research, is available, it will be very important either that it should be administered by the Medical Research Committee, or, if it be under a separate trust or management, that this should be in close relation to the Committee's work.[12]

He strongly objected to research organized under the new Ministry of Health. Scientists generally felt that the distribution of funds for the purpose of scientific research should be solely under their control and that only scientific men were suitably qualified to judge the validity of financial proposals for scientific work. Relations with the Ministry of Health were tense, in particular between Fletcher and Sir George Newman, Chief Medical Officer to the Ministry of Health (CMO). Competition continually occurred over areas of research, particularly relating to clinical research.

By informal agreement, the Ministry of Health was supposed to be concerned with aetiology, 'field' inquiries, and applied or health-related research, and the MRC was concerned with experimental clinical and laboratory research.[13] In practice it was difficult to sustain these boundaries.

[9] MRC PF3: R. Morant to A. J. Balfour, 28 October 1919.

[10] See Kohler, Walter Fletcher, F. G. Hopkins and the Dunn Institute of Biochemistry, pp. 338–40 (see note 1).

[11] See Austoker, J. (1988). *A history of the ICRF, 1902–1986*. Oxford University Press.

[12] MRC 1331/A: Walter Morley Fletcher, 'Endowment of medical research', 11 November 1918.

[13] MRC 1382 I: Fletcher to Gowland Hopkins, 21 November 1923; MRC 1382 I: George Newman, copy of minute to Secretary on Cancer Committee work, 30 November 1923.

The battle came to a head in bitter disputes over the establishment by Newman of the Ministry of Health's Departmental Cancer Committee in 1923. Much to Fletcher's annoyance this Committee frequently transcended these artificial boundaries. Discord was inevitable.[14] Disputes over the work initiated by the Committee exposed the lack of cohesion between the Ministry and the MRC. Caught in the middle of heated arguments, Sir Frederick Gowland Hopkins described himself as 'a poor little scientific Daniel surrounded by growling official lions'.[15] Constant assurances from Newman that he in no way wished to 'trespass in the smallest degree upon the perfectly proper preserves of the MRC', failed to placate Fletcher.[16] Ultimately it was necessary to draw up a scheme of differentiation between the inquiries of the Ministry and those of the MRC.[17] The dispute over cancer research thus led to an official concordat in January 1924 in which Newman and Fletcher were forced to set out precisely the respective spheres of influence.[18] The Ministry was to be concerned with 'applied research' relating to clinical problems, the MRC with initiating and organizing all new research in the basic biomedical sciences.

This division fitted in precisely with Fletcher's ideas for MRC patronage. It freed the MRC from any obligation to carry out a purely practical programme, enabling it to pursue its role in promoting fundamental research under the guidance and direction of those with a rigorous scientific training. Fletcher defined the primary function of the MRC as that of supporting fundamental scientific research, maintaining that progress in physiology, biochemistry, and pathology was essential to the development of clinical practice. He laid great emphasis on the practical applications that basic sciences could have in the prevention and cure of disease. This strong emphasis on the development of pre-clinical sciences had a far-reaching impact on the development of bacteriology, virology, and immunology, as well as on physiology, biochemistry, and pathology. These were all shaped according to the place they held in Fletcher's system of priorities. It is important to recognize this in order to understand how decisions were made and why certain fields of research were supported and others were not. Robert Kohler has convincingly demonstrated Fletcher's important contribution to the development of biochemistry, particularly at Cambridge

[14] MRC 1382 I: Newman to Fletcher, 5 December 1923; ibid. Walter Fletcher, minute upon the work of the Ministry of Health Cancer Committee, 13 December 1923. See also Chapter 3 in Austoker, *A history of the ICRF* (see note 11).

[15] MRC 1382 I: Hopkins to Fletcher, 22 November 1923.

[16] MRC 1382 I: Newman to Fletcher, 1 January 1924.

[17] MRC 1382 I: Newman to Fletcher, 7 January 1924; MRC 1190 I: draft document, 'Coordination of functions of the Ministry of Health and the Medical Research Council', 16 January 1924; ibid. 'Ministry of Health and Medical Research Council Research and Intelligence Services', 16 January 1924.

[18] MRC 1190 I: Concordat, 23 January 1924.

under the guidance of his friend Gowland Hopkins.[19] There Fletcher's high hopes were fully justified.

In implementing initiatives for the development of research and in considering the allocation of funds, Fletcher adopted an eclectic policy. Fellowships and research grants to individuals and university departments were complemented by the establishment of MRC research units to work on specific areas, and all these reinforced the work being developed in the Council's central research institute, the National Institute for Medical Research (NIMR). Another method introduced by Fletcher was to foster the election of small, specialized committees of what constituted a scientific elite.[20] These were able to exert control through the selective support of certain individuals and areas of research at the expense of others. The limitation of the membership of these committees to 'men with common objects' tended to define which skills were considered to be most relevant to a specific area and thereby provided them with the opportunity to actually define the area. Examples of these specialized MRC committees were the Radiology Committee, the Hormones Committee, the Human Nutrition Committee, the Bacteriology Committee, and the Human Genetics Committee.

The growth of the field of reproductive endocrinology exemplifies the approach of Fletcher and the MRC in the development of specific areas of research. This highly specialized branch of biomedical science began to gain international credence in the late 1920s. In 1930 Fletcher acknowledged its potential importance by setting up a Sex Hormone Committee to oversee all new work in this area. The few fellowships that the MRC had granted in the 1920s culminated in Guy Marrian's meticulous work on the isolation and structure of oestrogenic hormones from human pregnancy urine.[21] This work was reinforced with the establishment of an entire department at the NIMR, directed by Sir Alan Parkes and devoted to research on sex physiology.[22] This was followed by initiatives to determine international standardization of the oestrogenic hormones, carried out at the NIMR, by organized clinical trials, and by the production by Sir Charles Dodds of synthetic hormones such as diethylstilboestrol, which appeared at the time to have enormous clinical potential in gynaecology and obstetrics, but whose iatrogenic carcinogenic effects had not yet become apparent. Finally in 1946

[19] Kohler, R. E. (1982). *From medical chemistry to biochemistry*. Cambridge University Press.
[20] MRC 1381/1: Fletcher to Newman, 7 May 1918. Fletcher's 'instinct' was 'against the artificial formation of committees on logical grounds'. He believed in 'pragmatism' in the formation of these committees.
[21] See Grant, J. K. (1982). Guy Frederick Marrian 1904–1981. *Biographical Memoirs of Fellows of the Royal Society*, **28**, 347–78; Walsh, J. (1984). The Scientific work of Guy Marrian (1904–1981), mainly with respect to steroid hormones. Unpublished dissertation for the Final Honour School of Physiological Sciences. University of Oxford.
[22] See Chap. 3.

a Clinical Endocrinology Research Unit was established in Edinburgh, with facilities not only for clinical research, but also for 'extensive basic biochemical studies'.

Under Fletcher's shrewd guidance and persistent efforts, philanthropic interest in medical science was exploited to support not only basic biomedical research, but also clinical research and the promotion of specialized investigations in tropical medicine.[23] Increasingly he came to see the private endowment of university departments by patrons such as the Rockefeller Foundation and the Dunn Trustees as crucial to his overall mission.[24] He used all his powers of persuasion to convince the Dunn Trustees that biochemistry was 'a charity', leading to the relief of suffering. After successfully negotiating the establishment of a Dunn Institute of Biochemistry in Cambridge and a Dunn School of Pathology in Oxford, he proceeded to exhort the Rockefeller Foundation to establish an Institute of Biochemistry in Oxford and a School of Pathology in Cambridge as 'counterparts' to the Dunn establishments.[25]

This partnership between the MRC and the Rockefeller Foundation was crucial for the development of scientific medicine in Britain. In the inter-war period the Rockefeller Foundation provided approximately £2 500 000 for teaching and medical research in British universities. It was not until 1936, with the Nuffield benefactions at the University of Oxford for the development of clinical research and postgraduate medical education, that British philanthropy began to match the contributions of the Rockefeller Foundation.

The endowment of the pre-clinical sciences by the Dunn Trust and the Rockefeller Foundation reinforced the MRC's own funding policy and provided adequate testimony to Fletcher's remarkable negotiating ability and powers of coercion. In encouraging private patronage to develop certain areas of research, he was careful to ensure that the administration of these endowments remained in the hands of the MRC, thereby guaranteeing the co-ordination of these ventures with the MRC's wider programme.

Inter-war medical research was characterized by struggles between scientists and medical practitioners relating to the control of medical research. It was cancer research that brought Fletcher into direct confrontation not only with the Ministry of Health, but also with members of the medical profession. In 1923 he embarked on a crusade to ensure the

[23] Fisher, D. (1978). The Rockefeller Foundation and the British Empire: the creation of the London School of Hygiene and Tropical Medicine. *History of Education*, 7, 129–43.

[24] Fisher, D. (1978). The Rockefeller Foundation and the development of scientific medicine in Britain. *Minerva*, 16, 20–41; Fisher, D. (1977). The impact of American foundations on the development of British university education 1900–1939, pp. 123–321. Unpublished PhD thesis. University of California, Berkeley; Kohler, Walter Fletcher, F. G. Hopkins, and the Dunn Institute of Biochemistry, pp. 330–55 (see note 1).

[25] See the MRC series of files for information on the Dunn benefactions.

supremacy he sought for the MRC, providing tenacious and effective opposition to the founders of the British Empire Cancer Campaign (BECC, from 1970 the Cancer Research Campaign), who included such eminent men of medicine as Lord Horder, Sir John Bland-Sutton, Sir Charles Gordon Watson, Sir Bernard Spilsbury, and J. P. Lockhart-Mummery.[26] The resultant interaction between the MRC, the BECC, ICRF, and the Middlesex Hospital, was to have practical long-term implications for the organization and funding of cancer research in Britain.

Fletcher's reaction on hearing of this new organization was hostile, 'I ought I think, to remind you that the Medical Research Council is the body specially charged by the Government and Parliament with the duty of supporting and encouraging work in *all* branches of medicine.'[27] He saw the new movement as a threat, a challenge to the scientific hierarchy he was seeking to create and to the supremacy of the MRC within that hierarchy. A challenge, what is more, by a distinguished gathering of eminent men who Fletcher nonetheless felt were entirely unsuited to the task they had undertaken. Experimental research was remote from the experience of most clinicians who, in his opinion, should therefore have been excluded from participating in or at least supervising it. He proceeded to draw upon a number of resources and to use his very wide sphere of influence and contacts in an all out attack on the Campaign. What he sought to do was to enforce a scientific veto thereby bringing all scientific work carried out under the aegis of the Campaign effectively under MRC control. He criticized its domination by medical practitioners, claiming that 'A committee of eminent clinicians will . . . be perfectly useless, as well as highly embarrassing'.[28] The establishment of the BECC thus took place amidst angry arguments, acrimonious disputes, conflicting interests, and power struggles concerning the crucial question of who should control the direction of biomedical research. It was central to the fate of new initiatives in cancer research and in serving to reinforce the central role of the MRC in the complex mechanism of distributing financial resources for the promotion of research.

The MRC's reaction to the creation of the Campaign reflected the distrust that scientists had of clinical promotion of research. Scientists not primarily concerned with the relevance of their work feared that control of the medical profession would hinder their progress. Medical practitioners, Fletcher argued, were incapable of co-ordinating scientific activities. He believed for example that the development of experimental pathology was being hindered by its close association with clinicians. It was both his view and that of many pathologists that the problem of cancer had 'passed beyond the realms of

[26] This episode is described in detail in Austoker, *A history of the ICRF*, Chap. 3 (see note 11).
[27] Cancer Research Campaign archive, CRC X1/1071: Fletcher to Locker Lampson, 5 May 1923.
[28] MRC 1383 I: Fletcher to Hopkins, 12 April 1923.

clinical observation, and clinicians do not possess the requisite education
either to add to or even to supervise work which demands highly trained
biologists'.[29] He was concerned to ensure that resources were directed not
only to problems relating specifically to cancer, but also towards general
biological research. He believed that, in the long run, it would be detrimental
to cancer research if a broader approach was not adopted. Any committee
serving the interests of medical research should, he believed, not have 'its
scientific independence fettered in any way by restriction to *ad hoc*
problems'.[30]

In the period between the wars, medical practice witnessed a struggle
between the Royal Colleges and emerging specialist groups. The Royal
Colleges sought to retain medicine as 'a unified whole', whereas the specialist
groups wanted to raise the standards in their own fields.[31] Clinical research
was one means by which emerging specialist groups sought to improve their
status.[32] Medical research was therefore crucial to the process of
specialization. Lords Moynihan and Dawson saw the MRC as a potential
threat since it encouraged precisely those groups seeking to break away from
Royal Colleges' control. The traditional authority and supremacy of the
Royal Colleges as the great leaders of medicine was challenged by a new
young generation of medical practitioners who found themselves unable to
penetrate the 'charmed circle'. The self-perpetuating machinery of the Royal
College was geared to maintain autonomy. The Colleges were predictably
reluctant to see medicine becoming disunited.

The Royal Colleges regarded the divergence between scientific research
and clinical practice critically. Anxious about the deep-seated divisions
emerging within the ranks of the medical profession, they contemplated
the involvement of the MRC with suspicion and resentment. The MRC
was quite openly encouraging precisely those groups that were attempting
to disengage themselves from the stranglehold of the Royal Colleges.[33] As
far as the MRC was concerned it was crucial for it to gain a firm base of
support from the ranks of the anti-colleges lobby in that this assisted in its
ensuring that the pre-clinical sciences remained independent of practitioner
control.

The Royal Colleges refused to accept that they were 'not fit' to co-ordinate
or organize scientific research, and continued to express anxiety at the 'lack
of relevance' of much existing biomedical investigation being funded by the

[29] W. B. (1923). The problem of cancer. *Nature*, **112**, 101–2.

[30] MRC 1383 IV: Fletcher to Newman, 22 October 1924.

[31] Stevens, R. (1966). *Medical practice in modern England. The impact of specialization and
state medicine*. Yale University Press, Newhaven.

[32] Cantor, D. (1985). Resources for radiobiology: medical support for research into the
biological effects of radiation in inter-war Britain. *Society for the Social History of Medicine
Bulletin*, **37**, 72–5; see Chap. 9, this volume.

[33] See Austoker, *A history of the ICRF*, Chap. 5 (see note 11).

MRC.[34] In 1930 Moynihan, then President of the Royal College of Surgeons, persuaded his Council of the need to undertake 'surgical research' and to provide laboratories for this purpose.[35] This led to the establishment of an Institute for 'research relevant to surgery' at the Buckston Browne Farm, opened in July 1933. Moynihan persisted in recording his strong disapproval of what he referred to as the 'deplorable' and 'sinful indifference' of physiologists to clinical medicine, complaining somewhat bitterly that 'too much "medical research" was centred in the laboratory rather than the wards'.[36] He pointed to a 'grievous neglect' in biomedical research, so that the 'divorce of research from observation' was imminent. He detailed the distrust and antagonism felt by the Royal College, who strongly resented the MRC for remaining 'disdainful of clinical activities', and for deliberately having 'inadequate' clinical representation on the Council.[37]

In 1932 Leverhulme funds became available to the Royal Colleges enabling them to provide research scholarships.[38] This stimulated the Royal College of Physicians to contemplate the organization and direction of its own independent programme of research. The broader significance of such a move was immediately apparent to Fletcher. It prompted him to mount what was to be his final aggressive stand over the question of control of biomedical research.[39] In the last year of his life and in deteriorating health he resisted this threat to the MRC with all his characteristic energy and fervour. He was encouraged by Gowland Hopkins, who insisted that, 'the idiocy of the RCP pretending to start the control of research' ignored the tide of feeling against the 'Distinguished Clinicians'.[40] Hopkins assured his ailing friend that, 'Harley Street is feeling a new and more critical atmosphere. It is feeling chilly.'[41]

Fletcher's final and bitter clash in this unpleasant controversy brought him into direct confrontation with Lord Dawson, President of the Royal College of Physicians. Dawson, one of the profession's most distinguished and respected members, had in 1931 at Fletcher's suggestion agreed to serve on the MRC, hoping by this move to 'further co-operation between the Council's

---

[34] Ibid. p. 148.

[35] Berkeley Moynihan, Memorandum on surgical research, Meeting of the Council, Royal College of Surgeons, 14 June 1928.

[36] Lord Moynihan (1930). The science of medicine. *Lancet*, ii, 779–85; Editorial, (1930). Progress of clinical science. *Lancet*, ii, 805–6.

[37] Lord Moynihan (1930). The work of laboratories, letter to the Editor. *British Medical Journal*, ii, 979, 1103–4. See also Fletcher, W. (1930). The work of laboratories. *British Medical Journal*, ii, 928.

[38] Austoker, *A history of the ICRF*, p. 149 (see note 11).

[39] This is also referred to in Chap. 9 and 10. The episode is described in detail in Austoker, *A history of the ICRF*, Chap. 5 (see note 11).

[40] See Hopkins to Fletcher, 2 February 1933, in Fletcher, M. (1957). *The bright countenance. A personal biography of Walter Morley Fletcher*, p. 285. Hodder and Stoughton, London.

[41] Ibid. p. 285.

activities and the clinical field'.[42] Such optimism was in the circumstances scarcely realistic.

Dawson precipitated the crisis by criticizing the MRC's attitude to clinical research. He accused it of deliberately, 'minimising the value of practitioners' work in comparison with that of the research worker', by adopting a lofty or superior attitude to clinicians as of ' "highbrows" looking down upon "lowbrows" '.[43] In inquiring of Fletcher whether medicine was 'so inefficient that it requires the Royal Society [or MRC] to do its research', long years of acquaintance should have warned him as to the inevitable response. With characteristic bluntness Fletcher replied in the affirmative, reminding Dawson that the Royal College of Physicians, of which he himself was 'a loyal member', had no effective machinery for managing research work.[44] Further, Moynihan and Dawson had 'alienated scientific opinion' by stressing that headship amongst successful practitioners was a qualification in itself for leadership in scientific work. The Royal Colleges' insistence that it was their 'right' to assume a co-ordinating role over all aspects of medical research had invited 'discord and dissention'.[45] Past history, Fletcher pointed out, had shown how 'incompetent' they had been in managing research work, as demonstrated by the 'feeble' efforts to manage the affairs of the ICRF.[46] Until they did 'properly' what they had undertaken 30 years previously, with respect to the ICRF, they had 'no right to assume fresh responsibilities of a similar kind'.

Fletcher's interaction with the Royal Colleges provided another example of his overriding determination that it was the Council's responsibility to watch over the entire field of biomedical research in this country, irrespective of the agent involved. It also highlights his fervent commitment to the promotion of fundamental scientific research under the guidance and direction of those with a rigorous scientific training.

Fletcher can be considered as the architect of policy in the biomedical sciences in this country. His general plans for supporting basic research have undoubtedly had a profound influence on the overall development of medical research in this country. The central role of the fundamental biomedical sciences in the policy of the MRC in the inter-war period essentially confined initiatives in other areas. This emphasis, coupled with the various methods adopted by Fletcher and the Council to implement its research policy, essentially laid down the pattern of development of

[42] MRC PF 100/18: Dawson to Fletcher, 19 June 1931.
[43] See Fletcher to Dawson, 21 November 1932. MRC PF 100/18. See too the section on 'Clinical research' in the *Report of the MRC* (1931–32), pp. 9–11.
[44] MRC PF 100/18: Fletcher to Dawson, 9 January 1933, pp. 3–5.
[45] Ibid. p. 5.
[46] Ibid. p. 5.

institutional and university medical sciences which persisted far into the post-war years. Fletcher's influence cannot be ignored.

One should not lose sight, however, of the fact that Fletcher did believe in the ultimate utility of basic medical research to practical medical problems. He continually emphasized the need for the application of every 'discovery' to the problems of ill-health and disease.[47] He believed that the road to national health was 'along the advancing line of scientific progress'. How far this ideal has been realized is a matter for conjecture.

[47] See Contemporary Medical Archive Centre, CMAC PP/WMF/7: W. Fletcher, 'Medical research', 4 October 1926; CMAC PP/WMF/8: W. M. Fletcher, 'Research in relation to public health', Public Health Congress (1928), pp. 41–60; CMAC PP/WMF/8: W. M. Fletcher, 'The scope and needs of medical research', Royal Institution, 27 May 1932.

3

The National Institute for Medical Research and related activities of the MRC

JOAN AUSTOKER AND LINDA BRYDER

Following the allocation of a sum of money for medical research under the 1911 National Insurance Act, discussions commenced concerning whether the funds should go to existing research institutes including the universities, or whether a new central institute for medical research should be set up. Eventually a compromise was reached—a third of the research funds would be allocated to finance a central institute and the rest to finance research projects throughout the country. The central institute of the Medical Research Committee was set up in Hampstead in 1914 and became the National Institute for Medical Research (NIMR) in 1920. Initially it consisted of departments of bacteriology, applied physiology, biochemistry and pharmacology, and medical statistics. These departments expanded, contracted, or were amended in the following decades as new research opportunities were pursued, and the Institute also became involved in the area of standardization of drugs and other medicines at the behest of the Government. The Institute, under the directorship of Sir Henry Dale, became a world renowned centre for medical research and a jewel in the crown of the MRC.

Administration of the Institute, 1914 – 50

In 1914 the North London Hospital for Consumption, Mount Vernon, Hampstead (founded in 1880), was purchased freehold for £35 000, for the new research institute. It was situated near the summit of a hill in Hampstead, combining the advantage of ready access to the centre of London with those of 'freedom from the noise and vibration of London traffic, and elevation above the London smoke and dust'.[1] It was originally intended that part of the building should be used as a research hospital of 15–20 beds. Little was done to convert the hospital into a research centre initially, as negotiations

[1] NIMR Institute History: Sir Henry Dale notes, memorandum written for A. Flexner on the origin, development and activities of the NIMR, 19 May 1924.

were also underway with the Lister Institute, whose director, Charles Martin, had proposed handing over the Institute, complete with staff, to the Government for the purposes of the new research initiative. Lord Iveagh, already a generous benefactor of the Lister Institute, had also offered to provide money for the erection of a small research hospital on the Lister site. This attempt to 'rationalize the nation's research potential in medicine' proved highly controversial in the event, and was eventually rejected by the Ordinary Members of the Lister Institute, who preferred to retain the Institute's independence.[2]

At the commencement of war, the Medical Research Committee's central institute was handed over to the Army Medical Service as Hampstead Military Hospital, where work was done on the 'disordered action of the soldier's heart' under the direction of Thomas (later Sir Thomas) Lewis until 1917 when this work was transferred to Colchester (see Chapter 10). Hampstead Hospital was then used for Canadian war casualties, and later became the central hospital for officers of the Royal Flying Corps and the Royal Air Service, for the study and treatment of disabilities due to flying.

Directors of the departments of the Institute had been appointed by the outbreak of war. Sir Almroth Wright was to direct the Bacteriology Department, H. H. (later Sir Henry) Dale the Biochemistry and Pharmacology Department, L. E. (later Sir Leonard) Hill the Applied Physiology Department, and John Brownlee the Medical Statistics Department. During the war, the bacteriologists were based at the Inoculation Department of St Mary's Hospital, although much of their time was spent in France; the biochemists and pharmacologists were based at the Lister Institute; the applied physiologists were based at London Hospital; and the Department of Medical Statistics occupied a house in Guildford Street, Russell Square, London.

The Mount Vernon buildings were returned from the Army for the new Institute in April 1920, the same month that the MRC was established. A change which emerged after the First World War was the abandonment of the plan to incorporate a research hospital within the Institute. In his outline of the history of the Institute, Harington noted the abandonment of a research hospital 'on which so much stress had previously been laid . . ., although no reference to its formal abandonment is to be found in the Reports of the Council'.[3]

When the Institute had been founded in 1914, the appointment of a chief director had been discussed. It was rumoured that the post would go to Sir

[2] CMAC SA/LIS/H/10–19: for discussion relating to the merger proposal and its rejection. See also Morgan, N. (1986). A note of proposed amalgamation of the Lister Institute of Preventive Medicine and the Medical Research Committee: philanthropy and state support of medical research, 1914. *Annals of Science*, **43**, 287–9.

[3] *Proceedings of the Royal Society, Bulletin* (1949), **136**, 336.

Almroth Wright as one of the most distinguished scientists of the time. Wright was based at St Mary's Hospital where he was professor of pathology and where, during the previous decade, he had built up an international reputation as a result of his work relating to vaccines and vaccine therapy. Wright had fifteen assistants in the so-called Inoculation Department of St Mary's, including Alexander Fleming, who was appointed in 1906 and remained until 1948. It was there that Fleming discovered penicillin in 1929.[4] The rumour that Wright was to be offered the directorship of the new Institute had reached Wright himself. However, it was subsequently decided that no such appointment would be made, that each department would have its own director, of equal status, responsible to the Medical Research Committee and co-ordinated by a general secretary. 'Domestic affairs' would be in the hands of a staff committee, consisting of the directors and the secretary, and Wright was invited to become chair of this committee.[5]

In his history of the MRC, Landsborough Thomson surmised that personal considerations were largely involved in the decision not to offer the post to Wright, that the Medical Research Committee was finding it difficult to deal with this eminent scientist 'as a man of affairs'.[6] Wright was claiming the power of direction over all external workers in bacteriology supported by the Medical Research Committee, unless they were under local directors who were themselves of high standing. More importantly, he apparently wanted some influence in the management of the Medical Research Committee's general affairs. He believed that the directors of the departments should be made members of the Committee. Giving evidence before the Departmental Committee on Tuberculosis in 1912 he had been strongly in favour of a central institute for medical research, but had objected to an advisory committee as he felt it would interfere. Instead, what was required was a 'strong-minded director', and he cited the Lister Institute as an example, where Charles Martin was in 'supreme control'.[7] On the other hand, in 1914, before the appointment of Fletcher, Wright expressed his opposition to the idea of a secretary with wide-ranging powers, an opinion which he reiterated five years later.[8] Thus, according to Landsborough Thomson, 'One can sense that after the war it was not without relief that the Committee received, in March 1919, Sir Almroth Wright's request to be allowed, on terms to remain at St

[4] Macfarlane G. (1985). *Alexander Fleming: the man and the myth*. Oxford University Press.
[5] Landsborough Thomson, A. (1973). *Half a century of medical research*, Vol. I, *Origins and policy of the Medical Research Council (UK)*, p. 115. HMSO, London.
[6] Ibid. pp. 115–6
[7] Addison Box 32: Minutes of evidence before Inter-departmental Committee on Tuberculosis, 15 May 1912, p. 63.
[8] Landsborough Thomson, *Medical research*, Vol. I, p. 116 (see note 5).

Mary's Hospital.' He was given a personal grant supplementing his relatively small salary as director of the Inoculation Department of the hospital, an arrangement which continued until he was 65 in 1926. This needed to be stated, according to Landsborough Thomson, because Wright himself avoided public acknowledgement of this support, and his biographers tended to follow him in minimizing the connection.[9] Thus, more was involved than implied in Dale's explanation that 'Almroth Wright had wisely decided that it would no longer be worth his while to move from his familiar quarters and clinical contacts at St Mary's Hospital for a new and detached start at Hampstead, in view of the short term of service then left to him.'[10] In losing Wright, however, the MRC lost the services of a man regarded as a great scientist in his day and with the ability to inspire workers around him.[11] Of his staff, only Leonard Colebrook moved to the Institute (later becoming an external staff member) and Wright's assistant, S. R. Douglas became the director of the Department.

Eventually the Institute gained a capable and energetic director in Henry Dale, at that time the head of the Biochemistry Department and formerly director of the Wellcome Physiological Research Laboratories. When he was appointed overall director of the Institute in 1928 he expressed surprise at the appointment. Yet it was clear that the change was one of name only. Already in 1924, in an outline of the Institute for the benefit of Flexner, Dale had stated, 'For the purposes of administrative efficiency, . . . it has been found necessary to make one of the directors personally responsible for the ordinary administration of the Institute . . . this function is exercised by Dr Dale . . . For this purpose the Administrative Secretary and his office staff are directly responsible to Dr Dale, who acts as the normal medium of communication between the Council and the Institute as a whole.'[12] It appears that the 1928 appointment was merely formalizing an existing situation. Dale remained director until 1942, when he retired and was replaced by C. R. (later Sir Charles) Harington, formerly professor of Chemical Pathology and director of the Graham Medical Research Laboratories at University College Hospital Medical School. Harington directed the Institute until 1962, supervising the move of the Institute from Hampstead to Mill Hill in 1950.

[9] Ibid. p. 116.

[10] NIMR Institute History: Sir Henry Dale's notes for Landsborough Thomson, *c.* late 1960s, Early History, p. 2.

[11] See biographies of Wright: Cope, V. Z. (1966). *Almroth Wright. Founder of modern vaccine-therapy.* Thomas Nelson, London; Colebrook, L. (1954). *Almroth Wright. Provocative doctor and thinker.* Heinemann, London.

[12] NIMR Institute History: Dale's memorandum for Flexner, 19 May 1924.

Department of Bacteriology

The initial Bacteriological Department of the Medical Research Committee was in effect the Inoculation Department of St Mary's Hospital, under the direction of Sir Almroth Wright. In anticipation of arranging its own research hospital, the Medical Research Committee paid St Mary's Hospital a fee for the bacteriologists' use of research beds at the hospital. A fee of £2500 per annum was paid for the use of 25 beds, an arrangement which lasted until 1917. The main work undertaken in the Bacteriological Department during the war was the preparation of anti-typhoid and other vaccines for the use of the armed forces. Approximately 10 million doses of anti-typhoid vaccine were prepared at St Mary's Hospital during the war, with the Medical Research Committee providing the necessary staff at the cost of £1000 per annum.

Sir Almroth Wright himself was appointed Consulting Physician to His Majesty's Forces overseas in September 1914, and was sent to head an army laboratory in Boulogne. There he commenced research on the pathology and treatment of infected wounds. His main contribution was the development of a hypertonic saline solution for the treatment of grossly infected wounds, although there was some dispute over the efficacy of this treatment (see Chapter 4). Apart from Wright's hypertonic saline solution and the development of antiseptics for wound treatment, the production of a serum to combat gas gangrene was also being investigated. In November 1917 a British and American Joint Gas-Gangrene Committee was formed in France under the chairmanship of the surgeon Cuthbert Wallace. The problem of gas gangrene was at that time being actively studied under the direction of Simon Flexner at the Rockefeller Institute in New York. In 1917 he sent samples to Fletcher of a prospective serum against *Bacillus welchii*, the organism causing gas gangrene, for the Medical Research Committee to examine and conduct clinical trials. Collaboration between the Medical Research Committee and scientists at Boulogne, the Lister Institute, the Imperial Cancer Research Fund, the London Hospital, and the Wellcome Laboratories, resulted in supplies of protective serum against gas gangrene becoming available for the purposes of trial in France just prior to the Armistice.

S. R. Douglas, the new director of the Department of Bacteriology following the war, preferred the designation 'experimental pathology' to 'bacteriology' to describe his department, and both were incorporated into the title. In the 1930s it was further amended to become the Department of Experimental Pathology and Bacteriology with subdivisions of Protistology, Microscopy and Physical Methods. The area of research in which this department was largely absorbed after the First World War was virology, for which the Institute was to become famous. In 1932 D. P. O'Brien of the

Rockefeller Foundation described the NIMR as 'the most important center of research on viruses in England, and one of the most important in the world'.[13]

The suggestion that a useful line of inquiry would be the nature of infective agents which had been found to pass through bacteria-proof filters had come initially from Sir William Leishman, a member of the Council, and led to the proposal to conduct research into dog distemper. Dog distemper was considered suitable not only because of the availability of the research material, but also because an effective method of immunization or treatment was thought 'to make a useful appeal to a large proportion of the multitude of British keepers and lovers of dogs'.[14] Quite independently, J. B. Buxton, veterinary superintendent at the Wellcome Laboratories, had been approached by a group of titled Masters of Foxhounds who wished him to take charge of a special investigation of dog distemper, with the support of the fund for that purpose to be raised by *The Field* weekly journal and *The Daily Telegraph*. These funds were diverted into the NIMR effort, to finance research undertaken by S. R. Douglas, W. E. Gye, and P. P. Laidlaw.

While British lovers of dogs undoubtedly would have approved of a prospective vaccine or treatment for dog distemper, they did not appear so enthusiastic about the prospect of research being carried out on dogs. This was especially so for those in the neighbourhood of the Institute, described by Dale as 'so sniffy and snobbish a neighbourhood'.[15] Indeed when the research got underway, local residents began complaining of constantly howling dogs. Whether it was irritation at the noise of the dogs or pity for the dogs that led to the complaints remains unclear, but anti-vivisectionists quickly took up the cause and used it for a general attack on the MRC. The *Abolitionist* wrote in 1922 of 'a vast orgy of torture of sentient creatures and a heavy toll of animal life sacrificed in the interests of pinchbeck "science"'.[16]

It was local complaints that were largely responsible for the MRC's decision in 1921 to purchase a more remote site to accommodate dogs and ferrets (also susceptible to dog distemper and considered a convenient experimental animal). A derelict property known as Rhodes Farm, with frontage to the Ridgeway, Mill Hill, and consisting of 39 acres of agricultural land, was purchased in 1922 for £6000: accommodation for dogs and ferrets was constructed, as well as temporary buildings for laboratory research. Six acres on the east side of the plot were leased to the Imperial Cancer Research Fund (ICRF) in 1922, where it constructed the Stroud Research

---

[13] Rockefeller Archive Centre Archives: Box 21, 401, England, file 277, 5 August 1932.

[14] NIMR Institute History: Dale's notes for Landsborough Thomson, *c*. late 1960s, Researches at the Mount Vernon Institute, p. 3.

[15] Ibid. p. 16.

[16] NIMR press cuttings: *Abolitionist*, 1 March 1922.

Laboratory.[17] The MRC 'welcomed the association of the Fund on the farm at Mill Hill Park'.[18] Later, in 1934 a property known as Burton Bank, comprising 8 acres belonging to Mill Hill School and adjacent to the Stroud Laboratory, came onto the market.[19] In a decision later proved to be notable for its lack of foresight, the Fund decided not to buy the property but agreed to become the MRC's tenants if the MRC went ahead with the purchase.[20] Accordingly, following the purchase of the Estate by the MRC, the Fund was granted a lease from 1936 for fifty years, provided it vacated its existing premises in the Stroud Laboratory—the MRC had by this time laboratory plans to move the NIMR to Mill Hill and required the land on which the Stroud Laboratory was situated.

At Mill Hill from 1922 onwards, both the MRC and the Imperial Cancer Research Fund launched major programmes to resurrect tumour virology, which had been condemned to obscurity following Peyton Rous's seminal observations a decade earlier.[21] It was William Gye at the NIMR's farm laboratory who was to make a sensational impact on cancer research in Britain. Gye had moved from the ICRF Laboratories to the Department of Bacteriology at the NIMR in 1919. His work engaged him in the study of the causation of malignant fowl tumours by injection of cell-free filtrates from pre-existent tumours. Walter Fletcher regarded Gye's research as 'supremely important'.[22] In consequence, high-quality young research scientists sought the opportunity of working with Gye. Sir Frederick Andrewes, for example, requested that his talented son, Christopher (later Sir Christopher), be given permission to undertake research with Gye.[23] Christopher Andrewes' subsequent investigations in the field of virology were to establish him as a far greater authority in this field than Gye himself was ever to become.

In July 1925 Gye created a great stir when he reported the presence of malignant avian growths of hitherto undetected viral infectivity acting in conjunction with a specific chemical 'activator'.[24] His discovery involved elaborate biochemical and microscopic analyses of the neoplasms.[25] His collaborator came from another subdepartment of the Department of Bacteriology, that of Applied Optics, set up in 1919 and transferred in 1925 to the Council's Farm Laboratories at Mill Hill. There J. E. Barnard, a West

[17] ICRF Executive Committee minutes, 5 July and 14 October 1922; MRC 1170: Hallett to Fletcher, 6 July 1922.
[18] ICRF Executive Committee minutes, 22 July 1922.
[19] ICRF Executive Committee minutes, 10 October 1934; NIMR 588/2/4 and 588/2/4e.
[20] MRC 1170/41: Landsborough Thomson, memorandum, 16 October 1934.
[21] See Austoker, J. (1988). *A history of the Imperial Cancer Research Fund 1902–1986*, pp. 92–9. Oxford University Press.
[22] MRC 1115/GI: Fletcher to Hopkins, 9 January 1925.
[23] MRC 1115/GI: Andrewes to Fletcher, 25 March 1925.
[24] Gye, W. E. (1925). The aetiology of malignant new growths. *Lancet*, ii, 109–17.
[25] MRC 1115/GI: note to Press Agencies, 13 July 1925; Editorial (1925). 'The cancer virus'. *Lancet* ii, 183.

End hatter by profession and a leading figure among amateur microscopists,[26] had developed sophisticated new physical methods for the visualization of ultraviolet microphotography of the viruses cultivated from tumours of both fowls and mammals.[27] Using material provided by Reyton Rous in 1922, Gye claimed to have obtained two separate factors in tumour formation, one an extrinsic filter-passing infective agent, the other an unstable cell-specific chemical adjuvant. His interpretation of the 'cause of cancer' in terms of these two 'factors' was put forward as an all-encompassing hypothesis, serving to reconcile contrasting theories on the origin of cancer.

On the publication of their work, Gye and Barnard became instant celebrities. In what was regarded as 'the outstanding event of the period', the two men were widely acclaimed for their 'epoch-making' discovery.[28] Their conclusions were considered to be 'of first-class scientific and practical importance'.[29] In an unprecedented step, the King sought an audience with them to congratulate them on their 'significant achievement'.[30]

The irrefutable confirmation of Gye's theoretical assumptions and practical observations would have constituted a notable triumph.[31] At the ICRF, however, attempts to repeat Gye's fundamental experiments yielded 'specious results', and scientists were forced to concede that they could find 'no evidence' of the existence of a specific factor as postulated by Gye.[32] In the United States, Gye's work came to be regarded with suspicion as investigators reported negative results and negative conclusions when employing his techniques.[33] Gradually as repetition of his experiments failed to yield consistent results, Gye himself was reluctantly forced to concede that this early work on filterable viruses had 'fallen into disrepute'. He remained, however, resolute in his pursuit of fresh evidence to substantiate his ideas on the virus theory of cancer origin.

In 1931 Gye, with his collaborator W. J. Purdy, published a volume somewhat ambitiously entitled *The cause of cancer*.[34] In this Gye's logical

[26] NIMR Institute History: Dale's notes for Landsborough Thomson, *c*. late 1960s, Researches at the Mount Vernon Institute, p. 1.

[27] Barnard, J. E. (1925). The microscopical examination of filterable viruses. *Lancet*, **ii**, 117–23.

[28] ICRF: *Twenty-third annual report 1924–25*, p. 6; *The Sunday Times*, 6 December 1925.

[29] American Society for the Control of Cancer, 'The Barnard and Gye discoveries', *Campaign Notes*, 7 July 1925.

[30] MRC PF 123/1: Fletcher to Gye, 21 and 22 July 1925.

[31] Triola, V. and Shimkin, M. (1969). The American Cancer Society and cancer research: origins and organization, 1913–1943. *Cancer Research*, **29**, 1622.

[32] ICRF Executive Committee minutes, 2 June 1926 and 4 May 1927.

[33] MRC 1115/GI: Mueller to Gye, 9 and 14 May 1928. Mueller wrote that 'I have seen *no* evidence that your work and conclusions are right'. See also Mueller, J. H. (1927). An experimental study of Gye's cancer theory. *Journal of Experimental Medicine*, **45**, 243–62.

[34] Gye, W. E. and Purdy, W. J. (1931). *The cause of cancer*. Cassell, London.

exposure of many of the fallacies underlying orthodox theories of cancer aetiology, and his valuable description of the extent and importance of fundamental investigations, were offset by wild claims and speculations which others failed to confirm or refused to accept.[35] His inability to convince a 'sceptical pathological world' that viruses were concerned in the causation of tumours was not helped by the publication of preliminary, incomplete, and highly speculative results. He was forced to turn his attention to an immunological approach, obtaining results which were more reproducible.[36]

Despite the notoriety attached to Gye's work, the NIMR made an important contribution to the study of virology. The virus of dog distemper was, for example, eventually isolated, and a vaccine was produced by 1927 (commercially from 1928) which was so effective that the disease was soon practically eliminated. Researchers into dog distemper could therefore congratulate themselves on having a legitimate case against the anti-vivisectionists. Dale later described the dog distemper research as 'probably the most important contribution made by the MRC and the National Institute to the progress of medical knowledge, during my period there'.[37]

The researchers into dog distemper then turned their attention to influenza. In 1932 P. P. (later Sir Patrick) Laidlaw, C. H. Andrewes, and Wilson Smith succeeded in inducing a fever in ferrets by exposure to nasal washings from human cases of influenza. Confirmation that the ferret was really suffering from influenza came by chance when a feverish ferret sneezed violently in the face of C. H. Stuart-Harris who, 40 hours later, developed a typical attack of influenza.[38] In 1933 the influenza virus was isolated by Laidlaw, Andrewes, and Wilson Smith.

As work on the influenza virus continued, it was soon realized that the influenza virus strain varied from year to year. In 1947 the NIMR accepted responsibility for organizing a World Influenza Centre on behalf of the World Health Organization. This centre consisted of two small laboratories at the Institute. Every outbreak of influenza was reported, a sample sent to the centre, and the immunological character of the particular outbreak determined. It was hoped in this way to avoid a recurrence of the 1918–19 influenza epidemic which had caught the world totally unawares and in which an estimated 25 million people had died.

Andrewes proceeded to study the common cold. An isolation hospital was

[35] Andrewes, C. H. (1952). William Ewart Gye 1884–1952. *Obituary Notices of Fellows of the Royal Society*, **8**, 424.

[36] See Andrewes, C. H. (1934). Viruses in relation to the aetiology of tumours. *Lancet*, **ii**, 117–24.

[37] NIMR Institute History: Dale's notes for Landsborough Thomson, *c.* late 1960s, Researches at the Mount Vernon Institute, p. 5.

[38] Work, T. S. (1983). *Biologist*, **30** (2), 96.

set up in 1946 near Salisbury (Common Cold Research Unit, Harvard Hospital, Salisbury) where human volunteers would be infected and observed under controlled conditions.[39]

In 1928 Protistology was added to the Department to incorporate the work of Clifford Dobell. Indeed this subsection of the Department was entirely manned by Dobell, described as a perfectionist who preferred to work alone.[40]

By 1949 'Microscopy and Physical Methods', another subdepartment, had expanded considerably so that Harington wrote, 'One of the more remarkable developments in medical and biological research in recent years is the increasingly important part which is played by physical methods.' He described facilities for complicated procedures such as

phase contrast microscopy, electron microscopy, electrophoresis, high-speed centrifugation and ultrasonics. In addition to all this the introduction of the use of isotopes as valuable tools in biological research and particularly the almost unlimited availability of radioactive isotopes for this purpose has necessitated the undertaking of an amount of purely physical work which would have seemed fantastic for an institute of medical research even as little as ten or twelve years ago.[41]

At least half of the time of those in this Division was taken up with work in collaboration with those of other departments. Technology had entered the world of medical research and was there to stay.

Department of Biochemistry and Pharmacology

An early interest in this department was the study of insulin following its discovery by F. G. Banting and C. H. Best at the University of Toronto in 1921–2 (see also Chapter 8). In May 1922 the Board of Governors of the University of Toronto offered the patent rights for insulin in 'Britain and the rest of the Empire' to the MRC.[42] MRC scientists were 'interested but skeptical'.[43] In autumn 1922 Dale, together with H. W. Dudley, went to Toronto to report on the scientific status of insulin and to recommend whether, and if so how, arrangements could be made for its production and supply for the treatment of diabetes in Britain.[44] Their response was enthusiastic. 'The thing is undoubtedly a true story', Dale wrote to Fletcher,

[39] This is due to close down in 1990.

[40] Landsborough Thomson, A. (1975). *Half a century of medical research*, Vol. II, *The programme of the Medical Research Council (UK)*, p. 130. HMSO, London.

[41] Harington, C. R. (1949). *Proceedings of the Royal Society, Bulletin*, **136**, 344; *Nature* (1950), **165**, 150.

[42] See Bliss, M. (1983). *The discovery of insulin*, p. 139. Paul Harris Publishing, Edinburgh.

[43] Ibid. p. 165.

[44] MRC 1092/25: Fletcher memorandum, 7 July 1922.

emphasizing the importance of getting its production started by suitable manufacturers in Britain.[45] Dale and Dudley also conceded that patenting was probably necessary and that the MRC ought to accept control of the British patent. This, they claimed, would enable the Council to 'exercise a moral control over the manufacturers, and would induce the latter to submit to a system of supervision, as regards this product, which the law does not enable the Council at present to enforce'.[46] Accordingly the MRC instituted a programme whereby the organization of clinical trials could be supervised by the NIMR, while commercial production proceeded also in consultation with the NIMR. The Council later held a supplementary patent covering an improved method of purification devised by Dudley. Biological standardization of insulin was of vital importance—in appropriate doses it had life-saving effects, but the consequences of too much or too little were disastrous. The NIMR was to play a key role in its standardization. Dudley's new methods of purification and his production of a stable dry powder were put forward by Dale at an international conference in 1923.[47] After trial in various laboratories, this substance was standardized and formally adopted at a further conference 2 years later.

Other important work carried out in the Biochemistry and Pharmacology Department was Dale's own work on the chemical transmission of nervous impulses and acetylcholine, which gained him a Nobel prize in 1936 jointly with Otto Loewi of Graz. The first isolation of a vitamin, 'calciferol' or D2, occurred under the auspices of this Department, important because of its antirachitic activity. Work on the chemotherapy of malaria, kala-azar, and other tropical diseases continued at the Institute, and work was carried out on the modern use of curare and curare-like drugs in anaesthesia.

In 1926 the MRC set up a Chemotherapy Committee jointly with the Department of Scientific and Industrial Research, and chaired by Dale. This resulted from a desire to encourage co-operation between chemists, biologists and pathologists, and clinicians in the production of new compounds, in their experimental trials, and in the observations of their effects on human disease. The Committee provided fresh impetus to the MRC's involvement in the production and biological testing of new synthetic substances of potential therapeutic significance. From this Committee new synthetic compounds, many of them prepared at the NIMR, were put forward for biological study or for clinical trial. Other MRC committees, in particular the Sex Hormones Committee, were also expected to bring to notice biological products for which clinical appraisal 'under controlled

[45] MRC 1092/25: Dale to Fletcher, 26 September 1932.
[46] MRC 1092/25: H. H. Dale, H. W. Dudley, 'Report to the Medical Research Council of our visit to Canada and the United States', 30 October 1922. See also Bliss, *Discovery of insulin*, p. 166 (see note 42).
[47] Landsborough Thomson, *Medical research*, Vol. II, p. 247 (see note 40).

conditions' was called for.[48] The introduction of insulin for the treatment of diabetes, liver extracts for the management of pernicious anaemia, and Georges Dreyer's 'diaplyte vaccine' for the treatment of tuberculosis,[49] were tested accordingly.

In 1931 the MRC extended this interest by setting up a more regular machinery for the organization of clinical trials. After its Chemotherapy Committee had consulted with the Association of British Chemical Manufacturers, certain conditions were agreed to under which new substances, British and foreign, could be submitted to the MRC's newly formed Therapeutic Trials Committee (TTC) for clinical study. This provided the basis for co-operative effort between the MRC and many manufacturing firms, both in Britain and Europe.[50] Over the course of the next decade, trials of numerous and sometimes important new remedies were undertaken under the auspices of the TTC. Amongst the compounds clinically tested were calciferol, ephedrine and pseudoephedrine, amylsalicylate progesterone, oestrin, degroxin, ergotoxine, testosterone, and diethrol stilboestrol. The tests of the actions of sulphanilamide and related drugs in streptococcal and other infections were to prove of major medical significance.[51] Of particular note was the work undertaken in 1936 by Leonard Colebrook and Maeve Kenny which demonstrated the beneficial effect of prontosil in puerperal sepsis.

The TTC included a formidable array of clinical and pharmacological expertise. There were no statisticians on the Committee, although expert opinion was frequently sought from the MRC's Statistical Committee, in particular its director, Major Greenwood, and Austin (later Sir Austin) Bradford Hill. Although controls were used in these clinical trials, the evolution of the randomized controlled trial awaited the trial designed by Bradford Hill for the MRC in 1946 to measure the effect of streptomycin in respiratory tuberculosis.[52] Bradford Hill had in fact alluded to the importance of randomization in one of the early trials conducted by the TTC. Between 1931 and 1934 a trial was held in several centres in the UK to examine the therapeutic value of specific sera for lobar pneumonia.[53] In 1933 Bradford Hill questioned the methods used in allocating cases into serum and

---

[48] MRC: *Annual report 1930–31* (1932), p. 22.

[49] See Bryder, L. (1988). *Below the magic mountain: a social history of tuberculosis in twentieth-century Britain* , pp. 192–3. Oxford University Press.

[50] MRC 1523/1: TTC memo, 'Conditions under which the Therapeutic Trials Committee may be prepared to undertake clinical trials of new remedies, of British or foreign origin, submitted by the manufacturers', 1931.

[51] MRC 1523/33, I, II; MRC 1523/44; MRC 152, I, II, III.

[52] See Chapter 1; see also Hill, A. B. (1951). The clinical trial. *British Medical Bulletin*, 7, 278–82; Hill, A. B. (1963). Medical ethics and controlled trials. *British Medical Journal*, i, 5043–9.

[53] MRC 1487: TTC, 'The serum treatment of lobar pneumonia'. (1934) *British Medical Journal*, i, 241–5.

control groups. He noted in a detailed criticism of the provision of controls for this trial that greater effort should be taken 'that the division of cases really did ensure a random selection'.[54]

The concept of randomization when comparing different treatments originated in the pioneering work in agriculture of Ronald Fisher. The purpose of assigning treatments in a random arrangement was to avoid objective bias and to provide the basis for the standard methods of statistical analysis such as significance tests. As Fisher himself commented in his famous study of 1935, *The design of experiments*, randomization 'is necessary for the validity of [using] any test of significance'.[55] Despite his involvement with other MRC committees, in particular the MRC's Human Genetics Committee (set up in 1932), which undertook the organization of a large-scale statistical investigation of the question of consanguinity, and despite the fact that from 1935 the MRC fostered a detailed investigation into the genetic study of blood groups at University College Hospital under Fisher's direction, there is no evidence that Fisher interacted in any way with the TTC. This meant that his expertise was not utilized in order to translate his powerful ideas on experimental design into a clinical context. Only later was Fisher's work shown to be relevant to a range of theoretical and practical problems in experimental and clinical science.[56]

In 1937 a decision was taken to expand the research on chemotherapy undertaken at the NIMR.[57] There was, it was believed, 'great need for further research in Great Britain aimed at the discovery of new chemical substances of therapeutic value, and strong reason for developing a national scheme of investigation not unworthy of comparison with the work that is done abroad'. It was resolved to move the NIMR to new premises at Mill Hill, on the site of the ICRF's Stroud Laboratory. This move was occasioned partly by the Government's decision in 1936 to allocate an additional sum of £30 000 per annum for the MRC's work, with a special view to the development of research in chemotherapy.[58] It was anticipated that chemotherapy would be a rapidly developing field. This initiative followed in particular the discovery of the therapeutic action of the sulphonamides. The fact that many important discoveries in chemotherapy had occurred in Germany must have had some influence on the move to upgrade this research, with anti-German sentiment heightening with the imminent threat of war in the 1930s. However, the enormous expansion of drug research that

[54] MRC 1487, VI: A. Bradford Hill, 'Serum treatment of pneumonia', 22 December 1933.
[55] Fisher, R. (1935). *The design of experiments*, p. 51. Oliver and Boyd, London.
[56] Marks, H. (1987). Ideas as reforms: therapeutic experiments and medical practice, 1900–1980, p. 161. Unpublished Ph.D. thesis. Massachusetts Institute of Technology.
[57] MRC: *Annual report 1936–7* (1937), 9–15.
[58] NIMR 588/6: memorandum, 'The present position and future development of British research work in chemotherapy', 17 March 1936.

was to take place in industry was not anticipated, and in the event the NIMR contribution to chemotherapy research remained small; much of it related to tropical diseases. The TTC was disbanded soon after the start of the Second World War.[59] It had by this time become so large as to be unwieldy.[60] The success of its ventures had made the clinical trial of new products respectable in the eyes of the pharmaceutical industry, and manufacturers of new drugs began to make arrangements for their own trials directly with clinicians. The TTC had thus become in many ways a victim of its own success. The MRC's subsequent policy in this respect was to set up specific committees to organize trials of particular remedies when this was deemed appropriate. Notable among these were the Clinical Trials Committees for penicillin and tuberculosis vaccines, and the Poliomyelitis Vaccine Committee.

The Departments of Applied Physiology and Endocrinology

During the First World War Leonard Hill and Benjamin Moore, in the Department of Applied Physiology, were called upon by the Ministry of Munitions' Health of Munition Workers' Committee (see Chapter 7) to investigate a new chronic illness among workers, mainly female, in munition factories. They were filling shells with a new kind of high explosive— trinitrotoluene or 'TNT'. Dale wrote of the condition, 'The girls so employed acquired yellow complexions, and neither they nor their boys liked this . . .'[61] More seriously, however, the disease was sometimes fatal, and one of the aims of medical research was to attempt to recognize cases likely to progress to fatal illness. As many as possible of the 'safe' cases were to be kept on the work to maintain the production rate. The extent of serious illness eventually diminished, partly as a result of improved technology designed to increase the speed of the filling which also reduced the spillage and direct skin contact with the substance.[62]

The major contribution of the director of this Department following the war, Sir Leonard Hill, was the invention of what he called the 'kata-thermometer', an instrument for assessing conditions of ventilation or 'cooling power'—the composite result of the temperature, humidity, rate of

---

[59] Green, F. H. K. (1944). Clinical evaluation of new remedies in Britain. *British Medical Bulletin*, **2**, 58–60; Green, F. H. K. (1954). The clinical evaluation of remedies. *Lancet*, **ii**, 1085–90.

[60] Landsborough Thomson, *Medical research*, Vol. II, p. 238 (see note 40).

[61] NIMR Institute History: Dale's notes for Landsborough Thomson, Researches during the First World War and After (1914–1919/20), c. late 1960s, p. 1.

[62] Ineson, A. and Thom, D. (1985). T.N.T. poisoning and the employment of women workers in the First World War. In *The social history of occupational health* (ed. P. Weindling), pp. 89–107. Croom Helm, London; MRC *SRS* 58: *T.N.T. poisoning and the fate of TNT in the animal body* (1921).

movement of the air—in the open air and in artificially ventilated rooms. Hill was heavily involved in the open-air movement of the early twentieth century, claiming vast therapeutic powers of fresh air. Hill's work was used to give scientific respectability to the open-air school movement. With Hill's retirement in 1930, this department lapsed until the Second World War, when deep-sea diving, carbon monoxide poisoning in battle tanks, prevention of seasickness, and protective clothing against flames came under investigation. In 1949 the MRC re-established the Division of Applied Physiology under O. G. Edholm. The employees of this Division studied the effects of heat, cold, humidity, and light on human performance and efficiency.

Shortly after the Department of Applied Physiology ceased to exist as a separate division, the biological work of the Institute was extended in another direction by the establishment of a subdepartment of the Physiology of Sex Hormones under Alan (later Sir Alan) Parkes. Parkes had previously been at University College, London. There he collaborated with Guy Marrian who was supported by the MRC. They made major contributions to what was later called 'the heroic age of reproductive endocrinology'.[63] In particular the isolation and characterization of pregnanediol and oestriol were regarded by Parkes as 'a triumph for Marrian'.

Parkes' move to the NIMR followed a meeting at the Institute in the summer of 1932, held under the auspices of the League of Nations to establish an international standard for the oestrogenic hormones (see biological standardization below). Parkes' laboratory, which was treated as a subdepartment of Endocrinology, became widely recognized as a centre for the study of sex hormones. This work ranged from agricultural studies, in collaboration with J. (later Sir John) Hammond, to research undertaken with Solly (later Lord) Zuckerman on the endocrinology of the prostate gland in primates. Interest was also focused on 'the development of scientific methods for preventing fertility'.[64] Parkes' laboratory was responsible not only for advances in the knowledge of the fundamental physiology of the sex hormones, but also for practical discoveries which facilitated their therapeutic use. In this respect the MRC's Hormone Committee interacted closely with the TTC, helping to supervise the clinical trials of, for example, oestrin, progestin, and testosterone.[65]

Experimental work on hormones carried out at the NIMR was supplemented by a Clinical Endocrinology Research Unit, which was opened by the MRC in Edinburgh in 1946.[66] Research in this Unit, the first of its kind in Britain, was initially carried out on three sites: chemical hormone assay in

[63] Parkes, A. S. (1966). 'The rise of reproductive endocrinology, 1926–1940', The Henry Dale Lecture for 1965. *Journal of Endocrinology*, **34**, xx–xxxii.
[64] MRC 1644/5.
[65] MRC 1523/16, 13, 23a.
[66] MRC 403: Dunlop to Mellanby, 30 September 1946.

D. M. Dunlop's laboratory, bioassay in T. H. Gaddum's department, and clinical work in the Royal Infirmary. Under the direction of committee chaired by Gaddum, who had previously been at the NIMR, the Unit was to become one of the leading centres of hormone research in the country at that time. The department at the NIMR had by this time extended its interests beyond the limits of endocrinology. Parkes had become particularly interested in the broader implications of fertility and population, especially the fertilization and cultivation of mammalian ova *in vitro* and of the behaviour and preservation of mammalian and avian sperm *in vitro*. In 1950, after the move of the NIMR to Mill Hill, the Division was renamed 'Experimental Biology'.

Department of Medical Statistics

This Department was from 1914 under the charge of John Brownlee, a disciple of the eugenist Karl Pearson. At the beginning of the First World War the Medical Research Committee had placed its appropriate resources at the disposal of the War Office for medical statistical purposes.The compilation of medical and surgical statistics of war proved to be a formidable enterprise. The existing methods of collecting army medical statistics were 'imperfect and cumbersome'.[67] The project was not limited to the collection of information that would be useful after the war, but the material was made available to assess causes of illness or injury and the results of treatment. Thus, in addition to carrying out original statistical research, which was Brownlee's forte, his Department undertook routine sorting and classifying of the medical case sheets that were called in from military hospitals by the War Office. The work consumed so much space that rooms in the British Museum were also occupied for the purpose, and more than 100 clerical staff were employed. At the end of the war, the Statistics Department was receiving inquiries from the Ministry of Pensions at the rate of 1500 per month. It was later claimed that it was largely through the action of the Medical Research Committee in the war that the importance of medical-statistical organization in the fighting services had become established.[68]

Despite the importance of the Statistics Department to army medical statistics, Brownlee was not a good director of his own department. Dale later said of him that he 'had proved to be entirely useless to members of other Departments needing statistical advice or co-operation'.[69]   Major

[67] MRC 53A: reconstruction proposals relating to the conservation of health of the population, 28 December 1916.
[68] MRC 3016 V: Major Greenwood, Statistical Committee Report 1939–40, 12 August 1940.
[69] NIMR Institute History: Dale's notes for Landsborough Thomson, *c.* late 1960s, p. 9.

Greenwood, who was Statistical Medical Officer on the staff of the Ministry of Health, initially based at the Lister Institute but from 1920 at the NIMR, was even more disparaging. He saw Brownlee as 'a profound *thinker* [who] was constitutionally unfit to organise or effectively criticise'.[70] Greenwood, who was to become a major figure in the field of medical statistics and epidemiology, was himself not exempt from criticism. Described by Sir Leonard Hill's wife as 'a cynical little man',[71] and much later by Hill's son, Austin Bradford Hill, as having 'irreverent and ironic views',[72] he nonetheless provided the foundations of experimental and historical epidemiology.

Greenwood's transfer as a Ministry of Health employee to the NIMR in 1920 was seen to be 'of great value on both sides'.[73] The NIMR was well provided with costly statistical machinery, the use of which was, until Greenwood's arrival, 'only occasional'.[74]

In 1920 the future development of the Statistical Department was considered in relation to the MRC's general statistical requirements. In particular the Industrial Health Statistics Committee which was chaired by Greenwood was widening its activities (see Chapter 7).[75] This Committee linked up with the new Nutrition Committee of which Greenwood was also chair (see Chapter 5). In effect it became an advisory committee upon statistics for the whole field of the Council's work, thereby rendering Brownlee's Department to a large extent redundant, a fact which Greenwood frequently brought to Fletcher's attention. In 1925 the name of the Committee was changed to the Statistical Committee, to take cognizance of the range of its investigations.

A concordat of 1924 between the MRC and the Ministry of Health had not clearly defined the respective spheres of activities relating to statistical enquiry,[76] a factor further complicated by the presence of Greenwood, still a Ministry of Health employee, at the NIMR and as chair of the MRC's Statistical Committee. Indeed it made increasing sense to attempt to co-ordinate the respective statistical activities of the MRC and the Ministry of Health, although it was unclear how Brownlee's department would fit into such a scheme.[77] In 1927 circumstances arose which made it urgent for the

---

[70] MRC 3016 II: Major Greenwood, a memorandum on the present position and prospects of medical statistics and epidemiology, 11 February 1928, p. 1.

[71] Sir Austin Bradford Hill (1987). Introduction. In M. Greenwood, *The medical dictator*, p. vii. The Keynes Press, London.

[72] Ibid. p. xi.

[73] MRC PF 133: Buchanan to Newman, 24 June 1920.

[74] MRC 2080/4: Walter Fletcher, memorandum by the Secretary on the position of the Statistical Department and the Council's Statistical work in general, 9 February 1923.

[75] The Committee was originally the Statistics Committee of the IFRB, and was reconstituted by the MRC in 1921: MRC: *Annual report 1924–25* (1925), pp. 41–3.

[76] MRC 1190 I: Concordat, 23 January 1924.

[77] MRC 8/20: minutes of the Statistical Committee, 21 December 1926.

MRC to consider the whole future of its statistical work.[78] Greenwood was appointed to direct the Department of Epidemiology and Vital Statistics at the London School of Hygiene and Tropical Medicine (LSHTM). The Ministry of Health agreed to retain Greenwood in its service alongside his new post, and the MRC was asked to give similar approval to his transfer.[79] Brownlee's unexpected death facilitated the move of the MRC's statistical work to the LSHTM. Within days of his death and with characteristic bluntness, Greenwood observed that 'one very obvious difficulty in the way of co-ordination has, unfortunately and tragically, been removed'.[80] The Statistical Department at the NIMR was discontinued after Brownlee's death when the Council agreed to bring all its work under the direction of Greenwood and the Statistical Committee.[81] Furthermore the Ministry of Health agreed to bring all its own statistical work under the same Committee.[82] From 1928 the staffs of the NIMR Department, Greenwood's Ministry of Health Department, and the Statistical Committee were thus merged into one unit. From 1945, when Greenwood retired, this became the Statistical Research Unit under the direction of Austin Bradford Hill.

Under Hill the department enhanced its reputation, becoming heavily involved with the MRC's new clinical trials programme. The streptomycin trial (mentioned previously) was run parallel with large-scale trials of various vaccines. While the introduction of randomized controlled trials clearly represented a milestone in the revolution of clinical research, Hill was to make a crucial contribution to epidemiological research in another important respect. In 1947 the MRC embarked on a study of the relationship between the increasing incidence of lung cancer and cigarette smoking.[83] The retrospective trial, which commenced on 1 January 1948, was carried out by Hill assisted by Richard Doll. This culminated in their now classic observation in which they demonstrated that there existed a 'real association between carcinoma of the lung and smoking'.[84] This study, conducted under the auspices of the MRC and published in the *British Medical Journal* in September 1950, provided the basis of what remains to this day the single most reliably established and practicable means of reducing the proportion

[78] MRC 8/20: Walter Fletcher, Statistical work for the MRC; its future in relation to the Ministry of Health and the London School of Hygiene, 15 March 1927.
[79] Ibid. p. 1.
[80] MRC 3016 I: Greenwood to Fletcher, 24 March 1927.
[81] MRC 3016 II: Fletcher to Greenwood, 20 May 1927.
[82] MRC 3016 II: Greenwood, a memorandum on the present position of medical statistics and epidemiology, 11 February 1928; MRC 3016 III: Greenwood to Fletcher, 25 September 1931.
[83] For full details of the history of the MRC's involvement in the lung cancer and cigarette smoking debate, see Austoker, *History of the ICRF*, pp. 186–199 (see note 21); Webster, C. (1988). *The health services since the war*. Vol. 1, *Problems of health care. The National Health Service before 1957*, pp. 233–7. HMSO, London.
[84] Doll, R. and Hill, A. B. (1950). Smoking and carcinoma of the lung. Preliminary report. *British Medical Journal*, ii, 739–48.

of deaths from cancer. Yet the contribution of epidemiological surveillance to the formation of productive policies for the prevention of cancer required what has proved to be the confluence of essentially opposing interests.

Biological Standards

From 1914 onwards the Medical Research Committee believed that progress in many areas of the medical sciences was being delayed for want of fixed standards of measurement and of means for their ready application.[85] Many therapeutic and prophylactic substances called for special techniques in which potency could be determined in terms of biological effects compared with those of a recognized standard preparation. Britain had come to depend on foreign—in particular German—industry for potent new therapeutic substances whose activity was standardized by bioassay.

War accentuated not only the need for the production of potent therapeutic substances and the value of biological standards of measurement, but also highlighted 'our grave national deficiencies in this respect'.[86] Standardization thus assumed not just scientific or medical but also economic and political significance. The protection of patients was only one facet of a much wider debate. Certain companies such as Burroughs Wellcome had previously adopted biological standardization of their own products according to their own criteria. However, the absence of a central standards authority meant that British products were not marketable in other countries where there was strict regulation of potent medicines.[87]

In the early part of the war, the Medical Research Committee took charge of standardizing British-made salvarsan and neosalvarsan preparations as well as various sera and antitoxins which had been imported before the war.[88] Salvarsan and neosalvarsan preparations were prepared by Dale and G. Barger, working temporarily at the Lister Institute. Sera and cultures for the diagnosis of enteric and dysenteric infections were produced at the Standards Laboratory at the Dunn School of Pathology, Oxford, set up in 1915 under the direction of Georges Dreyer. In December 1916 the Medical Research Committee, in a memorandum prepared by request for Asquith's Reconstruction Committee, urged Government action towards the establishment of a National Biological Standards Laboratory.[89] The Medical Research Committee maintained that the absence of official standards of

[85] MRC. *Annual report 1919–20* (1920), pp. 119–120.
[86] Ibid. p. 120.
[87] Pfeffer, N. (1985). Biological standardisation and sex hormones. Paper given at the Annual Conference of the British Sociological Association Medical Sociology Group, September 1985.
[88] MRC: *Annual report 1914–15* (1916), pp. 42–44.
[89] MRC Reconstruction Files: memorandum on Reconstruction, December 1916, appendix II.

value was 'discreditable to our national position in the world of science and a source of grave danger to the community'.[90] This was followed by a fuller statement by the Committee to the Local Government Board in 1919, pointing out that standardization was not only 'an indispensable aid to scientific work but also for the practical purposes of national safety'.[91]

In 1920 the newly created MRC began to promote studies on biological standardization at the NIMR. A Committee for Biological Standards and the Methods of Biological Assay, chaired by William Bulloch, was appointed to advise on these studies, which were carried out under Dale's direction. In the same year the Minister of Health set up a Departmental Committee to advise on the administrative and legislative measures that might be necessary for controlling biological substances in medical use. Dale represented the MRC on this Committee, whose recommendations ultimately took effect in the Therapeutic Substances Act, passed in July 1925.

Initially workers were recruited from various departments of the NIMR to undertake work on biological standards as the need arose—in particular from the Biochemistry and Pharmacology and Bacteriological Departments. This included preparations of standards for diphtheria antitoxin (by Leonard Colebrook and then Percival Hartley) and the oxytocic hormone extract of the posterior lobe of the pituitary gland (by Dale and Burn), and the standardization of insulin, as has already been alluded to. In 1923 international standards for diphtheria antitoxin and posterior pituitary gland were set, and in 1925 an internal unit for the potency of insulin was adopted.

The Therapeutic Substances Act of 1925, which became effective in 1927, provided for the official control of therapeutic substances whose potency had to be determined by biological means. The MRC was given a statutory responsibility for the preparation and custody of British national standards. The exercise of this control fell largely to the NIMR, which was charged with issuing samples of appropriate standards to the manufacturers of scheduled substances, and for ensuring that products placed on the market by those manufacturers satisfied the requirements laid down in the Act. In several instances this involved the recurrent preparation, at short intervals, of solutions of the stable standards and the experimental verification of each of these before it was issued. In practice, the MRC was empowered not only to offer detailed scientific advice on the framing of regulations, but also to test and examine manufacturers' protocols, and scientists from the NIMR participated with medical officers of the Ministry of Health in the inspection of manufacturers' premises and methods.[92]

The Act meant that the Institute had not only new responsibilities, but a

[90] Ibid.
[91] Landsborough Thomson, *Medical research*, Vol. II, p. 245 (see note 40).
[92] See also MRC: *Annual report 1928–29* (1930), pp. 12–4.

greatly increased scientific burden. Up to 1927 the only NIMR scientist with a full-time commitment to standards work was Percival Hartley. With the Bacteriological Department now heavily preoccupied with virus research, it was no longer appropriate for the scientists in this Department to be involved in standards work on a part-time basis. Instead, from 1927 the determination of biological standards and the methods of biological assay and measurement became the responsibility of a newly constituted department under Percival Hartley's direction.

In various ways, and largely because of the influence of Henry Dale, the MRC acquired the responsibility not only for all British standards, but also for certain international standards. The Health Commission of the League of Nations had set up a Permanent Commission on Biological Standardization in 1924 in order to unify international standards. The standards agreed by the League of Nations were adopted as national standards for all member countries. The task of establishing standards was shared by the NIMR and the State Serum Institute in Copenhagen, who both entered into a formal contract with the League of Nations. The Danish Institute was allocated the standards for immunological products, initially diphtheria and tetanus antitoxins, while the international responsibility for maintaining the standards of other substances including insulin, pituitary extracts and other hormones and arsenics, fell to the NIMR. Later, during the German occupation of Denmark from 1940 to 1945, the NIMR at the request of the League of Nations, assumed responsibility for the supply of antitoxins and tuberculin which had also formerly been maintained in Copenhagen. This custody returned to the Serum Institute after the war.

The League of Nations sponsored conferences in certain areas in order to set international standards. International conferences on vitamin standards were held in London in 1931 and 1934, chaired by Edward Mellanby, and a series of conferences to establish standards for sex hormone preparations were held between 1932 and 1938. The first of these, to consider oestrogenic hormones, was held at the NIMR, the second, to establish standards for antrosterone and progesterone, was held in 1935 at the London School of Hygiene, and the last, which dealt with protein hormones, was held in Geneva. All three were chaired by Henry Dale. By 1939 no fewer than 21 different companies were supplying the British market with standardized sex hormone preparations.

Although Britain had moved towards biological standardization very late compared to its industrial competitors, the MRC and the NIMR in particular had assumed a position of national and international importance in this work. This largely reflected the involvement of Henry Dale. The concern of the MRC (as well as that of other interested groups such as lecturers in pharmacology in British universities and medical schools) with biological standardization was reflected in the first British Pharmacopoeia to be published by a Commission whose membership was dominated by scientists rather than medical practitioners. Amongst its radical innovations was the inclusion of information relating to biological standards that were legally binding according to the regulations of the Therapeutic Substances Act, together with information of many biological standards of imported substances that were not as yet legally binding. Significant therapeutic changes were thus apparent in Britain as potent substances gained in credibility, not necessarily because of a clear demonstration of their therapeutic value, but largely through recourse to biological standardization. It could be argued that the changes which took place owed little to developments in clinical medicine, but were largely the product of scientific ideas about the way to construct medicines.[93]

New Institute at Mill Hill

The move of the NIMR to Mill Hill was dictated not only by the anticipated extension of research into chemotherapy following the Government's allocation of an additional £30 000 per annum for chemotherapeutic research in 1936 (as discussed above), but also by expansion in other areas of research. The expansion of work described as 'Physical Methods', still a subdepartment of the Department of Experimental Pathology and Bacteriology, has been referred to. This was described at the time of the move of the Institute as one of the most rapidly expanding Divisions, and after 1950 became a separate Division in its own right, the Division of Biophysics and Optics. The desirability of expanding premises was also indicated by work related to biological standards, a growing concern at the NIMR, as has been discussed. One further advantage of moving the whole Institute to Mill Hill was given by Dale in 1937 who wrote of the Hampstead site, 'Together with other considerations . . . it should be borne in mind that we have a recurrent difficulty, due to the impossibility of keeping dogs here, without risking trouble with the neighbours'.[94]

The building of the new Institute commenced in 1937. By 1940 the outer shell was completed. The building was subsequently lent to the Admiralty to aid in the war effort from 1942 to 1946. The expansion of biophysical methods during the war necessitated revised planning of the internal layout of the new Institute, and the move was further delayed until the end of 1949. In May 1950 the Institute at Mill Hill was officially opened by Their Majesties King George VI and Queen Elizabeth. The new building was seven stories high and designed to accommodate approximately 100 qualified workers and

[93] N. Pfeffer (see note 86) provides a good argument to this effect.
[94] NIMR 588/3/1: Dale to Landsborough Thomson, 5 February 1937.

up to 300 assistants and others. The work on biological standards continued to expand so that it was necessary to reoccupy the old Hampstead laboratories and eventually to establish there, in 1972, a separate National Institute for Biological Standards and Control.

The work of the NIMR in the first 30 years of the MRC contributed greatly to the prestige of the MRC. Research was subsequently diverted away from the centre and the original allocation of a third of the MRC budget to the central institute was abandoned, so that the total share of the MRC budget directed to the Institute fell from 35 per cent in 1930, to 22.4 per cent in 1950, 17.4 per cent in 1960, 11.1 per cent in 1970, and 8.2 per cent in 1980.[95]

[95] Work, T. S. (1983). *Biologist* , **30** (2), 102.

4

Public health research and the MRC

LINDA BRYDER

The Emergency Public Health Laboratory Service (EPHLS) was set up during the Second World War as a wartime measure, but proved so useful that after the war 'Emergency' was dropped from the title and it became permanent. Its remit was the diagnosis, prevention, and control of infectious diseases in the community, and field work was incorporated as well as laboratory work and epidemiology. The MRC was made responsible for the new service. This was despite the delineation of the respective responsibilities of the Ministry of Health and the MRC in 1923 when the former had been given charge of public health research with practical application and the latter left to advance knowledge by 'pure research'. This chapter discusses the involvement of the MRC in research into microbiology and infectious diseases, and its relationship with the Ministry of Health; and considers the reasons why responsibility for the service devolved on the MRC rather than the Ministry of Health.

Public health and bacteriology

The bacteriological revolution of the late nineteenth century transformed public health work. The identification of the casual agents of most infectious diseases led to the new medical specialisms of bacteriology and immunology. Rather than focusing on sanitary engineering, public health now involved tracing and identifying the source of infectious diseases. Individuals thus traced would ideally be isolated and treated by vaccine therapy and their contacts vaccinated. Public health was thus becoming more concerned with the individual, and the laboratory was assuming a new importance.[1]

In 1898 *The Lancet* reported that Sheridan Delépine, professor of

---

[1] See also Fee, E. (1987). *Disease and discovery. A history of the Johns Hopkins School of Hygiene and Public Health 1916–1939* p. 19. The Johns Hopkins University Press, Baltimore. However, MOsH, in Britain at least, did not entirely abandon the sanitary approach: see Raymond, J. (1985). Science in the service of medicine: germ theory, bacteriology, and English public health, 1860–1914. Unpublished manuscript. Science in Modern Medicine Conference, Manchester, 19–21 April 1985, abstract in *The Society for the Social History of Medicine Bulletin* (1985), **37**, 43–5.

pathology at Manchester University, had set up a laboratory attached to Owens College, Manchester, which would transform the character of the work of the health department in the Manchester district.[2] He was said to be following the lead of Paris, Berlin, and Lille, where municipal authorities had come to financial arrangements with local pathological and bacteriological institutes, to their mutual benefit. These institutes were the Pasteur Institutes in Paris (founded in 1888) and Lille (1895), and the Institute Robert Koch, set up in Berlin in 1891. Bacteriological laboratories for disease analysis and control had also been established in the USA. Such a laboratory was set up in 1887 in the Staten Island Marine Hospital, which was moved to Washington in 1891 to become the Hygienic Laboratory with a Biologics Control Division, to test serums, vaccines, and other biological agents. In 1888, public health laboratories were founded in Providence (Rhode Island), and Michigan. In 1892, Hermann Biggs of the New York City health department, who was well known and much admired in Britain, set up a division of bacteriology and disinfection, with a laboratory under the charge of W. H. Park. The laboratory was originally established for the diagnosis of cholera and diphtheria, and in 1894 tuberculosis was added to its remit. It became an important research centre, and provided a model for other laboratories. By 1900 diagnostic laboratories existed in every state and in most cities in the USA. In the early twentieth century, the Hygienic Laboratory in Washington in particular gained a world-wide reputation for its research.[3]

In Britain, the Medical Office of the Privy Council under Sir John Simon had first authorized laboratory investigations into infective processes and physiological chemistry in 1865.[4] Parliament voted £2000 annual grants in support of the investigations from 1871. These studies were sponsored by the Local Government Board (LGB), although the LGB itself did not set up a laboratory until 1910. The Metropolitan Asylums Board (MAB) (set up in London in 1867 to provide institutional treatment for certain categories of the sick poor in London) also appointed a bacteriologist in 1913, accommodated first at the Lister Institute (originally the British Institute of Preventive Medicine, founded in London in 1891), and after 1920 at the NIMR. However, outside London, local authority laboratory facilities in Britain remained limited. Only a few local authorities appointed a bacteriologist and set up a laboratory, and when they did so they often combined it with the public analyst's laboratory. In some cases, medical officers of health did their own laboratory work, but they limited it to

    [2] *Lancet* (1898), **ii**, 883.
    [3] Harden, V. A. (1986). *Inventing the NIH. Federal biomedical research policy 1887–1937* pp. 25–6, 42. The Johns Hopkins University Press, Baltimore.
    [4] Brand, J. L. (1965). *Doctors and the State. The British medical profession and government action in public health, 1870–1912*, pp. 75–84. The Johns Hopkins University Press, Baltimore.

straightforward examinations, such as throat swabs for diphtheria, the Widal test for typhoid, and microscopic examinations for tuberculosis. Some medical officers of health actually opposed the appointment of a bacteriologist, as they feared that such an appointment would reduce their own powers.[5] They often delegated some or all of the laboratory work to commercial laboratories, hospital laboratories, or pathology and physiology departments in universities. Hospital laboratories undertook this work as a means of augmenting their income and showed little real interest in it.[6] As Matthew Hay, professor of forensic medicine and public health, University of Aberdeen, told the Departmental Committee on Tuberculosis in 1912 when discussing laboratory facilities, 'the requirements are so rapidly extending that it is not to be expected that universities will much longer allow their laboratories to be filled with a vast amount of routine work'. Hay regretted that Britain was 'at present without any organised and complete system to enable public health authorities, school authorities, poor-law authorities, hospital doctors, and private practitioners to obtain conveniently and reliably the bacteriological and cognate examinations that are now essential to the proper diagnosis, control, and treatment of infectious diseases in general'.[7]

Matthew Hay recommended that the research fund established by the sanatorium clauses of the 1911 Insurance Act be used to found 'State Bacteriological Institutes', with a central and local institutes. He explained that in his scheme, the local institutes would exist primarily for routine bacteriological examinations and investigations, and only secondarily for original research. The sole or main purpose of the central institute, on the other hand, would be original research. Besides a bacteriological department in the institute, there would be a biochemical department, a physiological–pharmacological department, and a statistical and sociological department. Certain other subdepartments, such as parasitology, would also be provided. Under his scheme, every town and county would have the resources of the whole organization available for the solution of special problems. The organization would, in turn, be able to place at the disposal of a central committee the whole bacteriological material of the country for research purposes.

Hay believed that the large body of highly trained and experienced bacteriological experts, brought into existence by his scheme and under the control of the State, would be particularly invaluable in times of war, pointing to the recent experience of the Boer War in South Africa, 1899–1902. He maintained that 'success in a prolonged campaign is now admitted

[5] Raymond, Science in the Service of Medicine, p. 12 (see note 1).
[6] Frazer, W. M. (1950). *A history of English public health 1834–1939*, p. 377. Bailliere, Tindall and Cox, London.
[7] *Final report of Departmental Committee on Tuberculosis*, Vol. II, Cd. 6654 (1913), p. 68.

to be in large degree dependent on the sanitary measures that are born of an application of bacteriological knowledge'. In his view, this would be the best purpose to which the research funds could be put.[8]

In its final report in 1913, the Departmental Committee on Tuberculosis recommended that a central research institute be established. Local laboratories were to be provided by local authorities.[9] The central institute of the Medical Research Committee followed closely the model proposed by Hay. That the original intention was to place much emphasis on bacteriology can be seen by the serious consideration given to the proposal to usurp the Lister Institute complete with staff for the new State-controlled institute. The Lister Institute had been set up by voluntary support in 1891 as the British Institute of Preventive Medicine, although the designation 'The Bacteriological Institute' had also been considered at the time, and bacteriology was given high priority.[10] Before negotiations between the Lister Institute and the Medical Research Committee were underway, a site had been purchased by the latter, and eventually the Lister Institute proposal was rejected by the governing body of the Lister Institute itself.

In 1914, David Lloyd George, Chancellor of the Exchequer, proposed that public money be made available for local authorities to set up public health laboratories; he suggested an additional £750 000 be allocated to local authorities for laboratory work, together with nursing and tuberculosis services. He pointed out that 'In Germany, in almost every town, and I think in France, you have pathological laboratories . . .'.[11] While the proposal appears to have had much support at the time,[12] it was buried with the outbreak of war. Thus a comprehensive system of local institutes that could be used by the central institute, as suggested by Hay, was not established. The only laboratory arrangements that local authorities were required to make were in relation to tuberculosis and venereal diseases.

Public health and the First World War

During the First World War the Bacteriological Department of the Medical Research Committee devoted its energies to the preparation of anti-typhoid

[8] Ibid. pp. 68–70.
[9] *Final report of Departmental Committee on Tuberculosis*, Vol. I, Cd. 6641 (1913), p. 16. The report recommended that laboratories be provided with funds other than those under the 1911 Act.
[10] Chick, H., Hume, M., and Macfarlane, M. (1971). *War on disease: a history of the Lister Institute* pp. 27, 30–1. Andre Deutsch, London; Hall, L. and Morgan, N. (1986). Illustrations from the Wellcome Institute Library: The Archive of the Lister Institute of Preventive Medicine. *Medical History*, **30**, (2), 212–5.
[11] *Parliamentary debates (official report) House of Commons*, 1914, LXII (4 May 1914), 79.
[12] *Public Health* (1914), **27**, (10), 326.

and other vaccines for the use of the armed forces. Approximately 10 million doses of an anti-typhoid vaccine, which had been developed by Sir Almroth Wright prior to the war, were prepared in the Inoculation Department of St Mary's Hospital where the bacteriologists were temporarily based. Other work sponsored by the Medical Research Committee and relating to typhoid was the supply of standardized preparations for differential diagnosis of typhoid and paratyphoid. This work was carried out by Georges Dreyer, professor of pathology, University of Oxford. It was the beginning of a permanent service that later became the Oxford Standards Laboratory and was housed in the Dunn School of Pathology, although independent of it. It later became part of the Public Health Laboratory Service (PHLS).

By 1916, although vaccination was voluntary, 98 per cent of the British troops going abroad had been vaccinated against typhoid. The effects are difficult to assess but appear to have been considerable. Estimates of how many deaths from typhoid would have occurred without the vaccine (based mainly on the experience of the Boer War) varied from three to ten times the number which actually occurred. The report of a survey, carried out after the war, of typhoid vaccination in the military personnel of several nations including Britain, France, Russia, Italy, Japan and the USA, concluded that there was little doubt that vaccination did protect against typhoid, but that the results were difficult to interpret because water and food supplies had also been controlled more than in previous wars.[13]

For the investigation of infectious diseases at the Front, motor vans were equipped as mobile laboratories. They were attached to clearing stations where medical officers examined and cultured morbid products from wounds, practised diagnostic serology (especially in relation to enteric and cerebro-spinal fevers), and searched for contacts and carriers of infectious diseases.

Wound infections were soon perceived as a major problem, specifically tetanus and gas gangrene which flourished in the highly cultivated and well-manured fields of France and Flanders where wounded men often lay for several hours before being rescued. In 1914, at the request of the Director-General of the Army Medical Service, Sir Alfred Keogh, the Medical Research Committee sent Sir Almroth Wright to an army hospital laboratory in Boulogne, to direct a research unit on the bacteriology of wound infection and the best methods of overcoming it. Wright's assistants included S. R. Douglas, Alexander Fleming, Leonard Colebrook, Parry Morgan and John

[13] Macpherson, W. G., Leishman, W. B. and Cummins, S. L. (eds.) (1923). *History of the Great War, Medical services, pathology*, pp. 211, 248–59. HMSO, London; MRC *SRS* 6, IV: *Reports upon investigations in the United Kingdom of dysentery cases received from the Eastern Mediterranean* (1917), p. 22; Spink, W. W. (1978). *Infectious diseases: prevention and treatment in the nineteenth and twentieth centuries*, p. 63. Dawson, University of Minnesota. (1978).

Freeman. They developed a 'physiological' approach to treatment of wound infection, encouraging the body's natural defensive mechanisms against infection without the use of antiseptics. They claimed that antiseptics were not only useless but dangerous, and published their results in the MRC's Special Report Series after the war. However, there was some dispute over the efficacy of Wright's treatment of wound infection by a hypertonic salt solution as opposed to H. D. Dakin's antiseptics (the latter also sponsored by the MRC at Manchester). It is not known how widely either method was adopted by army surgeons. Sir Henry Dale later claimed that Wright's hypertonic salt solution was useless.[14] Landsborough Thomson, on the other hand, wrote that Wright's method of irrigation of wounds by a hypertonic salt solution without antiseptics was widely adopted immediately.[15] One medical historian maintained that, except for those who worked with Wright, army medical officers continued to use antiseptics, although by the Second World War Wright's method had become standard practice.[16] Another medical historian held that at the end of the war, only a few old-guard 'Listerians' clung to antisepsis.[17] At any rate, the incidence of gas gangrene declined considerably during the war, probably largely because of more prompt surgery. Tetanus infection, however, was an undisputed success story for bacteriology in the First World War. In 1914 tetanus occurred in eight per thousand wounded, with 85 per cent mortality rate; by 1918 the rate had dropped to 0.6 per thousand wounded, a change attributed to the availability of ample antitoxin for all to receive prophylactic injections soon after being wounded.[18]

Attention was also directed to other public health problems of the armed forces. For example, during the war John Freeman was sent to Galicia by the Medical Research Committee to study cholera, and anti-cholera vaccine was produced at St Mary's Hospital. R. T. Leiper and two assistants were sent to Egypt to study bilharziasis. They demonstrated that Egyptian bilharziasis could only be communicated to humans through a freshwater snail. They showed that transient collections of water were safe even if recently contaminated, but that all permanent collections of water, such as the Nile, canals, and marshes, were dangerous because of the possible presence of that snail as the intermediary. As a result, special precautionary measures were devised for the treatment of water, which were sufficient to safeguard the military forces from immediate infection. Thus it was reported that 'Apart

[14] NIMR Institute History: Dale's notes for Landsborough Thomson, *c.* late 1960s.

[15] Landsborough Thomson, A. (1975). *Half a century of medical research*, Vol. II. *The programme of the Medical Research Council (UK)* p. 280. HMSO, London.

[16] Macfarlane, G. (1985). *Alexander Fleming: the man and the myth* p. 88. Oxford University Press.

[17] Cartwright, F. F. (1977). *A social history of medicine* p. 147. Longman, London.

[18] Parish, H. J. (1965), *A history of immunization*, pp. 170–1. Livingstone, Edinburgh; MRC: *Annual report 1938–39* (1940), p. 27.

from the humanitarian and romantic aspects of freeing the Egyptians from this age-long plague . . . preventive work for the Army must have saved us millions . . . The few cases from the South African War are still costing about £6000 a year.'[19]

Bacillary and amoebic dysentery were also studied, and it was later claimed that knowledge of the symptoms, causes, treatment, and prevention of amoebic dysentery was placed upon 'a firm scientific foundation' largely owing to work done during the war.[20] The concentration of large bodies of troops in billets and camps led to outbreaks of cerebro-spinal meningitis and 'spotted fever' (cerebro-spinal fever). In January 1915 the Medical Research Committee was consulted by Sir Alfred Keogh about an outbreak of cerebro-spinal fever among troops in Britain. He was even more concerned for the troops abroad who were congregated in large numbers under housing conditions and in a climate thought to favour the spread of this disease. A central laboratory to study the disease was established at the Royal Army Medical College, Millbank, and Mervyn H. Gordon, assistant pathologist at St Bartholomew's Hospital, was appointed by the Medical Research Committee as a bacteriologist to the War Office. It was found that the meningococci present in the cerebro-spinal fluid of cases fell into four antigenic groups of which two were particularly prevalent. The Medical Research Committee was responsible for supplying diagnostic sera and for arranging tests. This was considered of great importance in the war effort as it appeared to be necessary to place in quarantine only carriers of the organism causing the current epidemic. Specific bacteriological examinations eliminated or shortened the periods of quarantine which would have been imposed based on previous procedures.[21] Landsborough Thomson claimed that knowledge of meningococcal groups was even more important in treatment, as group-specific antisera were found to be efficacious.[22] However, the efficacy of the antisera was disputed; according to one bacteriologist, a 'definite treatment of meningitis still had not been achieved' by the outbreak of the Second World War,[23] although sulphonamide treatment was soon introduced with successful results.

In 1916 the Medical Research Committee assisted in the work of J. W.

[19] Addison Papers Box 67: notes for MRC *Annual report 1923–24*, p. 5; MRC 1472, I: Fletcher to Addison, 29 October 1919, p. 3; *British Medical Journal* (1915), ii, 755.

[20] Macpherson *et al.*, *History of the Great War*, p. 277 (see note 13).

[21] MRC *SRS* 2: *Report of the Special Advisory Committee upon bacteriological studies of cerebro-spinal fever during the epidemic of 1915* (1916); MRC *SRS* 3: *Bacteriological studies in the pathology and preventive control of cerebro-spinal fever among the Forces during 1915 and 1916*; (1916); MRC *SRS* 50: *Cerebro-spinal fever. Studies in the bacteriology, preventive control, and specific treatment of cerebro-spinal fever among the military forces 1915–19* (1920).

[22] Landsborough Thomson, *Medical research*, Vol. II, p. 284 (see note 15).

[23] Spink, *Infectious diseases*, p. 291 (see note 13).

(later Sir John) McNee on trench fever, a form of 'pyrexia of unknown origin' that was temporarily incapacitating up to a million men in France and Belgium, although causing no deaths. It was first recognized in Flanders in the spring of 1915, and the name 'trench fever', which first came into use among the soldiers themselves, was accepted in the official nomenclature for the disease. McNee and his colleagues were the first to demonstrate its infective nature, although the infecting organism remained unknown. Experiments carried out by the War Office under American auspices on 82 volunteers from the American army proved that the infection was louse-borne and therefore preventable by de-lousing measures.[24]

In 1915, the Medical Research Committee was asked by Sir Alfred Keogh to assist in investigations of a condition variously known as 'acute nephritis' (epidemic dropsy), 'acute (trench) nephritis', and 'trench (war) nephritis'. This form of kidney inflammation was another common illness among the troops in France, with an incidence of one per thousand troops in December 1916. The Medical Research Committee sent a chemical pathologist, Hugh Maclean, to France to see whether it was infective in origin or due to exacerbation of some latent deficiency in kidney function. Maclean assessed the kidney efficiency of 50 000 fit young men, but the ultimate cause of war nephritis was not discovered. All that could be said was that it appeared to be 'a result of a specific infection of unknown natures and origin'.[25] Maclean's work together with other contemporary work for the Medical Research Committee did succeed in proving that the 'clinical' guesses at prognosis and the right treatment for nephritis cases were almost meaningless. He worked out kidney function tests from which an estimate of existing damage could be made, and which could guide treatment and indicate prognosis. This test was used by the Ministry of Pensions after the war, and Fletcher estimated that the number of assessments for pensions was halved by its use, and the number of lowest assessments (including 'no disability') quadrupled, saving £150 000 in the first year, or, as he hastened to add, double the amount proposed by the Treasury for medical research on all subjects.[26]

Great advances occurred in bacteriology as a result of the war. As was explained in the *British Medical Journal*:

War makes experiments on man on a huge scale, horrible to contemplate, but the horror is mitigated when the opportunity is taken to institute inquiries into means of prevention or alleviation; such inquiries serve not only the immediate practical needs of

---

[24] MRC 1472, I: Fletcher to Addison, 29 October 1919; *British Medical Journal* (1918), **ii**, 577–8; Macpherson *et al.*, *History of the Great War*, p. 485–512 (see note 13).

[25] Macpherson *et al.*, *History of the Great War*, pp. 541–65 (see note 13).

[26] MRC 1472, I: Fletcher to Addison, 29 October 1919; Addison Papers Box 33: memorandum by Fletcher, 17 February 1920.

the army by saving the life and health of the troops now engaged, but also the civil population of to-morrow, while hastening the progress of medicine throughout the world.[27]

Sir Clifford Allbutt, Regius Professor of Physic at the University of Cambridge, also pointed to the importance of war in carrying forward research by giving 'opportunities for disciplined study and for consistent and extensive observation', which in time of peace 'would have been obtained far more slowly, if at all'.[28] Infectious diseases were a well-known invisible enemy in warfare, and the Medical Research Committee had contributed substantially to the national effort through its work in this area. Intent on not losing the support achieved during the war, Fletcher argued in 1920,

The present impoverishment of the country seems greatly to increase the urgency of further remunerative expenditure upon medical research. The money waste due to present ill-health and disease is so gigantic that relatively small advances in knowledge in any one of a number of different numerous directions are likely to bring gain out of all proportion greater than the whole expenditure upon medical research.[29]

Was the MRC now to focus its attention more directly on civilian health, which, apart from some work on tuberculosis, nutrition, and TNT poisoning in munition factories, had been largely neglected during the war?

Co-operation between the Ministry of Health and the MRC

Research during the war by the Medical Research Committee was thus of immediate practical application, but it was largely restricted to non-civilians. Following the war, as a result of a dispute over responsibilities relating to cancer research, an agreement was drawn up between the Ministry of Health and the MRC defining their respective research responsibilities.[30] The Ministry of Health was to undertake research with direct applicability to public health administration, using methods of research already established. The MRC was to investigate new methods of research, 'to promote new knowledge by the initiation of an organisation of research in the medical sciences'. Epidemiology fell into both departments. That there were two separate departments responsible for medical research seemed surprising to Sir Alfred Mond, Minister of Health in 1921, for one. The Permanent Secretary to the Ministry of Health, W. A. (Sir Arthur) Robinson had also thought that research would have been one of the first duties of a health department.[31] However, medical scientists had argued in favour of, and

---

[27] *British Medical Journal* (1915), **ii**, 757.
[28] *British Medical Journal* (1916), **ii**, 785.
[29] Addison Papers Box 33: memorandum by Fletcher, 17 February 1920.
[30] MRC 1190: concordat, 1923, 16 January 1924; see also Chapter 2.
[31] MRC 1190: 25 May 1921, W. A. Robinson to Fletcher.

won, unfettered academic freedom.[32] Fletcher stressed that there would be some overlap and close co-operation with the Ministry of Health. He was indignant when Sir Watson Cheyne suggested that the Minister had to come 'cap in hand' to the MRC.[33] Co-operation was evident, according to Fletcher, by the contact of the Ministry of Health with the MRC's work on statistics, nutrition, tuberculosis, and syphilis, and by the representation of the MRC on the Ministry's Influenza Committee, its Cancer Committee, and its involvement in encephalitis work.[34]

Research into infectious diseases was one area in which some degree of co-operation between the two departments was indicated. Yet co-operation in this area, when attempted, was far from smooth, as illustrated by the experience of the Vaccine Committee, a joint committee of the Ministry of Health and MRC set up in January 1926, with Sir Humphry Rolleston as chair and J. R. Hutchinson as secretary, to investigate brain and other nervous diseases as a complication of smallpox vaccination (superseding an earlier Vaccinia Committee set up by the MRC in 1923). In 1927 Sir George Newman, Chief Medical Officer of the Ministry of Health, objected that he had not been consulted about the plans of one member of the committee, J. R. Perdrau, to publish his research independently and shortly before the committee's report was to appear. Fletcher described in vivid detail his meeting with Newman over this matter in September 1927. Newman had apparently forgotten that it had been set up as a joint committee. Newman 'shouted aloud that the Ministry had never had a joint committee [with the MRC] on any subject, and certainly not in this'.[35] The subsequent correspondence was hostile, with Fletcher accusing Newman of causing 'unnecessary alarm', and Newman retorting that the unnecessary alarm was Fletcher's own manufacture. Fletcher declared himself bewildered by the change when Newman permitted Perdrau to publish independently, and Newman replied that he was annoyed by all the 'potter and heavy weather about this simple episode when I was extremely busy and trying to catch a train'. Fletcher then took up the matter of whether the committee was joint, repeating Newman's own correspondence of the previous year to him.[36] When the committee's report was completed Fletcher complained that it was not sent to the MRC for comment. The Permanent Secretary to the Ministry of Health, W. A. Robinson, replied to an accusation from Fletcher in June 1928, 'Frankly I do not think that there is any evidence of a lack of desire on our part to

---

[32] Addison Papers Box 67: notes for MRC *Annual report 1923–24*, p. 19; *British Medical Journal* (1919), **ii**, 715; see also Harden, *Inventing the NIH*, p. 71 (see note 3).
[33] MRC 1190: Fletcher to Sir Watson Cheyne, 25 May 1921.
[34] MRC 1190: Fletcher to Newman, 17 January 1924.
[35] MRC 1297: Fletcher, Report of Meeting with Newman, 30 September 1927.
[36] MRC 1297: correspondence, Fletcher and Newman, October 1927.

treat seriously the co-operation we invited.'[37] Fletcher suggested that the committee should be disbanded following its report in 1928, although in the event it sat for another two years and was disbanded following a second report in 1930. The clash of personalities at the top level did little to aid effective co-operation of the two departments.

Thomas Carnwarth, a senior medical officer in the Ministry of Health, had commented on a lack of co-operation in 1922 relating to research into encephalitis. He wrote to Fletcher concerning the Ministry of Health's report on encephalitis lethargica, that negotiations with the MRC 'left an impression—unfortunate, and I am sure unintentional—of a disposition on the part of the MRC to do less than justice to work issuing from the Ministry'. He was acting as deputy Permanent Secretary to the Ministry of Health in Robinson's absence and constantly heard 'rumblings of discontent' relating to co-operation between the two departments. In his opinion the most serious defect was that the MRC contained no official representative of the medical staff of the Ministry of Health, 'the Department of State most closely interested in the work of the MRC and most directly concerned in exploiting the practical results of any research carried out under its auspices'.[38]

The division of responsibilities between 'pure' and 'applied' research might have worked, despite strained relations, had there been attached to the Ministry of Health an equivalent of the American Hygienic Laboratory and National Institutes of Health as part of the Public Health Service, concerned with epidemic and infectious diseases and nutrition-related diseases.[39] The British Ministry of Health's own research facilities consisted of a small central pathological laboratory which had been taken over from the Local Government Board in 1919, where three bacteriologists were employed. These were Arthur Eastwood (in charge of the laboratory until his retirement in 1933), F. Griffith, who was the first to describe type transformation in pneumococci and also developed a serotyping method for haemolytic streptococci, and W. M. Scott (later the first director of the EPHLS). The work undertaken was described as 'of a very high order both in the field of research and routine investigation'.[40] However, conditions under which the bacteriologists worked were said to be 'primitive'.[41] The activities of the laboratory were later outlined by the MRC as 'restricted to a few special types of work; the Ministry also regularly collected epidemiological information, but not necessarily supported by laboratory reports, and

[37] MRC 1297: correspondence, Fletcher and Robinson, June 1928.
[38] MRC 1190: T. Carnwarth to Fletcher, 2 November 1922.
[39] See Harden, *Inventing the NIH* (see note 3).
[40] Frazer, *History of English Public Health*, p. 378 (see note 6).
[41] Foster, W. D. (1970). *A history of medical bacteriology and immunology*, p. 169. Heinemann, London.

from time to time conducted special investigations'.[42] Indeed, it seems that the MRC had little idea of what went on at the Ministry of Health's laboratory. In 1928, when the lease for the laboratory premises was due for renewal, the Treasury wrote to Sir Henry Dale, director of the NIMR, asking whether the Institute would consider accommodating the Ministry of Health's bacteriologists. Dale wrote,

I do not know with sufficient accuracy what their duties are, how far they are occupied with routine work of a diagnostic type, or to what extent their work is really research. I have the feeling that it would be bad policy on the Council's part definitely to allot a part of this building to the use of a staff wholly appointed by another organisation, and engaged in work having no real contact with our own.[43]

This does not imply any degree of co-operation.

Research at the Ministry of Health

The Ministry of Health's report on encephalitis lethargica, referred to above, was produced by Arthur Eastwood at the Ministry's laboratory and published in its series on public health and medical subjects,[44] a series of reports on medical research which it had inherited from the Local Government Board. Between 1920 and 1939 a full 90 reports were published in the series, although many of them were admittedly brief. In the early days the series served as a publication outlet for work done at the Ministry's laboratory by Eastwood, Scott, and Griffith, with three reports entitled 'bacteriological studies' appearing in 1922 and 1923; thereafter the reports were more selective. It is clear, however, that the Ministry of Health did not entirely neglect its medical research function. There appeared in this series short reports of local outbreaks of diseases such as scarlet fever, diphtheria, enteric fever, paratyphoid fever, and a number of reports dealing with food poisoning. Five reports on maternal mortality were produced between 1922 and 1932 by Janet Campbell, who was in charge of the maternal and infant welfare services in the Ministry of Health. Three reports dealt with tuberculosis, and 14 reports dealt with cancer, many of the latter being written by Janet E. Lane-Claypon. There was also a report on unemployment and health, written in 1938 by E. Lewis-Faning, a member of the MRC's statistical staff.

Apart from reporting occasionally on local outbreaks of infectious

[42] MRC: *Medical research in war. Report of the Medical Research Council for the years 1939–45* (1947), p. 165; *British Medical Bulletin* (1943), **1**, (4), 38.

[43] NIMR 588/1(v), 1928: Dale to Thomson, 17 February 1928.

[44] Ministry of Health: A. C. Parsons with contributions by A. S. MacNalty and J. R. Perdrau, (1922). *Report on encephalitis lethargica*, Reports on Public Health and Medical Subjects no. 11. HMSO, London.

diseases, in 1932 the Ministry of Health set up a Committee on Immunisation, a committee which had originally been conceived as a possible joint committee with the MRC, and with a strong research component. The Ministry of Health retained full control of the committee but Newman asked Dale to act as chair, which was interpreted by Fletcher as an attempt to pass over responsibility for the work to the MRC.[45] Dale declined owing to his already numerous responsibilities. Sir George Buchanan was nominated as chair and J. R. Hutchinson as secretary (who had also been secretary of the Vaccinia Committee). Its brief was 'to advise the Ministry from time to time on administrative action in connection with the application of methods of immunization against diseases other than smallpox'.[46] It was responsible for issuing a Ministry of Health memorandum in 1932 on 'The production of artificial immunity against diphtheria', although it achieved little else before 1940. In this the Committee on Immunisation reflected the inertia of the Ministry of Health itself, which followed the policy of leaving decisions relating to immunization to local authorities, as will be discussed further.

Public health and the MRC

The original Department of Bacteriology of the Medical Research Committee became after the First World War the 'Bacteriology and Experimental Pathology Department', and in the 1930s the 'Experimental Pathology and Bacteriology Department' with subdivisions of protistology, microscopy, and physical methods. Virological research absorbed most of the attention of the Department of Bacteriology and Experimental Pathology in the 1920s, and by the 1940s the subdivision of physical methods was one of the most rapidly expanded divisions of the NIMR. Research during this period included work on the salmonella group and cholera, carried out by P. Bruce-White, and work on the streptococcus and puerperal infection, carried out by Leonard Colebrook at Queen Charlotte's Hospital, Hammersmith, as an external worker of the Department. The Bacteriological Committee of the MRC published bacteriological textbooks under the guidance of P. (later Sir Paul) Fildes: *Diphtheria: its bacteriology, pathology and immunology*, 1923, and *A system of bacteriology in relation to medicine*, a monumental reference book of nine volumes, published between 1929 and 1931. However, these provided a consolidation of knowledge rather than a contribution to new knowledge.

The failure of the MRC to undertake major research into infectious diseases such as diphtheria was commented on by W. W. C. Topley,

[45] NIMR 591/11(a): Newman to Dale, 10 June 1932.
[46] MRC 2119: Minutes of Ministry of Health Committee on Immunisation, 1932–34.

professor of bacteriology at the London School of Hygiene and Tropical Medicine in 1938. He wrote to Mellanby, 'I'm becoming more and more convinced that nothing will really be done to put public health work on its scientific side, on a proper footing until we hit on some way of getting it fertilised by the research spirit.' He claimed that this required 'a closer and different liaison between the Council and the Ministry of Health, because it's impossible, except on paper, to separate the two aspects of the work'. He suggested setting up a National Public Health Laboratory, run by a joint executive committee of the MRC and the Ministry of Health, combining the Ministry's Pathological Laboratory and the MRC's Standards Laboratory and with a few subsidiary provincial laboratories. He also suggested that a Public Health Problems Committee be set up by the MRC, containing one or more representatives of the Ministry of Health. He wanted greater communication between those studying public health problems in the field and in the laboratory. In his opinion, 'the creation and growth of the MRC has, in fact, reacted unfavourably on the Ministry, by removing the scientific side of medicine more and more from the Ministry's activities, and so weakening the position of the medical as compared with the lay staff'. He thought that there were all kinds of activities, such as diphtheria immunization, where the Ministry was an essential factor because of its relation to the local authorities.[47]

In January 1939 Topley wrote a confidential report for the MRC. He pointed out that while the MRC was supporting research in sciences ancillary to medicine and clinical research, it did almost nothing to promote research in the field of preventive medicine, as represented by public health activities. Yet he maintained that this field was at least as promising as any other, and was at that time in urgent need of an effective stimulus. He described the long lag that occurred between the discovery in the laboratory of a potentially effective method of prevention and its successful application in the field as 'one of the most striking phenomena of the present time'. He maintained that the record of Britain in this respect was 'peculiarly humiliating', giving the example of diphtheria prophylaxis, which had been developed 'on a wide scale, and with striking success' in Canada and the USA, and had become compulsory in France and Hungary. Effective immunization agents had been available since the early 1920s, and reports of successful, large-scale trials in Canada and the USA had been published by 1930. Deaths from the disease in Ontario, Canada, where mass immunization had been introduced, had been reduced from 25.7 per thousand in 1920 to 0.9 in 1939; while in Britain the rate showed no decline in that period. Immunization in Britain was left to the initiative of the local authorities, and, as Topley pointed out, only a limited number of local authorities had taken any steps to introduce diphtheria

[47] MRC 477: Topley to Mellanby, 6 December 1938.

immunization, and in most areas where something had been done, the scale had been small. As Jane Lewis has pointed out, large numbers of medical officers of health, who were responsible for immunization in their respective localities, were preoccupied with more traditional approaches to the control of the disease, particularly after the expansion of their clinical and hospital-administrative responsibilities following the 1929 Local Government Act. They tended to be distrustful of diphtheria immunization as a method of control, as also of tuberculosis immunization (see Chapter 1). For diphtheria control, attention was focused on swabbing throats (and sometimes noses) in an effort to identify carriers and on confining victims in isolation hospitals.[48]

Public health officials were thus not recognized innovators. Topley believed that the formation by the MRC of a Public Health Problems Committee, or a Preventive Medicine Committee, would supply just the stimulus required to push local authorities into action. Areas to be explored included not only diphtheria, but also whooping cough, influenza, cross-infection in fever hospitals, and nutritional problems of childhood. He added that there were many other problems in which the school medical service, the venereal diseases and tuberculosis services, administered by local authorities, provided opportunities for field research that were at that time largely neglected: 'In all such matters a Preventive Medicine Committee, backed by the Council in co-operation with the Ministry of Health and with members in personal touch with medical officers of health throughout the country, could obtain information, and initiate inquiries, that would be of great value to medical research as a whole.'[49] Such a Committee would include one or more whole-time professors of hygiene, a representative of the Ministry of Health, a few more active medical officers of health, a clinician interested in public health problems, a statistician, a bacteriologist, a nutrition expert, and perhaps a physiologist.

A Preventive Committee was set up by the MRC in 1939 with Sir Wilson Jameson (Chief Medical Officer of the Ministry of Health from 1940 to 1950) as chair and D. K. M. Chalmers as secretary, and including Topley and Bradford Hill among others. Accepting an invitation to join the committee, R. M. F. Picken, professor of preventive medicine at the University of Wales, wrote that he had thought for a long time that inadequate use had been made of the material available for studying problems of applied hygiene, and that insufficient guidance had been given to those who were in a position to carry

[48] MRC 477: Topley, 9 December 1938, 11 January 1939; Lewis, J. (1986). *What price community medicine? The philosophy, practice and politics of public health since 1919*, pp. 28–9. Wheatsheaf Books, Brighton, Sussex; Lewis, J. (1986). The prevention of diphtheria in Canada and Britain 1914–1945. *Journal of Social History*, **20**, (1), 168–76; see also Foster, *A history of medical bacteriology and immunology*, pp. 148–54 (see note 41), and NIMR 591/11(a): Newman to Dale, 10 February 1932.

[49] MRC 477: Topley, 9 December 1938, 11 January 1939.

out such investigations.[50] Sir Edward Mellanby was unable to attend the first meeting of the Committee in April 1939, but sent his apologies to Jameson, regretting that he could not greet the committee on behalf of the MRC. He wrote, 'It seems to me that the setting up of this Committee is one of the most promising projects the Council have ever undertaken. The tardiness of this action is only another indication that the subject of preventive medicine has never received proper recognition, although it is obviously the most important of all in medical practice.'[51]

By 1940, six subcommittees had been formed: a mass immunization committee against diphtheria, a subcommittee on whooping cough vaccination, a subcommittee on cross-infection in hospital wards, a subcommittee on measles, a subcommittee on infant mortality due to enteritis, and a subcommittee on the control of school infections. Topley intended to utilize the facilities set up under the newly created EPHLS for the Committee's work.[52]

The Emergency Public Health Service

Besides a Preventive Medicine Committee, Topley had also advocated a central public health laboratory and subsidiary laboratories as a necessary part of the new public health initiative. The creation of such laboratories was already being discussed in the context of the war. As early as 1934, the secretary of the Committee of Imperial Defence, Maurice (later Lord) Hankey, consulted the MRC secretary on precautions to be taken in case of outbreak of war, relating to prospects of bacteriological warfare in particular and the spread of infectious diseases under war conditions. Three bacteriologists were appointed to review the situation—J. C. G. (later Sir John) Ledingham (formerly director of the National Collection of Type Cultures, 1920–31, and director of the Lister Institute, 1931–42), S.R. Douglas, and Topley. In 1936 a subcommittee of the Committee of Imperial Defence under Hankey's chairmanship, with Landsborough Thomson as secretary, issued a report, recommending certain precautions. These included preparation for various hygienic measures, the stockpiling of certain immunological substances not usually available in large quantities, and arrangements for the instant mobilization of an emergency public health laboratory service. The first task was allocated to the Ministry of Health, the other two to the MRC (under the charge of Ledingham and Topley respectively), and the cost until the outbreak of war was to be met by civil

[50] MRC 477: Picken, 17 February 1939.
[51] MRC 477: Mellanby to Jameson, 28 April 1939.
[52] MRC 477/1: Topley to Ryle, 16 January 1940; MRC 477: G. B. Wilson, 25 August 1949.

defence funds. The stockpiling of certain substances was designed to prevent a repetition of the situation that had arisen during the First World War when drugs from Germany, specifically salvarsan and neosalvarsan, were suddenly in dangerously short supply. The emergency public health laboratory service was to include reference laboratories and an intelligence service to assist in preventing the spread of epidemic diseases. The control of infectious diseases was once again recognized as crucial to a successful war effort.

An investigation of public health laboratories showed just how inadequate facilities were at that time. The London County Council (LCC) ran a bacteriological laboratory service which had been taken over from the MAB on the latter's abolition in 1929. When in 1921 the MAB had attempted to pass the responsibility for bacteriology research to the MRC, the MRC had replied that the amount of money spent in London by municipal authorities on research was far less than the 'equivalent authorities of great cities in other civilised countries'. It pointed to the New York City which was 'conducting at great expense a very important inquiry' into immunization of children against diphtheria. Not only did the MRC dissuade the MAB from abandoning its commitment to research, but it persuaded the Board to appoint an assistant bacteriologist as well.[53] This was inherited by the LCC in 1929, and by 1937 the LCC supported seven laboratories. Outside London at this time, only 40 public health laboratories had been provided by local authorities, and seven by universities. There was, moreover, a 'disconcerting irregularity' in the distribution of the services. In some places, laboratory services were simply non-existent. While some universities provided facilities, public health work was subordinated to the claims of teaching and research, not necessarily in public health. Hospital laboratories were generally more interested in the diagnosis and treatment of individual cases, concentrating on clinical pathology rather than bacteriology. Commercial laboratories used by local medical officers of health were often expensive, deterring them from extensive use.[54]

Preparations for the new Public Health Laboratory Service, organized mainly by Topley, were begun in early 1938. Premises in schools, technical colleges, and universities were designated as future laboratories; scientific and technical staff were recruited from the bacteriological staff departments of medical schools, research institutes, and the Ministry of Health's laboratory in London. Apparatus was bought and stored at convenient centres, and provision was made for transport at the different laboratories. There were in total three central laboratories (Oxford, Cambridge, and Cardiff) and sixteen subsidiary laboratories in different parts of England and

[53] MRC 101/C: MAB Infectious Diseases Research, 1921.
[54] MRC: *Report 1939–45* (1947), p. 165; Wilson, G. S. (1948). *Journal of the Royal Sanitary Institute*, **68**, (4), 221; *British Medical Bulletin* (1951), **7**, (3), 147.

Wales under the direct control of the MRC, as well as ten subsidiary laboratories on the outskirts of London and six university laboratories in the Midlands and North England. Similar arrangements were made by the Department of Health for Scotland, in consultation with the MRC. Four depots were set up for the collection, storage, and supply of blood for transfusion purposes. When the call for mobilization came at the end of August 1939, the staff moved rapidly to their allocated posts, and within a week or so were ready to cope with any emergency that might arise.

Topley envisaged using the new service for work other than that related to the war effort, for example research into dysentery and gastro-enteritis in children.[55] John Ryle, Regius Professor of Physic at the University of Cambridge, who was in charge of the laboratory set up under the EPHLS in Cambridge, predicted that the use of the laboratory service under the control of the MRC for other than war emergencies would antagonize local medical officers of health (MOsH). He claimed, 'They [MOsH] naturally take a pride in their own organisations, and except in the case of large outbreaks would not, I fancy, feel really pressed or in need of extra help.'[56] The Ministry of Health was asked to send a circular to local medical officers to ward off potential hostility, using the war to explain the new initiative. The circular pointed out how, shortly before the outbreak of war, the MRC had appointed a small subcommittee to investigate the problem of dysentery and gastro-enteritis in children, a problem which was likely to become more urgent under war conditions. It was explained that the MRC was anxious to take advantage of any opportunities that presented themselves for studying such outbreaks as might occur, both on the bacteriological and clinical sides. The circular referred to the emergency laboratories that had been established under the direction of the MRC, together with larger central laboratories at Oxford, Cambridge and Cardiff. The facilities provided by the service were to be used for the bacteriological side of the inquiry, and were regarded by the Council not as a supplement to the ordinary diagnostic laboratory work of the various public health authorities, but as part of a definite research programme, undertaken in the hope of attaining new and useful knowledge in regard to an important problem of preventive medicine.[57] In the event, they had no need to tread so carefully, as local MOsH, far from resenting the new facilities, soon began to utilize them in their own routine work. The main reason for this was that the EPHLS services were provided free of charge, while they formerly had to pay for services.

The Ministry of Health's memorandum relating to the EPHLS at the outbreak of the war, emphasized that the services of the emergency

---

[55] MRC 477/1: Topley to Ryle, 16 January 1940.
[56] MRC 477/1: Ryle to Topley, 10 November 1939.
[57] MRC 477/1: Draft of Circular, 11 November 1939.

laboratories were available without charge to the civil and military health authorities for help in the control of infectious diseases. The MRC was to be reimbursed for the cost of the service from Ministry of Health funds. Subsequently, when it became clear that the laboratories were not experiencing the envisaged war emergency calls, but that they were actively participating in laboratory work on behalf of local health authorities, the Ministry of Health felt that such work should be paid for by the local authorities themselves. The MRC, however, resisted any suggestion of a 'fee per specimen' charge, on the grounds that it would inhibit the use of the laboratories. Eventually a compromise was reached, by which local authorities reimbursed the MRC with a block grant at a rate equivalent to the sum that local authorities had spent on laboratory services before the war. In return, the EPHLS gave unlimited service within an agreed schedule. This proved satisfactory to the local authorities, and many of them discarded their peacetime arrangement and transferred all their work to the emergency laboratories. By 1941 the block grants arrangements had been agreed by seven counties, three county boroughs, 97 urban districts and municipal boroughs, 71 rural districts and seven joint hospital boards. There was, however, some resentment at the intrusion of the free service into an area that had previously offered a source of earnings to a number of individuals and hospitals.[58]

Sir Wilson Jameson, the Chief Medical Officer of the Ministry of Health, reported during the war that active participation of the emergency laboratories in the investigation of outbreaks of diphtheria, dysentery, and scarlet fever, was one of the most fruitful developments of public health during the war. These field investigations were always conducted at the request, or with the consent, of the local MOH, and 'for the first time it was possible to apply methods of modern bacteriology and immunology in the field, unhampered by considerations of cost'.[59]

The MRC's Preventive Committee, unlike the laboratories, was not set up in relation to the war. Indeed, the subcommittee on cross-infection in hospital wards reported in 1940 that much of its work had been curtailed since the outbreak of the war, although Hedley A. Wright's investigation into cross-infection in diphtheria wards was being continued. However, the war was indicating other areas of research. The subcommittee reported that it worked in close co-ordination with the EPHLS in investigating infectious diseases in residential and day nurseries set up in the early years of the war, and in nurseries of maternity homes. The war also made the work of the whooping cough immunization subcommittee

---

[58] Williams, R. E. O. (1985). *Microbiology for the public health: the evolution of the Public Health Laboratory Service 1939–1980*, pp. 16–7. Public Health Laboratory Service, London.
[59] Ibid. p. 25.

appear more urgent as a result of expected epidemics relating to gas attacks and in day nurseries.[60]

Several outbreaks of diphtheria were reported in village schools following the evacuation of children from cities to rural areas in 1939. The diphtheria subcommittee worked on methods of protection, devising a method based on swabbing and combined active and passive immunization, which enabled authorities to bring the outbreaks of diphtheria under control without closing the institutions. Mass immunization of children against diphtheria was finally introduced in 1940 in the context of the war. It was organized by the Ministry of Health's Immunisation Committee, and the EPHLS laboratories took part in a number of trials of different makes of toxoid. By 1949, nearly 5.5 million children had been vaccinated and the annual number of deaths had declined to 934, from the 1940 figure of 2480. By 1959, although there were 102 cases, none were fatal.[61]

The EPHLS had been charged with responsibility for meeting the demand for vaccines and sera that might be required on an unusually large scale in the war for the control of possible epidemics of typhoid and paratyphoid fever, bacillary dysentery, and cholera in the civilian population. In the event, no serious epidemics occurred, but typhoid–paratyphoid vaccine was used widely for general prophylaxis. Problems of food hygiene arose in canteens and communal feeding centres set up during the war, which were also studied by the EPHLS. Imported foodstuffs of unusual kinds, such as dried eggs, which were suspected of causing food poisoning, were investigated. The EPHLS made a special study of the increased incidence of bovine tuberculosis among children of school age, and came out firmly in favour of pasteurization of all milk.[62] Thus much bacteriological research during the Second World War, unlike the First World War, was directed to the civilian population.

The MRC's involvement in research related to the non-civilian population during the war included investigations of sulphonamides in controlling wound infection, and later penicillin, and research into jaundice, malaria, and typhus. An important area of activity was involvement in the Emergency Blood Transfusion Service. The limited use of blood transfusion during the First World War had indicated its potential value, and its value was further demonstrated in the Spanish Civil War of 1936–9, when an efficient blood transfusion service was held responsible for saving many lives among the wounded. In 1939 four blood transfusion depots were set up in London, and a Depot Committee established. The MRC set up a Blood Transfusion

[60] MRC 477/2: Preventive Committee minutes, 8 March 1940; on the subcommittees, see MRC 477/3, and NIMR 588/2/24, 18 March 1942.
[61] Williams, *Microbiology for the public health*, p. 20 (see note 58); Chick, Hume and Macfarlane, *War on disease*, p. 184 (see note 10).
[62] MRC: *Report 1939–45* (1947), pp. 171–2.

Research Committee into which the original Depot Committee was merged, with Topley as chair until 1940, when he was succeeded by A. N. (later Sir Alan) Drury. Blood transfusion was organized in pathology departments of hospitals and remained separate from the EPHLS. From 1946 the Lister Institute housed two MRC units working on blood and blood products: the Blood Group Research Unit directed by R. R. Race, and the Blood Group Reference Laboratory under the direction of A. E. Mourant.[63] The MRC also ran a Bacterial Sabotage Reference Laboratory during the war, under the direction of P. Bruce-White, which examined 'suspicious objects', although it did not find any of enemy origin.[64]

The Public Health Laboratory Service

The bacteriologists who had previously worked in the Ministry of Health's central laboratory were involved in running the new service, with one of them, W. M. Scott, as director. In 1941 Topley himself left the service to become secretary of the Agricultural Research Council (until his death in 1944), and G. S. (later Sir Graham) Wilson was appointed director of the EPHLS following the death of Scott in 1941 (in an air raid which also killed Griffith).

By 1944, when the new National Health Service (NHS) was being planned, the emergency service had established itself so firmly in the public health organization of the country, and was so widely used by local authorities, that it was decided to make provision for its continuance in the permanent post-war structure. Section 17 of the NHS Act of 1946 empowered the Minister of Health to provide a bacteriological service.[65] The PHLS as established in 1946 consisted of one central laboratory at Colindale in north-west London in premises that were originally designed for the Government Lymph Laboratory (that is for the preparation of smallpox vaccine). The central laboratory included an epidemiological department, and four reference laboratories (the Central Enteric Reference Laboratory and Bureau, the Salmonella Reference Laboratory, the Streptococcus and Staphylococcus Reference Laboratory, and the Virus Reference Laboratory). Also in the central laboratory was a food hygiene laboratory, a reference laboratory for food poisoning, and a standards laboratory for serological reagents, which had previously been the Oxford Standards Laboratory, preparing

---

[63] MRC 2181/I: Emergency Blood Transfusion Service. General VI, 24 August 1946; Chick, Hume and Macfarlane, *War on Disease*, p. 194 (see note 10).

[64] MRC: *Report 1939–45* (1947), p. 164; Williams, *Microbiology for the public health* p. 15 (see note 58).

[65] Webster, C. (1988). *The health services since the war*, Vol. I, *Problems of health care. The National Health Service before 1957* pp. 316–19. HMSO, London.

suspensions and antisera used for the diagnosis of infectious disease. It also included the National Collection of Type Cultures, housed for many years at the Lister Institute. The Central Public Health Laboratory became virtually an institute of public health bacteriology. Five regional laboratories were also set up, and 49 area and associated laboratories, which grew out of the emergency service (by 1961, there were 59 public health laboratories, but by 1986 the total had fallen to 54 as a result of closures of several small laboratories).[66] The director of the Service from 1943 until 1963 was Sir Graham Wilson. The PHLS was separated from the MRC in 1960, when it was placed under an independent Public Health Laboratory Service Board. The separation was largely a result of pay disputes. The MRC found itself in the embarrassing situation whereby MRC workers in the PHLS, who were paid on NHS-salary scales at the same rate as hospital pathologists and based on an agreement reached in 1949, received more pay than other MRC workers, who were on university pay scales. The PHLS workers were also eligible for 'distinction awards' under the NHS, which meant that some senior MRC staff with administrative duties received lower salaries than more junior staff in clinical work. Attention was drawn to the discrepancies in 1954 and the MRC began to negotiate with the Ministry of Health to take over the PHLS, but this proposal was rejected by the Treasury. Finally in 1960 the PHLS Act was passed which established and incorporated a new PHLS Board as a statutory body capable of acting in its own right as an agent for the Ministry of Health.[67]

Matthew Hay had predicted that war would highlight the importance of public health bacteriology, and indeed it was war which eventually provided the impetus for the service which he had advocated in 1912. The First World War had provided a stimulus for the development of bacteriology as a medical specialism, but bacteriology and the control of infectious diseases had not attracted the interest of the MRC following the war. The subsequent agreement between the Ministry of Health and the MRC left the Ministry of Health in charge of public health research, but it showed itself to have neither the resources nor perhaps the interest and ability to undertake major research projects. Research into infectious diseases was thus neglected by the Ministry, as was research into nutritional problems (see Chapter 5). The former was not as politically sensitive as the latter, yet neither did it have so many champions, with the majority of MOsH wedded to a less interventionist approach to the control of infectious diseases. Isolation of infected individuals (in public hospitals which MOsH were in charge of after 1929), education in preventive hygiene, and the more traditional preventive

[66] Wilson, G. S. (1951) *British Medical Bulletin,* **7**, (3), 147–52; *Public Health Laboratory Service year book 1962*, p. 1; *Annual Report. The Public Health Laboratory Service 1985/86* (1987), p. 10–11.
[67] Williams, *Microbiology for the public health*, pp. 79–81 (see note 58); see also Webster *Health services since the war*, Vol. I. pp. 318–9 (see note 65).

measures of sanitary reform remained their brief. Little interest in research into infectious diseases, bacteriology, and immunology arose from the Ministry of Health and its officials. Thus research into infectious disease fell between two stools. Topley reproached the MRC for its neglect of this area and Mellanby, as already noted, claimed that the setting up of the Preventive Medicine Committee in 1939 was 'one of the most promising projects the Council have even undertaken'. Leaving research into public health, bacteriology and immunology to the Ministry of Health had implied that such research was of low status, for it was the MRC and not the Ministry of Health which had the medical expertise and facilities to do the investigative work. While it was the Second World War that provided the impetus for the creation of the PHLS, one must suspect that those pressing for research into public health bacteriology used the Second World War as a convenient pretext to establish the laboratories. The rhetoric of war urgency was a powerful clarion call.

In his history of the PHLS, Sir Robert Williams, director of the PHLS from 1973 to 1981, claimed that the MRC was the appropriate body to manage the service, as it could provide the scientific support and guidance needed for the practical application of bacteriological methods to epidemiological problems, which would itself constitute a major research topic. Yet, while under the control of the MRC, the PHLS remained largely isolated from other departments of the Council, and in 1960 it became totally separate. Although several members of the PHLS staff went on to become research workers with the MRC,[68] and the Council called on the PHLS to provide an organizational base for some of its field trials of immunizing agents, such as measles, whooping cough, and rubella, there were relatively few collaborative projects with MRC staff in the 1950s, as Williams pointed out. Perhaps, he suggested, this was in large part because the MRC's interests at that time were directed more to 'basic' than to 'applied' research.[69] The MRC's Preventive Committee had been disbanded in 1949. War had acted as an interlude in the MRC's programme, when it responded to an immediate national crisis.

[68] Williams, *Microbiology for the public health*, p. 27 (see note 58).
[69] Ibid. pp. 26–7.

5

Primary research and public health: the prioritization of nutrition research in inter-war Britain

CELIA PETTY

In 1904 the Committee on Physical Deterioration,[1] which was convened in response to revelations of low standards of physique among Boer War recruits,[2] reported that incorrect choice of food was 'prominent among the causes to which degenerative tendencies might be assigned'.[3] Outbreaks of concern about the effects of poor diet on health have punctuated the public health debate of the present century.

Developments in nutrition science have, however, produced a series of changes in the definition of what constitutes a 'correct' diet, and these changes are reflected in shifts both in public health propaganda and in nutrition intervention strategies. This chapter is concerned with the upheaval in nutrition science, which was known to contemporaries as the Newer Knowledge of Nutrition, and it considers the impact of the Newer Knowledge on the public health debate of the inter-war period.[4]

The Newer Knowledge of Nutrition was based on discoveries in the field of micronutrient biochemistry and was funded in the UK chiefly by the Medical Research Council (MRC). In addition to primary research, the MRC also sponsored a series of nutritional surveys during the 1920s and early 1930s, and it campaigned vigorously for the application of nutrition science in public health practice. The most important aspect of the Newer Knowledge of Nutrition for the public health movement lay in the new definition of dietary quality that it produced. Whereas the 1904 Committee on Physical

---

[1] *Report of the Interdepartmental Committee on Physical Deterioration*, Cd. 2175 (1904).
[2] For a detailed account of the public outcry which accompanied the publication of Boer War recruiting statistics see Gilbert, B. B. (1966). *The evolution of national insurance in Great Britain. The origins of the welfare state.* Michael Joseph, London.
[3] *Report of the Interdepartmental Committee on Physical Deterioration*, Cd. 2270 (1904), para. 216.
[4] The Newer Knowledge of Nutrition was the title of a book published in 1918 by the American vitamin researcher, E. V. McCollum. It documented the origins of work on the micronutrients and gave a comprehensive account of current research. The Newer Knowledge of Nutrition became a standard text, which was regularly up-dated throughout the inter-war period.

Deterioration had argued that the diets of the poor were deficient in protein and fat,[5] during the 1920s and 1930s vitamin and mineral deficiencies were widely believed to be the chief nutritional causes of ill health and inferior physique. This shift in opinion formed the basis for Boyd Orr's assertion in *Food, Health and Income,*[6] which was published in 1936, that over 50 per cent of the UK population was consuming a diet which was inadequate for good health.

In response to the far reaching public health applications that were claimed for the new science of nutrition, the government turned to leading researchers for guidance in matters relating to food and health, and in 1931 the Ministry of Health's first expert advisory committee on nutrition was convened. The government did not question the credentials of scientists to act as policy makers, nor was their analysis of social and economic data derived from nutrition surveys questioned. However, this analysis merits a critical re-examination. Similarly, the appropriateness of the nutrition intervention strategies recommended by expert scientific commentators deserves further scrutiny.

Scientific origins of inter-war nutrition policy

The origins of the revolution in human nutrition on which the 'expert advice' of the inter-war years was based, can be traced to observations made in the course of a series of controlled animal feeding experiments that were carried out during the first two decades of the present century. Gowland Hopkins's seminal investigations, undertaken in the period 1900–12,[7] provided a protocol for these experiments. Hopkins's work appeared to demonstrate the presence in various foods of 'accessory' substances or 'vitamines' that were essential for normal growth, but were required only in minute quantities. For example, Hopkins's results of 1912, shown in Figures 5.1 and 5.2, compared the growth of young rats fed a semi-purified basal artificial ration that lacked vitamins with the growth of rats fed the same basal diet plus 3 cm³ milk. Growth failure occurred on the basal diet, but was resumed on the addition of milk. Hopkins postulated a biochemical explanation for these results and suggested that they were caused by the presence in milk of a 'catalytic or stimulative growth factor'.[8]

His belief that growth stimulation—or normalization—was a

[5] *Report of the Interdepartmental Committee on Physical Deterioration*, Minutes of Evidence, Cd. 2210 (1904): see for example Hutchison, Q. 9995.

[6] Orr, J. B. (1936). *Food, health and income* Macmillan, London.

[7] Hopkins, F. G. (1906) *Analyst*, **31**, 395; Hopkins F. G. (1912). *Journal of Physiology*, **44**, 425–60.

[8] Hopkins, F. G. (1912) *Journal of Physiology*, **44**, 425–60.

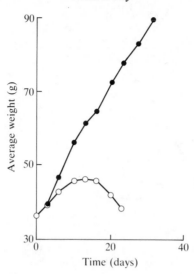

Fig. 5.1. Results of Gowland Hopkins's feeding trials, 1912. Lower curve, six rats on artificial diet alone. Upper curve, six similar animals receiving in addition 2 cm³ of milk each per day. Reproduced by permission from the *Journal of Physiology* (1912), **44**, 432.

micronutrient effect was apparently corroborated by further research undertaken during the period 1913–18. Studies funded by the MRC and carried out at Cambridge and the Lister Institute seemed to demonstrate that laboratory animals showed greater alertness, vitality, and resistance to disease, as well as better growth, when they were fed dietary supplements such as butter, fruit, green vegetables, and yeast: similar findings were reported in the United States.[9] This work convinced many physiologists and biochemists that the adequacy of human diets could no longer be judged by the old criteria; whereas nutrition science had traditionally taught that a diet containing adequate quantities of protein, carbohydrate, and fat was sufficient for health,[10] research on the micronutrients soon produced a view that 'unknown organic substances' were the chief source of dietary deficiency and a major cause of national ill health.[11]

The belief that micronutrient deficiency was responsible for growth failure appears to have been based on an initial misinterpretation by Hopkins of its cause, and although Hopkins's results of 1912 are difficult to replicate, it

[9] See for example MRC *SRS* 38: *Report on the present state of knowledge concerning accessory food factors (vitamines)* (1919) and McCollum, E. V. (1922). *The newer knowledge of nutrition* (2nd edn). Macmillan, New York.

[10] McCollum, *Newer knowledge*, p. 354.

[11] See McCollum, *Newer knowledge*, and MRC 1500: Fletcher to Macfadden, 20 September 1921.

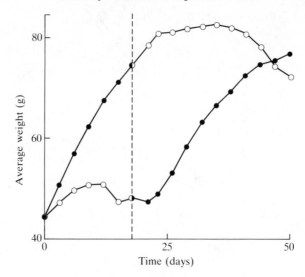

Fig. 5.2. Results of Gowland Hopkins's feeding trials, 1912. Lower curve (up to 18th day), eight male rats upon pure dietary. Upper curve, eight similar rats taking 3 cm³ of milk each per day. On the 18th day, marked by vertical dotted line, the milk was transferred from one set to the other. Reproduced by permission from the *Journal of Physiology* (1912), **44**, 433.

now seems clear that they reflect a reduced food intake in rats fed a purified, deficient diet, rather than a lack of a 'catalytic or stimulative growth factor'. This assertion can be made with confidence since animals eating normal amounts of energy must somehow dissipate the calories they consume in order *not* to grow; they can only do this by increasing their metabolic rate. However, with the exception of Essential Fatty Acid (EFA) deficiency, vitamin deficiency does not produce such an effect,[12] and EFAs were available in the artificial ration used by Hopkins. Sodium deficiency[13] can also increase metabolic rate, but this nutrient was also available in the artificial ration.

Subsequent research, including that of Harriet Chick, acknowledged the problem of food intake variations, but her attempts to allow for this again produced confusing results. In 1942, Chick published data which showed that rats fed brown bread grew faster than those fed white bread.[14] These rats also ate more food, but Chick showed that their weight gain per gram of food or protein consumed was higher—and therefore, presumably, that brown bread with its higher micronutrient content, was better than white bread.

[12] Rivers, J. P. W. and Frankel, T. L. (1981). *British Medical Bulletin*, **37**, (1), 59–64.
[13] Miller, D. S. and Parsonage, S. R. (1971). *Proceedings of the Nutrition Society*, **30**, 76A.
[14] Chick, H. (1942) *Lancet*, **i**, 405.

Widdowson and McCance considered this effect in later work[15] and Widdowson recently wrote that Chick's results 'showed clearly that the increase in weight per gram of protein eaten was greatest for the wholemeal flour. Something in the wholemeal flour made it better food than white flour for the weanling rats'.[16] However, there is a simple arithmetical explanation for these results. Animals have basic daily requirements of protein and energy that are needed simply to avoid weight loss, and growth can only occur when intake is above this level. Consequently, the more that is consumed, the greater is the gain per unit of consumption: the gross efficiency of the diet rises with intake, even though the net efficiency remains constant, because the importance of the maintenance quotient is reduced as intake rises.

The reason why loss of appetite occurred in animals fed purified artificial rations and why recovery took place on the addition of milk or other 'natural' foods is obscure. Increased palatability or possibly a physiological response to the deficient diet may have been responsible. Nevertheless, the cause of growth inhibition was unquestionably a deficiency in total food intake, rather than a deficiency in vitamin intake. But many contemporary observers, including Sir Walter Fletcher, drew the opposite inference from these experiments. For them, the case that growth inhibition was a qualitative effect seemed proven beyond reasonable doubt.

Public health inferences of the Newer Knowledge of Nutrition

Kohler has pointed out that Fletcher was an early enthusiast for the medical applications of vitamin biochemistry[17] and certainly by 1915 he was also convinced of its general public health importance as well as having more specialized clinical applications.[18]

The practical significance of nutrition research was enhanced by Mellanby's work in 1917 on rickets.[19] Mellanby demonstrated that rickets was a dietary deficiency disease, and his initial hypothesis was that it was caused by a lack of 'Fat soluble A'—Hopkins's 'growth factor'—the chief dietary source of which had been identified as milk fat. Fletcher used Mellanby's results to strengthen his case for the state funding of medical

---

[15] MRC *SRS* 287: Widdowson, E. M. and McCance, R. A. (1954). *Studies in the nutritional value of bread*.

[16] Widdowson, E. M. (1975). Extraction rates—nutritional implications. In *Bread* (ed. A. Spicer), pp. 235–46. Applied Science, London.

[17] Kohler, R. E. (1982). *From medical chemistry to biochemistry*. Cambridge University Press.

[18] MRC PF106: Fletcher to Hopkins, 23 June 1915. The first clinical applications of nutrition science were for the deficiency diseases beri beri and scurvy, neither of which presented a public health problem in the West.

[19] MRC *SRS* 61: Mellanby, E. (1921). *Experimental rickets*, and MRC 99 files for details of MRC rickets research.

research. For example, in his annual report for 1918 he commented on recruiting statistics, which, like those published in the aftermath of the Boer War, revealed the poor physical status of working-class recruits, and wrote that 'The recent revelations of our low national standard of physique made by the telling figures now emerging from . . . the National Service Ministry . . . give fresh force to the demand for the knowledge by which alone right action can be guided'.[20]

Fletcher's case was strengthened by further investigations into the dietary aetiology of rickets, which included Chick and Gribbon's clinical studies in post-war Vienna.[21] Their work showed that rickets, which had a reported prevalence rate of up to 80 per cent in some industrial cities,[22] could be prevented, as well as cured, by the use of the 'antirachitic vitamin', which was known to be present in both milk fat and cod liver oil.

Fletcher was confident that work on the vitamins would eventually lead to the eradication of many of the problems of 'defective growth' that drained the armed forces of manpower resources. However, he also stressed that nutrition science could contribute to peacetime health and prosperity, and during the early 1920s he drew attention to its wide-ranging applications. For example, in 1921 he wrote of the 'economic value' of vitamin research, which, he informed the Ministry of Health's Food Division, was 'becoming almost monthly more apparent, affecting as it does at a thousand points the food of the population, its choice, its preparation in manufacturing processes and in the kitchen, its production by agriculture'.[23]

Fletcher's belief in the immediate applications of the Newer Knowledge pushed forward research on the micronutrients in the UK, and secured for human nutrition around one sixth of MRC research grants throughout the inter-war period.[24] Nutrition research was, he wrote in his annual report of 1921 'a good example of work of the kind which it is highly proper to support from public funds'.[25]

The Newer Knowledge of Nutrition produced a belief that micronutrient deficiency was the chief nutritional problem facing the UK. This view influenced welfare feeding strategies, particularly during the 1930s when, ironically, concern about the effects of mass unemployment on the health of

---

[20] MRC: *Annual report 1917–18* (1918), p. 73.

[21] MRC *SRS* 77: Chick, H. (1923). *Studies of rickets in Vienna, 1919–22*; Gribbon, M. R. and Fergusson, M. I. H. (1921). Nutrition in Vienna. *Lancet*, **i**, 474–7.

[22] See Report of the School Medical Officer for the County of Durham, 1920; MacIntosh, J. W. (1935) *Journal of State Medicine*, **4**, 187–98.

[23] MRC: *Annual report 1920–21* (1921), p. 12.

[24] See for example MRC 1200/1: Fletcher to Dawson. 15 April 1931.

[25] MRC: *Annual report 1920–21* (1921), p. 12. Currently, nutrition receives between 1%–2% of the MRC's annual research budget. Rivers, J. P. W. (1985). Social constraints on nutritional knowledge. In *Advances in diet and nutrition* (ed. C. Horowitz), pp. 389–95. John Libbey, London.

the nation's schoolchildren led increasingly to a policy of providing malnourished schoolchildren with milk rather than high calorie dinners. The emphasis that was placed on the importance of the vitamin-rich 'protective foods' also reinforced the case for nutrition education as a welfare intervention strategy, and nutritional surveys carried out by the MRC during the 1920s were seen as proof that the poor could be taught to gain 'greater physiological value' from their diets. In the following sections the evidence that led to the adoption of these policies is reconsidered and an alternative view of the nutrition problem in inter-war Britain is suggested.

The MRC and the public health administration: A policy for diet and health?

Both Fletcher and his successor as MRC Secretary, Edward Mellanby, urged the public health administration to take action on nutrition, and in 1919 Fletcher looked to the newly established Ministry of Health to adopt a positive nutrition policy. The Ministry had a statutory obligation to advance and encourage preventive medicine,[26] and Fletcher believed that nutrition science could make a major contribution in this endeavour. One of his first initiatives as Secretary of the MRC was therefore to set out proposals for public health action on nutrition, and in 1919 he presented Sir George Newman, the Chief Medical Officer (CMO), with a memorandum that was intended to guide the Ministry in matters of nutrition policy and research.[27]

This document called for collaboration between the MRC and the Ministry in field research, and co-operation from the Ministry's Medical Officers in the application of scientific discoveries in public health practice. Initially, the prospects for a 'combined attack' on the nutrition question seemed favourable. For example, in 1920 the Ministry proposed studies on the nutritive value of milk and on dental decay.[28] The first of these proposals led to Corry Mann's controlled feeding trial at Dr Barnardo's Home in Woodford, Essex,[29] and the second led to May Mellanby's work on predisposing dietary factors in dental disease, which the MRC continued to support throughout the inter-war years.[30] However, relations between the Ministry and the MRC deteriorated rapidly:[31] proposals for a study of nutrition during pregnancy and infancy, to be carried out in collaboration

[26] See CMO: *Annual report 1919–20* (1920), Appendix IX, p. 389.
[27] MRC 1500: Fletcher to Newman, 25 November 1919.
[28] MRC 1500: Newman to Fletcher, 3 December 1920; MRC 1381/1, Fletcher to Newman, 7 December 1920.
[29] MRC *SRS* 105: Mann, H. C. (1926). *Diets for boys during the school years*.
[30] See for example MRC *SRS* 140: Mellanby, M. (1929). *Diet and teeth*.
[31] See for example MRC 1958: Fletcher to Carnwarth, 3 November 1922.

with the Maternal and Child Welfare services, were put forward unsuccessfully by the Council in 1922 and a subsequent request by the Ministry for assistance in a similar project was turned down by Fletcher.[32] The tensions which arose between the Ministry and the MRC can be traced to conflicts over the demarcation of research interests and, although a concordat defining their respective responsibilities in relation to research was drawn up in 1924,[33] there was little co-operation in studies relating to problems of human nutrition during Fletcher's tenure of office.

During the 1920s, Fletcher's initial vision of a united attack on the problem of dietary deficiency remained unfulfilled and he became increasingly outspoken in his criticism of the Ministry's attitude to nutrition. This criticism was not confined to the public health administration, but extended to its Medical Officers of Health (MOsH) who, Fletcher claimed, had failed to grasp the true significance of the 'Newer Knowledge'. A lack of intellectual vision had, he maintained, condemned a generation of children to preventable disease,[34] and in a lecture delivered in 1928 at the Public Health Congress and Exhibition he urged MOsH to familiarize themselves at first hand with experimental evidence of the effects of vitamin deficiency.[35] Similarly, in one of his last printed works, Fletcher argued that by looking at research that was taking place in the laboratory, public health workers would be convinced of the ' "threshold" for adequate nutrition, of the actuality of a veiled malnutrition'.[36]

Fletcher placed his trust in experimental evidence which suggested that the internal chemical environment, rather than the external physical environment, determined the success of physiological functioning; the Newer Knowledge of Nutrition taught that the most effective defences against disease lay within the organism itself and that 'Highly satisfactory nutritive conditions are capable of protecting young animals to a surprising degree against physical and hygienic handicaps'.[37] This view of the underlying biochemical cause of poor physique and 'sub-optimal health' led Fletcher to criticize the priority that the Ministry of Health gave to housing, and objections to official housing policies were a persistent theme in his public and private statements throughout his term of office. Thus, in 1921 he wrote to the Ministry's Food Division that 'dietetic deficiency is overwhelmingly more important than the housing question'.[38] In 1931 he told Lord Dawson, who had recently accepted a seat on the MRC, that

---

[32] MRC 2070/25: Fletcher to Paton, 10 July 1922; MRC 1190: Fletcher to Newman, 16 December 1924.

[33] MRC 1190: Fletcher to Newman, 17 January 1924.

[34] See for example MRC PF 133: Fletcher to Greenwood, 27 October 1931.

[35] *Medical Officer* (1928), **ii**, 253.

[36] Fletcher, W. M. (1932). The urgency of nutritional studies. *Nutrition Abstracts and Reviews*, **I**, (3), 357.

[37] McCollum, *Newer Knowledge*, p. 396 (see note 9).

[38] MRC 1500: Fletcher to MacFadden, 20 September 1921.

'. . . the medical administrators have delayed inexcusably to use the abundant new knowledge that has been pouring out of the laboratories in the last fifteen years . . . Physiology teaches that faulty nutrition is far worse for our population than faulty housing. We waste untold millions a year by not using the new knowledge we have'.[39]

In the same year he endorsed the work of M'Gonigle, MOH for Stockton on Tees (who had undertaken a study into the effects of rehousing on nutrition and mortality), and wrote that modern physiological knowledge pointed conclusively to 'the importance of diet, rather than that of better housing, in the interest of national health'.[40]

Antagonism between the Ministry of Health and the MRC over the official attitude to nutrition reached a climax in 1931 when Newman wrote in his annual report that the diet of the pregnant woman was a matter of 'common sense'.[41] In a furious reply, Fletcher pointed out that this both challenged the results of 'much brilliant recent British work' and undermined the MRC's case for Treasury support in nutrition research—a subject which was, he maintained, 'of vital and immediate practical value'.[42] According to Fletcher, it might be inferred from Newman's report that nutrition was neither a suitable subject for scientific investigation nor a proper part of medical research, yet, he maintained, it had been shown conclusively that improving dietary quality was far more important than 'increasing quantity ignorantly (or by common sense) as wages rise and far more important than improvement in housing'.[43] This report confirmed Fletcher's belief that, despite his assurances to the contrary, Newman condoned the Ministry's policy of putting housing first, thereby withholding action on nutrition.

Although Fletcher failed to convince the administration that action on nutrition deserved the highest prioritization, public health officials endorsed the new dietetics with considerable enthusiasm. From the early 1920s the view that health and vitality could be improved by eating more of the 'vitamin rich protective foods'[44] was set out in Ministry of Health and Board of Education publications and this message soon appeared in public health propaganda at local authority level.[45] The enthusiasm of public health professionals for the dietary prescriptions of the Newer Knowledge is also reflected in the public health press and in the reports of local authority Medical Officers,[46] which

[39] MRC 2100/1: Fletcher to Dawson, 15 April 1931.
[40] MRC 1741: Fletcher to M'Gonigle, 26 October 1931.
[41] CMO: *Annual report 1930–31* (1931), p. 163.
[42] MRC 1190: Fletcher to Newman, 22 October 1931.
[43] Ibid.
[44] See for example Chief Medical Officer of the Board of Education, *Annual report: health of the schoolchild (HOSC) 1920* (1921), p. 146; *HOSC 1923* (1924), p. 98; *HOSC 1927* (1928), p. 7.
[45] For reports of these activities, see for example *Public Health* (1925), **ii**, 333–4; *Medical Officer* (1925), **ii**, 217; *Medical Officer* (1926), **i**, 75–6; *Medical Officer* (1927), **i**, 123.
[46] See *Medical Officer* (1920), **i**; 80; ibid. (1925), **i**, 112, 000; ibid. (1926), **i**, 200, 214. See also Petty, E. C. (1987). Unpublished PhD thesis, pp. 137–40. University of London.

indicate that discoveries in nutrition science merely reinforced existing views about working-class ignorance and incompetence in matters relating to the 'correct' choice of food. The precise nature of these prejudices was recorded in evidence presented to the Committee on Physical Deterioration of 1904; witnesses placed the blame for bad nutrition on the inability of working-class wives to manage their budgets wisely, on their incorrect choice of food, and on their lack of domestic skills.[47]

A series of nutritional surveys conducted by the MRC's Committee on Quantitative Problems of Human Nutrition during the 1920s and early 1930s[48] seemed to confirm the view that nutrition education, combined with domestic training for elementary schoolgirls, was the way to reform the national diet and improve standards of nutrition.[49] These studies, which have been overshadowed by fundamental research on vitamin biochemistry carried out during the same period, had a decisive impact on the debate about the applied possibilities of nutrition science. Just as the Newer Knowledge taught that the diets of the poor were deficient in quality rather than in quantity, so the MRC's dietary surveys were interpreted as proof that nutritional defects could be remedied by education rather than by increasing family income.[50]

The Committee on Quantitative Problems of Human Nutrition was convened in 1922 and it was hoped that, in addition to food supply data, the new Committee would also provide information relating to the diet and health of various social and economic groups.[51] The Committee selected mining communities as the subject for its first dietary survey, and its 'Report on the Nutrition of Miners and their Families'[52] seemed to confirm many well established prejudices concerning working-class spending patterns.

Although the Committee asserted that its aim had been to collect

---

[47] For a full discussion of these aspects of the Report, see Petty, unpublished PhD thesis, Chap. I (see note 46).

[48] MRC *SRS* 87: *Report on the nutrition of miners and their families* (1924); MRC *SRS* 151: *An inquiry into the diet of 154 families of St Andrews* (1931); MRC *SRS* 165: *An inquiry into the diet of families in Cardiff and Reading* (1932). See also *Report of the Committee on Physical Deterioration* (1904) paras 310–14 for recommendations concerning domestic education. The Quantitative Committee was fused with the Vitamin Committee in 1926 to form a single Nutrition Committee. Members of the new Nutrition Committee included Cathcart (chairman), Greenwood, Hopkins, Mellanby, Boyd Orr, and J. C. Drummond.

[49] The MRC's Child Life Committee also published a study, *Poverty, nutrition and growth* which included nutritional survey data and considered the relationship between diet and health. Its authors, D. Noel Paton and Leonard Finlay, concluded that maternal efficiency, rather than income, was the chief factor influencing nutritional status among the poor. For a discussion of issues raised by this report see Petty, unpublished PhD thesis (see note 46).

[50] See for example MRC 2100: Fletcher to Newman, 20 June 1924; *Public Health* (1937), **50**, 175–6; *British Medical Journal* (1937), **i**, 334.

[51] MRC 2100: Greenwood to Fletcher, 30 October 1921: MRC 2100/1: Committee on Quantitative Problems of Nutrition, preliminary memorandum, 7 June 1922.

[52] MRC *SRS* 87: *Report on the nutrition of miners and their families*.

observations on the 'single issue of nutrition' and it disclaimed any interest in economic aspects of the problem,[53] the nutrition of mining communities was unavoidably linked with matters of political and economic concern. The survey was conducted in the wake of the 1921 coal strike, which left the mining industry with reduced rates of pay and continuing high levels of unemployment; these were conditions which had led to accusations in the House of Commons that there was 'actual starvation' in the mining districts and that 'the vast mass of the mining population' was in a state of 'semi starvation'.[54]

The Report addressed two issues: the composition and physiological value of the diet available in different coal-fields, and the physical status of the child population. Its criteria for assessing physical status were crude; the average heights and weights of children in mining communities were compared with the average for elementary schoolchildren in the same area.[55] It was found that heights and weights fell below the average for the district in only one mining community,[56] and this of course implied that reports that miners' children were starving were inaccurate. Having dismissed the view that there was actual starvation in the coal-fields, the committee focused on the efficiency of family budgeting. For example, it had been suggested that miners' wives who had been in domestic service might be better domestic managers than those who had not. Although numbers proved to be too small for statistical analysis, this hypothesis is indicative of the kind of relationships which the Committee thought could be usefully explored.

Discrepancies were found in the 'nutritional value for money' achieved by miners' wives, and an analysis of these discrepancies was undertaken. In order to evaluate the 'adequacy of return for expenditure', linear regressions of a range of variables, which included calorie intake and calories purchased per penny on income, were made.[57] These produced correlations that appeared to support the hypothesis that more efficient marketing would increase the food intake of the poor, and the Committee concluded that 'by better education and organisation more adequate physiological results can be obtained . . .'. The Committee explained that by education they meant 'knowledge of the factors which ought to be taken account of in marketing'.[58]

But, although the Committee used linear regression analysis, in many cases the actual relationships were curvilinear. For example, whilst linear regression assumed a constant relationship between differences in income

[53] Ibid. p. 6.
[54] Ibid. p. 5.
[55] Ibid. Section VIII, pp. 33–46.
[56] Ibid. Section VIII, pp. 33– 46.
[57] Ibid. Section VII, pp. 25–33.
[58] Ibid. p. 29.

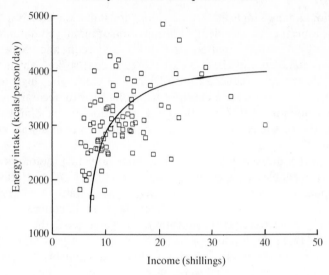

Fig. 5.3. Relation of energy intake to income. Data from MRC survey of miners' families (1924).

and changes in food intake over the whole range, the data showed no such constancy. Thus, Figure 5.3 shows that energy intake changed rapidly with income at very low income levels, while above a threshold of 8s. to 10s. per head it changed only very slowly, if at all, with changing income: the relationship between income and calorie intake was not linear and linear regression distorted the true relationship, which Figure 5.3 shows was curvilinear. In fact, as income fell, purchasing became far more efficient. Figure 5.4 shows that families with incomes of around 16s. per man value per week purchased only 250 calories per penny, whereas families with incomes of between 8s. to 10s. per man-value purchased 400–500 calories per penny. Similarly, at lower levels of income, a higher fraction of income was used for food: this is Engels' law, which had been known to economists since the nineteenth century. In the poorest families, almost the entire income was spent on food, and again the relationship is best described as a curve (see Figure 5.5). Bread and flour came to dominate food expenditure in the poorest families and Figure 5.6 indicates that there was a critical income threshold of around 10s. per man value per week, below which the percentage of total family income spent on cereals rose steeply.

The Committee's analysis of these budgets led it to conclude that the poor could be taught to make better use of their incomes,[59] and when the report was published in 1924, Fletcher urged Newman to take positive action on its

---

[59] Ibid. p. 47.

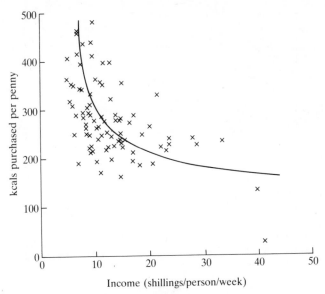

Fig. 5.4. Relation of calories purchased per penny to income. Data from MRC survey of miners' families (1924).

findings. The report was, he told the CMO, further evidence of the need for a 'really big campaign in this fundamental business of nutrition and the right use of money and of cooking methods',[60] particularly among the working classes.

However, the data actually demonstrate that working-class wives already made extremely efficient use of inadequate resources and had a better grasp of economic realities than their academic critics. Nevertheless, the Report on the Nutrition of Miners and their Families appeared to put on an objective basis attitudes concerning working-class ignorance and inefficiency, which had been current in the public health movement since the beginning of the century.

Clearly, theoretical objections can be raised against retrospective analysis of this kind. However, its purpose is *not* to belittle the statistical achievements of the Committee with the advantages of hindsight and modern technology. The Committee's aim was to apply modern scientific methods to improve the well-being of an economically disadvantaged group, and their technical skills cannot be faulted. But in order to carry out the extremely laborious task of statistical computation, a series of arbitrary—although rational—choices were made. By reconsidering the choices made by the

---

[60] MRC 2100: Fletcher to Newman, 20 June 1924.

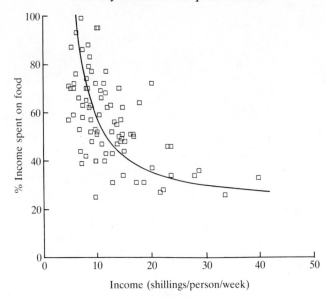

Fig. 5.5. Relation of percentage income spent on food to income. Data from MRC survey of miners' families (1924).

Committee, valuable social and moral insights can be gained into the kind of relationships it was believed would be found. This is not only of historical interest, but also of considerable importance for contemporary public health practice, since the Committee's analyses have provided a scientific rationale for much health education work in the UK and in developing countries up to the present time.

Further evidence that appeared to support the case for nutrition education was gathered by E. P. Cathcart, Chairman of the Committee on Quantitative Problems of Human Nutrition, who carried out a series of nutritional surveys on behalf of the MRC between 1926 and 1932.[61] Since Cathcart adopted the same methodology as earlier surveys had used, this is hardly surprising. Cathcart believed that his nutritional surveys were proof that: 'when the housewife is skilled in marketing and in cooking an excellent return per penny spent can be obtained, even with abnormally small incomes'.[62] Furthermore, he claimed that inadequate feeding could not simply be ascribed to inadequate income but that 'Bad buying and bad cooking' accounted for a great deal.[63]

[61] Cathcart, E. P.; MRC *SRS* 165: Cathcart, E. P.; MRC *SRS* 151: MRC *SRS* 218: Cathcart, E. P. and Murray, A. M. T. (1936). *A dietary survey in terms of actual foodstuffs consumed* .

[62] Cathcart, E. P. (1931). The foundations of the national diet. *Medical Officer*, i, 143–6.

[63] Cathcart, E. P. (1931). 42nd Congress of Royal Sanitary Institution, reported in *Medical Officer*, ii, 90–1.

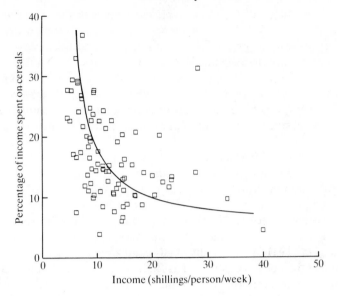

Fig. 5.6. Relation of percentage food expenditure spent on bread and flour to income. Data from MRC Survey of Miners' Families (1924).

This view was fully endorsed by Fletcher, who saw in Cathcart's work, ammunition to convince the Ministry of Health that it should take a more active role in promoting nutrition education. In the same way Mellanby (who disagreed with Cathcart over almost everything else[64]) shared Cathcart's belief that an improvement in nutrition was 'as much a matter of improved education as of increased wages'.[65]

The public health administration and the Medical Research establishment did not argue about the need to change dietary habits, and throughout the inter-war period both the administration and MRC continued to claim that improvements could be made in both the choice and the 'economical use' of food. However, during the 1930s it became increasingly difficult to justify the view that an adequate diet could be secured simply by improving budgeting efficiency. This development in the debate about food and health can be traced to the publication of official nutritional guidelines which were laid down by government committees.

---

[64] Cathcart, like Paton, disagreed with the inferences for human nutrition which were derived from discoveries in the field of vitamin biochemistry. However, this debate is beyond the scope of the present chapter. For a full discussion see Petty, unpublished PhD thesis. (see note 46).

[65] Cathcart (1931). *Medical Officer* ii, 90–1 (see note 63). See also PRO MH 56/44: 16 April 1931, for Mellanby's comments on 'laziness' and 'apathy' among working-class housewives.

In 1931, the Ministry of Health convened an Advisory Committee on Nutrition which proceeded to recommend standard dietaries. However, these dietaries were beyond the means of the low paid and unemployed,[66] and despite their attempts to keep nutrition out of politics,[67] the Ministry's panel of experts put the nutrition question at the centre of a bitter standard-of-living controversy.[68] Edward Mellanby, who succeeded Fletcher as MRC Secretary in 1934, was a keen advocate of the expert advisory committee, and so played a vital role in a reorientation of the nutrition debate that occurred during the 1930s.

Although Mellanby's appointment did not change the MRC's prioritization of nutrition research, the tactics he adopted in dealing with the public health administration were very different from Fletcher's. Whereas Fletcher had preferred to restrict the discussion of scientific matters to the MRC's own committees and had been scathing of the Ministry's belated interest in nutrition, signalled by the appointment of the Advisory Committee in 1931,[69] Mellanby had campaigned vigorously for the establishment of such a committee. His first move in this campaign had been to outline a programme for State action in relation to food,[70] which was published by the *British Medical Journal* in 1927, and this was followed immediately by discussions with Newman, the CMO.[71]

Like Fletcher, Mellanby argued that action by the State and local government in relation to nutrition would bring about improvements in health equal to those of the sanitary revolution of the nineteenth century, and that 'correct feeding' was of even greater importance than good hygiene in combatting the problem of disease. He too believed that the public health movement was hopelessly ignorant of the discoveries of nutrition science, but he argued that a Board of Nutrition, composed of experimental scientists, should be convened by the Ministry of Health to translate these discoveries into public health policies and that this body should also be used to guide the public through the 'morass of conflicting statements' that were being made about diet and health.[72] This approach represented a departure from previous MRC policy. Whilst Fletcher had believed that the place for scientists was in the laboratory and not in committee rooms (especially when these were the

---

[66] Rathbone, E. (1934). *Memorandum on the scale of needs suitable for adoption by the Unemployment Assistance Board.* Children's Minimum Committee, London.

[67] PRO MH 56/43: Greenwood, 30 November 1933; PRO MH 56/40: Carnwarth to Newman, April 1933; MRC 2106/1: Greenwood to Hudson, 21 November 1933.

[68] PRO MH56/55: Labour Party 'Notes for Speakers', 1 December 1933.

[69] MRC 1190: Fletcher to Robinson, 5 December 1930.

[70] Mellanby, E. (1927). Duties of the State in relation to the nation's food supply. *British Medical Journal*, ii, 66.

[71] PRO MH56/43: minute of meeting between Newman and Mellanby, 6 December 1927.

[72] Mellanby, E. (1927). *British Medical Journal*, ii, 66.

Ministry's rather than those of the MRC),[73] Mellanby, by contrast, preferred to work directly with Whitehall.

The membership of the Nutrition Advisory Committee that was eventually summoned by the Ministry of Health virtually duplicated the MRC's own Nutrition Committee. It included Hopkins and Mellanby from the vanguard of the Newer Knowledge; Major Greenwood, Professor of Epidemiology and Vital Statistics at the London School of Hygiene and Tropical Medicine; Cathcart, Chairman of the MRC's Nutrition Committee—who held the minority view that diet should be assessed on the basis of quantity rather than quality; and Mottram, a former pupil of Fletcher and Professor of Physiology at King's College for Women. This group of experts had been gathered by Fletcher and his immediate advisors in the early 1920s when Hopkins had been called on to identify key workers in the field of vitamin biochemistry[74] and Major Greenwood had recommended a team of prominent physiologists to sit on the Committee on Quantitative Problems of Human Nutrition.[75] The only 'outsiders' to be appointed to the Ministry's Advisory Committee were a domestic economist and a representative of the Society of Medical Officers of Health.

It was the administration's intention that this committee should direct a health education initiative, guiding the public to better health through dietary self-help.[76] From the Ministry's point of view, the Newer Knowledge presented a prospect of low cost welfare at a time of mass unemployment and financial crisis: for example in 1932 Janet Campbell, who was responsible for the Ministry's Maternal and Child Welfare services, wrote of the 'special need for attention to nutrition at a time when it is difficult or impossible to obtain additional money for this purpose'.[77] Carnwarth, a Medical Officer in the Food Division, described the 'importance of maintaining a proper standard of nutrition where unemployment is widespread and of long standing'.[78] Both the Ministry and the MRC believed that nutrition education was a viable method of achieving these ends. For example, at an early meeting of the committee, V. H. Mottram asserted that the solution to the nutrition problem was in 'the better education of the housewife and the potential housewife',[79] and Cathcart made the observation that 'Very often

[73] MRC 1200/1: Fletcher to Dawson, 15 April 1931; MRC 1190: Fletcher to Robinson, 5 December 1930.
[74] See Kohler, *From medical chemistry to biochemistry*, pp. 77–8 (see note 17); also Platt, B. S. (1956). Sir Edward Mellanby. *Annual Review of Biochemistry*, 25, 1–28.
[75] MRC 2100: Greenwood to Fletcher, 30 October 1921.
[76] PRO MH56/44: Advisory Committee minutes, January 1931; MRC 2106/1: Robinson to Fletcher, 9 December 1930.
[77] PRO MH 56/52: Campbell to Wrigley, May 1932.
[78] PRO MH/52: Carnwarth to Newman, 15 November 1932.
[79] PRO MH56/44: Advisory Committee minutes, April 1931.

combined with inadequate income there is ineffective spending'.[80] which was not, apparently, challenged by other members of the committee. The Secretary to the Minister of Health, A. W. Robinson, confirmed the administration's commitment to this view in 1933 when he informed the Minister that 'Malnutrition is ignorance quite as much as insufficient resources and it is the ignorance on which I want to organise the attack'.[81]

However, despite the common ground that existed between the experts and the administrators over the importance of education in raising nutritional standards, nutrition education in fact came very low on the Committee's agenda, and discussion focused increasingly on questions of nutritional requirements. In response to official requests for authoritative information on healthy eating, a series of statements on minimum needs were produced that attempted to translate nutrient requirements derived from laboratory experiments into dietary guidelines for free living populations.

The first of these statements, *The criticism and improvement of diets*, [82] which appeared in 1932, prompted the British Medical Association (BMA) to produce its report on the minimum cost of a 'physiologically adequate' diet.[83] The disagreement between the BMA and the Advisory Committee over the definition of minimum requirements provoked by this report cast a shadow over the subsequent proceedings of the Advisory Committee.[84] However, the BMA document was welcomed by welfare campaigners and it became a touchstone in the standard of living debate until the outbreak of the Second World War.[85] In 1935 the first internationally agreed dietary requirements were produced by the League of Nations (the *Report on the physiological basis of nutrition*[86]), and in 1936 the UK Interdepartmental Advisory Committee produced further dietary recommendations in its 'Nutrition report'.[87] In the same year Boyd Orr claimed in *Food health and*

[80] PRO MH56/44: Advisory Committee minutes, January 1931.

[81] PRO MH56/52: Robinson to Minister of Health, 27 June 1933.

[82] *The criticism and improvement of diets* (1932). HMSO, London; see also *Diets for children in poor law homes* (1932). HMSO, London.

[83] *Report of Committee on Nutrition, To determine the weekly expenditure which must be incurred by families of varying size if health and working capacity are to be maintained and to construct specimen diets* (1933). British Medical Association, London.

[84] MRC 2106/2: Greenwood to Landsborough Thomson, 3 August 1935, 'I haven't forgotten the nightmare of the last advisory committee . . . I take it that directly a scientific question becomes of political interest, the science begins to evaporate'. See also Petty unpublished PhD thesis, Chap. 3, Part II (see note 46), for a discussion of the Ministry of Health's first Advisory Committee on Nutrition and its deliberations.

[85] The BMA standard was used in many local enquiries in order to establish the extent of malnutrition. See for example Sheffield Social Survey Committee: *A study of the standard of living in Sheffield* (1933); Ipswich Campaign Against Malnutrition: *An enquiry into malnutrition* (1938); Birmingham Social Survey Committee: Soutar, M. S. (1939). *Nutrition and size of family*; see also Rathbone, *Memorandum* (see note 66).

[86] League of Nations Technical Commission: *Report on the Physiological Basis of Nutrition* (1935). London.

[87] UK Interdepartmental Advisory Committee on Nutrition: *First report 1936* (1937).

income that, according to current scientific criteria, up to half the population of the UK was malnourished.[88] The process of producing recommended nutritional requirements has continued relentlessly throughout the post-war period—although it is now generally agreed that inflated protein requirements laid down by panels of experts in the 1950s and 1960s led to misguided intervention strategies during this period.[89]

The Ministry's first Nutrition Committee therefore established a precedent which has had a lasting influence on both the theory and practice of nutrition science. Mellanby was a key figure in this process for he saw in the expert committee a means of pressurizing the government to adopt a positive nutrition policy,[90] and leading nutritionists have continued to use the Committee structure for the same purposes. For Mellanby, a positive nutrition policy meant advocating a vast increase in the consumption of fat-soluble vitamins, especially among a target population of pregnant and lactating women, and children in the first years of life: his success is reflected in the dietary standards set by the Nutrition Committees that sat in the period 1931–9.[91]

These standards were challenged by E. P. Cathcart, who sat both on the MRC's Nutrition Committee and on the Advisory Committee, and who argued that generations of healthy highlanders had been raised on diets which were, according to the Newer Knowledge, 'inadequate in almost every respect'.[92] However, the tide of opinion ran in Mellanby's favour: as early as 1932, Ministry officials endorsed Mellanby's belief that there was a need to

[88] Orr, *Food health and income* (see note 6).
[89] See McLaren, D. S. (1974). The great protein fiasco. *Lancet* , ii, 93–6; Waterlow, J. C. and Payne, P. (1975). The protein gap. *Nature*, **258**; 113.
[90] See for example MRC 2127: minute of a meeting between Mellanby and Hankey, 23 February 1934; MRC 2127: Hankey to Baldwin, March 1934; MRC 2110/14b: Meeting of Economic Advisory Committee Scientific Research Committee, 11 May 1934; EAC (SR) 74: *Report on the need for improved nutrition of the people of Great Britain*, 30 June 1934.
[91] See PRO MH56/45: 12 February 1933, for Mellanby's 'ideal' nutritional standards, which included 1 pint milk per day for all children under 5 years, and 1–2 teaspoons of cod liver oil; the League of Nations: *Report on the physiological basis of nutrition* (1935) (chaired by Mellanby); Interdepartmental Advisory Committee on Nutrition: *First report 1936* (1937). HMSO, London. Mellanby was an active member of this committee, which was set up on his initiative.
[92] PRO MH56/47: Advisory Committee minutes, 14 January 1934; PRO MH56/46: Carnwarth to Becket, 18 April 1932. Little was heard of the opposition view during the war years. However, in the course of the 1930s, Cathcart had continued to express his disagreement with the teachings of the Newer Knowledge of Nutrition on public platforms as well as on panels of experts. For example, his London School of Hygiene and Tropical Medicine Lectures, delivered in 1931, set out the case against the public health inferences which were being drawn from experimental work on the micronutrients. Cathcart argued at a time when nutrition science was increasingly concerned with the precise definition of dietary requirements, that, although it was a truism to say that 'the welfare of the race, its health, energy, resistance to disease, etc., is largely a function of its state of nutrition . . . Fortunately . . . the organism is not too delicately balanced where food is concerned. . .' . For an account of objections raised by both 'traditional' physiologists such as D. Noel Paton and E. P. Cathcart, and by the public health administration, see Petty, Unpublished PhD thesis, (see note 46).

improve dietary quality, particularly, according to Carnwarth, 'when the organism is subjected to severe stress'.[93] This assumption formed the basis for wartime welfare feeding policies and the debates of the pre-war Nutrition Committees undoubtedly prepared the way for the massive programme of nutritional supplementation, which was undertaken from 1940–5.[94]

Milk and school feeding

Despite his success in setting up panels of experts whose pronouncements received official endorsement, Mellanby, like Fletcher, felt that the discoveries of nutrition science had made no real impact on the 'life of the people'[95] and that the Ministry had been negligent in its failure to implement the Newer Knowledge. The Newer Knowledge of Nutrition did, however, make its mark in one important area of public policy, for throughout the inter-war years School Medical Officers were urged to apply the new dietetics in school feeding practice. From the early 1920s, Newman stressed that the supplementation of qualitative dietary factors was the main objective of school feeding,[96] and it is clear from their annual reports that School Medical Officers during the 1920s and 1930s understood the nutritional problem to be one of micronutrient deficiency.[97] The prevailing view was summarized by the School Medical Officer for Stoke on Trent, who wrote in 1928 that 'deficiencies in the diets of poorer elementary school children resolve themselves practically into deficiencies of foodstuffs . . . containing the essential vitamins . . . the vitamin deficiencies can be remedied by supplying auxiliary meals of milk and cod liver oil'.[98] It had become a truism that shortage of food was no longer a problem, even among poor schoolchildren, and for this reason, milk feeding was advocated by the CMO as the 'ideal supplementary ration'.[99]

However, neither clinical, anthropometric, nor dietary survey data support this view. For example, dietary surveys of low-income families consistently show that calorie intake did not meet requirements, and by analysing nutrients present per calorie in these low-income diets it can be

[93] PRO MH56/51: Carnwarth to Newman, 1 December 1931.

[94] See *How Britain was fed in war time, food control 1939–45* (1946). HMSO, London; Chief Medical Officer of the Ministry of Education: *Report for 1939–45* (1946). HMSO, London.

[95] MRC: *Annual report 1934–5* (1936), p. 9.

[96] *HOSC 1920* (1921), p. 146 (see note 44); *HOSC 1923* (1924) (see note 44), pp. 97–8; *HOSC 1925* (1926) (see note 44), p. 183; CMO: *Annual report 1925* (1926), pp. 159–60; CMO: *Annual report 1926* (1927), p. 184.

[97] See Petty, unpublished PhD thesis, Chap. 4 (see note 46).

[98] *HOSC 1928* (1929), p. 69 (see note 44).

[99] *HOSC 1925* (1926), pp. 110, 123 (see note 44). Substantial milk surpluses also added to the attractiveness of milk as a welfare food and in 1934 the Treasury subsidized a Milk Marketing Board initiative which supplied milk to schools at half price.

demonstrated that had calorie intake been adequate to meet energy requirements,[100] qualitative deficiencies would have been eliminated.[101]

The high reported prevalence of rickets (associated with vitamin D deficiency) was cited as evidence that inadequate vitamin intake was a widespread problem. Owing to the unknown contribution of skin synthesis of cholecalciferol, dietary data do not provide a satisfactory guide to the estimation of vitamin D status in the population, and simple calculations of nutrient densities for vitamin D can be misleading. The interaction of rickets and general undernutrition can, however, be deciphered by considering growth data rather than dietary survey data, and four investigations appear in the literature of the period which can be used to calculate differences in height and weight between rachitic and non-rachitic children of matched ages.[102] Results show that on average, rachitic children were both shorter and lighter than the non-rachitic controls. Although bowing of the legs accounted for some of this deficit in height, a comparison of trunk lengths in rachitic and non-rachitic children suggests that this accounted for no more than 60 per cent of the shortfall in height[103] and that the rest was due to 'genuine' stunting. Rickets would not of course introduce noise into the measurement of body weight. The most plausible explanation for the poor growth recorded among rachitic children is that qualitative malnutrition was caused by extreme underfeeding rather than by a bad choice of food.

Evidence of other deficiency diseases was rare. Beri beri and pellagra simply did not occur in the UK at this time, and scurvy was virtually unknown: it was only reported then, as now, among adults with eccentric eating habits.[104] Although iron deficiency anaemia was reported in infants and was a problem among women of child-bearing age (as it remains today),[105] it is unclear how far this reflects impaired absorption of iron due to other items in the diet, rather than simple deficiency. Population surveys show that anaemia was rarely found among either adult males or children of school age.[106]

---

[100] Target standards are derived from Department of Health and Social Security: *Recommended daily amounts of food energy and nutrients for groups of people in the UK. Report on health and social subjects No. 15* (1979). HMSO, London. For a full methodological explanation and discussion of results see Petty, unpublished PhD thesis, Chap. 6 (see note 46).

[101] See Petty, unpublished PhD thesis, Chap. 6 (see note 46).

[102] Tully, A. M. T. (1924). The physique of Glasgow school children. *Journal of Hygiene* **23**, 186–97; Rose, G. (1924). The incidence and effect of rickets. *Medical Officer, 297; Rose, G. (1926). Factors influencing the growth and nutrition of children. Medical Officer*, 271. For a full discussion of this phenomenon see Petty, unpublished PhD thesis (see note 46).

[103] Tully *Journal of Hygiene* **23**, 186–97 (see note 102).

[104] See for example Wood, P. (1935). A case of Adult Scurvy. *Lancet* **ii**, 1405–6.

[105] MRC *SRS* 157: Mackay, H. (1931). *Nutritional Anaemia in Infancy*; Davidson, L. S. P., Fullerton, H. W., and Campbell, R. M. (1935). Nutritional iron deficiency anaemia. *British Medical Journal* **ii**, 195–8.

[106] Davidson *et al.* (1935). *British Medical Journal*, **ii**, 195–8 (see note 105); Research done by the Carnegie Foundation, 1937, published as Carnegie Foundation: *Diet and health in pre-war Britain* (1952). Carnegie Foundation UK.

Vitamin A deficiency was also rare, despite the claims of contemporary nutritionists. A one-year survey of 4100 patients who attended an ophthalmology department at Newcastle Royal Infirmary, published in 1931, showed that only four had clinical signs associated with Vitamin A deficiency,[107] but like the rachitic children they too were underweight and presumably, therefore, underfed. L. J. Harris of the MRC's Dunn Nutrition Laboratory later claimed that his surveys of dark adaptation suggested a high prevalence of nyctalopia (secondary to vitamin A deficiency) among schoolchildren. However, his results must now be seen as suspect, reflecting a misinterpretation of the physiology of dark adaptation.[108] Other evidence of vitamin A deficiency, such as skin signs, would not now be accepted as evidence of the disease.[109]

Clinical, dietary survey, and anthropometric evidence all corroborate the view that underfeeding, rather than qualitative dietary deficiency—which was the focus of so much discussion—was the real nutritional problem facing inter-war Britain. An estimate of the extent of this problem can be made by assessing the anthropometric status of individual children: by comparing heights and weights with the mean values of a standard reference population, it is possible to calculate the number of children who would today be classified as malnourished. This technique is currently used in developing countries to assess the need for nutritional intervention.[110]

For example, data from a survey of over 2000 children who were measured in 1937 by the Rowett Research Institute as part of an extensive clinical and dietary survey[111] reveal a prevalence of low weight age of 10 per cent and a prevalence of stunting of 24 per cent among elementary schoolchildren. Similar prevalence rates are found today in developing countries[112] and would be seen by nutritionists as evidence of a need for intervention designed to increase food supplies at the community level.

But, ironically, in inter-war Britain the emphasis placed by nutrition science on micronutrient deficiency led to a *reduction* in the calorie value of supplementary meals fed to poor malnourished schoolchildren. Throughout the 1920s and 1930s, public health officials were encouraged to promote milk feeding in schools, and the main nutritional initiative of the period, which involved the introduction of subsidized school milk in

[107] Spence, J. C. (1931). A clinical study of nutritional xerophthalmia and night blindness. *Archives of Disease in Childhood*, **vi**, 17 26.

[108] See Petty, unpublished PhD thesis (see note 46).

[109] See for example Carnegie Foundation: *Diet and health in pre-war Britain* (see note 106).

[110] World Health Organisation: *Measuring nutritional status* (1983). WHO, Geneva.

[111] Aggregated data from this survey appear in Carnegie Foundation: *Diet and health in pre-war Britain* (see note 106); unpublished raw data are held by Rowett Research Institute.

[112] For contemporary prevalence rates for malnutrition in developing countries, see World Health Organization, Nutrition Unit, Division of Family Health, *Global nutritional status. Anthropometric indicators* (1987). WHO, Geneva.

Table 5.1 Calculated nutritional analysis of the impact of subsidized milk on school feeding

	Meals per child fed	Percentage of meals as milk	Calories	
			per meal	per child fed
1930–1933 (A)	148	55	356	52,600
1934–1937 (B)	178	71	272	48,600
B % A	120%	130%	76%	92%

Data derived from *Annual Reports* the Chief Medical Officer to the Board of Education, *1930–1937.*

1934, actually produced a fall in the energy value of free meals (see Table 5.1).[113]

Official enthusiasm for milk feeding was fuelled by a series of milk feeding trials that were undertaken during the 1920s[114] in order to demonstrate that the growth-inducing effect of milk on Hopkins's laboratory rats could be reproduced in human populations. The most important of these trials was Corry Mann's experiment, which was carried out on behalf of the MRC at Dr Barnardo's Home in Woodford between 1922 and 1925.[115] Corry Mann's results seemed to confirm the view that milk feeding had a preferential effect on growth, compared with other dietary supplements. These results were interpreted by Fletcher as 'absolutely conclusive evidence . . . of . . . the unwisdom of giving a policy of better housing . . . priority over better nutrition'.[116]

However, by assessing the nutritional status of each boy involved in the experiment, and his response to feeding, it has been possible to challenge the validity of Corry Mann's conclusions.[117] When height increments were re-analysed and children were subdivided according to initial height for age status, it was found that non-stunted milk-fed children

[113] Data for this analysis are derived from the Chief Medical Officer to the Board of Education, *Annual reports 1930–1937*. For a fuller discussion of the nutritional impact of the subsidized milk in schools scheme see Petty, unpublished PhD thesis (see note 46).

[114] MRC *SRS* 105: Mann, H. C. (1926). *Diets for boys during the school years*; Orr, J. B. (1928). Milk consumption and the growth of school children. *Lancet*, **i**, 202; Scottish Board of Health: *Annual report, Milk and the school child* (1929); Leighton, G. and McKinlay, P. (1930). *Milk consumption and the growth of school children.* HMSO, London. It was accepted by the MRC's Nutrition Committee that the trials carried out on free living populations were poorly controlled and that results were of little scientific value.

[115] MRC *SRS* 105: Mann, H. C. (1926). *Diets for boys during the school years.*

[116] Fletcher, W. M. (1932). The urgency of nutritional studies. *Nutrition Abstracts and Reviews*, **I** ,(3), 357.

[117] See Petty, unpublished PhD thesis, Chap. 5 (see note 46).

did not grow significantly better than children fed other supplements; in fact, they did not even grow better than children fed the basal unsupplemented diet. The milk group did, however, include a disproportionate number of children who were stunted (i.e., whose height for age was below the third centile) and among these children, growth was significantly better than among the other groups. Corry Mann was therefore recording 'catch-up' growth in a group of chronically malnourished children, rather than super-growth in an adequately fed group, as it was claimed at the time. This reinterpretation of results challenges the hypothesis that growth in the study population was limited by a non-caloric factor and reveals that the real parallel between Hopkins and Corry Mann was misinterpretation of data. However, Corry Mann's results were used to support the view that the findings of laboratory experiments could be directly applied to human populations, which in turn influenced the level at which nutrient requirements for human populations were set.

On the basis of these requirements, Boyd Orr maintained in *Food health and income* that half the population of the UK was malnourished since they could not afford to buy a 'minimum diet' and these claims received a sensational press coverage.[118] But, despite the public outcry these assertions provoked, the application of economic criteria in the assessment of the prevalence of malnutrition did not have the effect the welfare reform lobby had anticipated. Although welfare campaigners—as well as many nutritionists—hoped that an 'objective' measure of the cost of a minimum diet would force the government to increase benefit levels accordingly,[119] the economic standard in fact had the reverse effect, for in the absence of any evidence of widespread nutritional deficiency disease, government ministers argued that existing levels of welfare spending must necessarily be adequate.[120] And so the trump card in the reformers' pack turned out to be a joker. The high micronutrient requirements endorsed by official committees during the 1930s did not produce welfare benefits linked to the cost of the 'physiologically adequate diet' and moreover these requirements led to a nutrition intervention strategy that was totally inappropriate for the target population. Among poor elementary schoolchildren, anthropometric analysis shows that underfeeding remained prevalent throughout the inter-war years.

[118] See for example the *Daily Worker*, 5 March 1936; *Sunday Dispatch*, 16 March 1936; *Evening Standard*, 12 March 1936 and Ritchie Calder's *Daily Herald* reports, 1936.

[119] See for example Rathbone *Memorandum* (see note 66); *Medical Officer* (1933), *50*, 212; ibid. (1934), *52*, 15; ibid. (1937), *58*, 145–8.

[120] PRO MH 56/215: Briefing papers prepared for the Minister of Health prior to the House of Commons debate on malnutrition, 8 July 1936.

Applications of primary nutrition research in public health practice

In his final years, Fletcher felt that the public health administration had neglected the findings of primary research in nutrition and had thereby failed the cause of preventive medicine. He believed that the public health administration was shackled to an anachronistic set of health priorities by a lack of intellectual vision which left it unable to grasp the full implications of advances in pure science. In correspondence with Major Greenwood, Fletcher accused Newman and the administration of negligence and ignorant complacency;[121] but Greenwood (who was Chairman of the Ministry of Health's Advisory Committee on Nutrition from 1931–4 and was a friend and colleague of Fletcher) put a different interpretation on the nutrition problem. He argued that poverty, not micronutrient deficiency, was responsible for poor growth and ill-health among the working classes, and in response to Fletcher's complaints he wrote, 'My emotion boils over quite as much as yours, but not because the powers that be don't read the latest news from the research front . . . but because people are told to use their common sense and economically are stopped from doing so'.[122] He maintained that 'the people of this country are in no pressing need of any kind of preaching, what they are in need of is an economic organisation enabling them to do what they for the most part knew suited them long before the Ministry of Health or Medical Research Council existed'.[123]

Greenwood rejected the notion that any simple, inexpensive change in the diet could bring a fundamental improvement in national health and he asked Fletcher whether, in his eagerness to claim practical applications for nutrition research, he was not 'unconsciously afraid' of defending research on grounds other than the directly utilitarian.[124]

This was a sound critique of Fletcher's position. Where steps were taken to 'apply' the Newer Knowledge of Nutrition, the results were either irrelevant or counter-productive. The policy of mass prophylactic dosing of Vitamin D, which was finally adopted during the Second World War in order to prevent rickets—after more than a decade of lobbying from the MRC, resulted in many unnecessary deaths from hypercalcaemia.[125] The need for mass dietary

---

[121] MRC PF 133: Fletcher to Greenwood, 27 October 1931 and 2 November 1931.

[122] MRC PF 133: Greenwood to Fletcher, 31 October 1931.

[123] MRC PF 133: Greenwood to Fletcher, 31 October 1931. The preaching continues and the view that social class inequalities in health can be attributed to the 'incorrect' eating habits of the poor has remained popular with government and public health officers up to the present time: for example in 1986 the Junior Health Minister, Edwina Currie, made her memorable criticisms of the dietary preferences of families in the North of England.

[124] MRC PF 133: Greenwood to Fletcher, 31 October 1931.

[125] Lightwood, R. (1952). Idiopathic hypercalcaemia and failure to thrive. *Proceedings of the Royal Society (Med)*, **45**, 401; Passmore, R. A. and Eastwood, M. A. (1986). *Nutrition and dietetics*, pp. 111–12. Churchill Livingstone, London.

vitamin D supplementation was extremely dubious, since clean air legislation had already led to a steady decline in both the prevalence and virulence of the disease. Similarly, the drive to promote milk drinking in schools led to a reduction in the supply of food to underfed children.

Scientifically, however, the work was a success: for example, the fundamental research in vitamin biochemistry undertaken during this period laid the basis for the modern subject of metabolic biochemistry, and McCance and Widdowson's studies of dietary intakes were seminal in the development of the present understanding of the variability of nutritional requirements. Fletcher can claim the credit for fostering advances such as these, since under his leadership the MRC developed a strong research basis for nutrition science; this tradition was of course continued by Mellanby, who had won distinction early in his career for his work on rickets and vitamin D. Thus, during the 1920s and 1930s the MRC funded work on a comprehensive range of nutritional problems which included research on the nature of the chemical composition of the vitamins, the elucidation of functional failure caused by vitamin deficiency, and the determination of the vitamin composition of foods. This extensive research programme bears witness to Fletcher's success in achieving one of his primary objectives; throughout the inter-war period, the United Kingdom remained a 'world leader' in nutrition research and however self-deluded nutritionists may have been about the immediate significance of their work, it did establish a scientific edifice which has led to a greatly enhanced understanding of both physiology and biochemistry.

Acknowledgements

I am extremely grateful to John Rivers of the Department of Human Nutrition, London School of Hygiene and Tropical Medicine, for his incisive comments and guidance in the analysis of nutritional data. I also wish to thank colleagues in the Department of Human Nutrition who have shared their scientific and technical knowledge, and Charles Barber for his unwavering support and encouragement. Finally, I should like to acknowledge the assistance of the Wellcome Trust in financing this research.

6

The inner world of imperial sickness: the MRC and research in tropical medicine

JENNIFER BEINART

The first half of the twentieth century has been commonly regarded among medical historians as the period when tropical medicine conquered tropical diseases. In a fairly typical expression of this 'optimistic' view, one author wrote that 'Western medicine has utterly changed the outlook of the inhabitants of the tropics' and 'consigned the myth of the "White man's grave" to legend.'[1] Such statements, expressed 20 years ago without reservation, might be modified now, in the light of the AIDS epidemic, the drug resistance developed by disease organisms, and the wider recognition that the majority of the population of tropical countries, especially in rural areas, has little access to medical services. However, many experts in tropical medicine still regard the history of their speciality in terms of a series of discoveries leading to great advances in prevention and treatment. This is the way that textbooks in tropical medicine tend to present history, and it is embodied in museums and the medical literature. In such presentations, the history of research in tropical medicine is unproblematic—merely a matter of cataloguing the places and agencies involved.

This chapter attempts to give a rather different account, centred on the MRC's contribution to research in tropical medicine. A set of historical problems, or questions, rather than a series of achievements, dominates the narrative. Foremost among these is the relationship between the MRC and the Colonial Office, and the question of how colonial policy with regard to medicine and medical research was formulated. It might be expected that the Colonial Office would turn to the MRC for advice on these matters, giving the MRC a dominant role in the forging of medical research policy for the British Empire. What actually seems to have happened is almost the contrary. The MRC was involved in policy-making only marginally, took few initiatives, and seems to have expressed an interest in tropical medical research in response to promptings from the Colonial Office. But the Colonial Office was oriented towards developing medical services rather than

---

[1] Garnham, P. C. C. (1968). Britain's contribution to tropical medicine 1868–1968. *Practitioner*, **201**, 153–61.

promoting research. Thus, at least up to the Second World War, there was more rhetoric than real policy making; and the MRC persistently interpreted tropical medicine as a branch of medicine to be researched mainly in the metropolitan country.

The phrase 'inner world of imperial sickness' is used here in several different senses. In the area of policy-making, which is its chief focus, the narrative involves a succession of committees which were formed within or between the MRC and the Colonial Office. The formation and dissolution of these committees tended to reflect the fluctuating fortunes of Britain and its Empire; hopes for expansion in the 1920s, economic depression and contraction after 1930, slight recovery in the later 1930s, and post-war reconstruction. The functioning of the committees was an inner world, often remote from the realities of life and disease among millions of Britain's colonial subjects. Throughout this period, Britain's Empire was itself increasingly ailing, so that the growing efforts towards development, including research in tropical medicine, can be interpreted partly as belated medicine for its ills. One of the main lines of research backed by the MRC and discussed in this chapter, chemotherapy for specific tropical diseases, involved an examination of the inner world of disease organisms. The other, nutritional investigations, apparently involved greater integration of factors within and outside the sick individual. However, the MRC tended to back an approach which enabled the medical problems associated with nutrition to be divorced from the social, economic, and political problems. Its devotion to basic research permeated much of its response to issues raised in relation to tropical medicine; its role could be summarized as the promotion of laboratory research in a spirit of colonial isolationism. How far this was altered by changes in the MRC leadership, by the war, by Colonial Office development policies, and by the evolution of tropical medicine, is open to question. These are among the central themes considered in the course of this chapter.

The MRC, the Colonial Office and research
in tropical medicine to 1939

Looking at the whole body of research in tropical medicine from the beginning of the century to the beginning of the Second World War, the part played by the MRC does not appear to have been very large. Most research in the field had resulted from work begun by colonial government medical officers, or had emerged directly from the few medical research establishments in the Colonies, while most tropical medical research in the UK was closely associated with the Liverpool and London Schools of

Table 6.1 Committees on tropical medical research under the Colonial Office and/or the Medical Research Council, 1927–1960

Dates	Title	Appointed by
1927–1930	Colonial Medical Research Committee	Joint Colonial Office and MRC
1936–1939/40	Tropical Medical Research Committee	MRC
1945–1960	Colonial Medical Research Committee	Joint Colonial Office and MRC
1960–	Tropical Medicine Research Board	MRC

Tropical Medicine.[2] Where outside bodies provided funding to assist medical research projects in British colonies, the most generous donor was the Rockefeller Foundation (which had also provided the main funding to establish the London School of Hygiene and Tropical Medicine (LSHTM)),[3] while the Wellcome Trust (a private charity) rivalled the MRC among British sponsors.[4] Nevertheless, the MRC regarded itself as the most expert body on all matters relating to medical research, and the Colonial Office shared this view to a varying extent, as reflected in the series of committees set up by the two bodies (Table 6.1). The Colonial Office had its own Colonial Advisory Medical and Sanitary Committee, established in 1909, but this had very little interest in research.[5]

References to work connected with tropical medicine in the early Reports of the Medical Research Committee/Council are scattered and few. There was an expedition to Egypt during the 1914–18 war to study bilharzia (headed by Leiper); work on quinine (cinchona) at Liverpool (Professor Ramsden's Department of Biochemistry) and at the National Institute for Medical Research (NIMR) (Acton and H. King); and work on trypanocides at the NIMR (also King). A White Russian exile, Korentchevsky, was working on beri beri in 1919–20. From 1920 onwards, there are references to the work of Dr Keilin at Cambridge in the field of metazoan parasitology, but this does not take on a tropical hue until after 1926. His Molteno Institute of Parasitology was later to become one of the key centres for the work on malaria. The early MRC Reports mention work on malnutrition, but not in

[2] Worthington, E. B. (1938). *Science in Africa: a review of scientific research relating to Tropical and Southern Africa*, pp. 463–9. Oxford University Press, London, gives a useful overview for Africa; the best historical analysis is Worboys, M. (1979). Science and British Colonial Imperialism, 1895–1940. D.Phil. thesis, University of Sussex.

[3] Fisher, D. (1978). Rockefeller philanthropy and the British Empire: the creation of the London School of Hygiene and Tropical Medicine. *History of Education*, 7, 129–43.

[4] Wellcome Trust: *First report 1937–56* (1957), esp. pp. 14, 32–3.

[5] This was originally constituted by the Colonial office in 1909 as the Advisory Medical and Sanitary Committee for Tropical Africa and in 1922 became the Colonial Advisory Medical and Sanitary Committee, with wider scope.

the colonial context; these early studies were conducted in Glasgow (cocoa butter for marasmic children, 1919–20), Vienna (1919–22), and Edinburgh (1923–4). The only major publication with a clear tropical relevance was a 1925 report comparing quinine and quinidine in the treatment of malaria.[6]

A change took place in 1926 with the decision to appoint a Colonial Medical Research Committee (Colonial MRC) jointly between the MRC and the Colonial Office. This followed the Imperial Conference of 1926 and the recommendations of its Research Subcommittee.[7] The initiative seems to have come from the Colonial Office rather than the MRC; at the same time the Secretary of State for the Colonies was added to the Committee of Privy Council which oversaw the MRC. In any case, Walter Fletcher now took up the notion with enthusiasm, and the issue of research relating to 'the Empire' was given pride of place in the MRC Report for 1926–7. The new joint committee was intended to co-ordinate medical research in relation to the Colonies, Protectorates and Mandated Territories (not the mainly white Dominions, nor India which had its own research service), but clearly it had a major problem—it had no special funds. In regard to funding, Fletcher made an extremely revealing comment when he noted that the Colonial Office held funds contributed by various Colonial Governments for research, and that 'the effectiveness of the work of the Committee in future will be measurable by the augmentations that come to these funds'.[8] Colonial medical research would be not only self-funded, but a way to extract extra resources from the colonies for workers in this country. The latter point is implicit in Fletcher's discussion of the indivisibility of medical research—a unitarian philosophy which reclaimed colonial medical science for the metropolis. He said: 'For many, if not most, of the diseases peculiar to the tropics the preliminary observational studies of field and clinical enquiries have already been made, and the stage is set for intensive laboratory investigation wherever that can best be done', which would be 'wherever the man best fitted for it can most easily find his opportunities for progress'.[9] While work in laboratories or the field overseas was not ruled out, Fletcher clearly had in mind opportunities in UK research institutions.

Fletcher himself undertook a five month trip to India in the autumn of 1927, serving as chairman on a committee looking into the organization of medical research in India.[10] One of the other members of this committee was

[6] MRC *SRS* 96: Committee on Cinchona Derivatives and Malaria, *Clinical comparisons of quinine and quinidine* (1925).

[7] *Imperial Conference 1926, Summary of Proceedings*, Cd. 2768 (1926); see also the earlier *Report of a Committee on Research in the Colonies*, Cd. 1472 (1921), with reservation by Fletcher advocating working-parties of scientific men to advise government bodies on research spending in relation to colonial subjects.

[8] MRC: *Annual report 1926–27* (1928), p. 10.

[9] Ibid. pp. 10–11.

[10] MRC: *Annual report 1927–28* (1929), p. 10.

Sir Rickard Christophers, an FRS whose work on malaria was regarded as outstanding. It may be that his later appointment to an MRC unit at the LSHTM stemmed in part from this contact with Fletcher.

By 1929, the Colonial MRC was able to report on a number of trials of bismuth compounds in the treatment of yaws, for which the co-operation of several Colonial governments had been secured, as well as on investigations of trypanosomiasis treatment in Tanganyika, of dietetic problems in the West Indies, and of the etiology of blackwater fever at the Tropical Diseases Hospital in London. It is of interest that the publication cited in the section on tropical medicine in the MRC report for 1928–9 is a paper on tuberculosis in the tropics by H. H. Scott;[11] as Fletcher had pointed out, diseases like tuberculosis and measles were now possibly more prevalent in the tropics than in England, and could profitably be studied in the Colonies. The following year's report recorded a heightened level of research into chemotherapy to counter trypanosomes, spirochaetes, and malarial parasites, at several different centres including Cambridge. There were also clinical investigations into the efficacy of some of these compounds in various territories, and field studies of tuberculosis in Zanzibar and the Sudan.[12]

However, one of the most significant pieces of work to emerge from this period was conducted under the auspices not of the Colonial MRC, but of the Dietetics Committee of the Economic Advisory Council; and it was funded by the Empire Marketing Board. This was a study by John Boyd Orr, then Director of the Rowett Research Institute at Aberdeen, and J. L. Gilks, Director of Medical and Sanitary Services in Kenya, of the health of two tribal groups, the Kikuyu and the Masai. It was published by the MRC in its Special Report series in 1931.[13] The MRC publication followed a series of investigations in Kenya, which had been selected by the Dietetics Committee as the first area in which to study 'native dietetics'; work had been published from 1926 on, in various journals, but the findings of interim papers were included in the MRC publication with the aim of making the work accessible to as many workers in the field as possible. In spite of substantial caveats offered at the beginning of the report, it was likely that readers would be most impressed by the striking differences in physique and health between the tribes; the meat- and milk-eating Masai were shown to be taller and stronger than the cereal- and vegetable-eating Kikuyu. That these physical differences might be partly hereditary was suggested but not brought out. Although the report recommended that both peoples should eat more green vegetables, and the Kikuyu should consume more milk, the view seemed to be that both diets were badly balanced. The link was made between nutrition and health, with

[11] Scott, H. H. (1929). Tuberculosis in the tropics. *British Journal of Tuberculosis*, **23**, 179.

[12] MRC: *Annual report 1928–29* (1930), p. 111.

[13] MRC *SRS* 155: Orr, J. B. and Gilks, J. L. *Studies in nutrition: the physique and health of two African tribes* (1931).

the Kikuyu diet seen as predisposing to a greater degree of ill-health than the meat and milk Masai diet.[14]

The problem of hunger—and the Kikuyu were arguably suffering from land hunger leading to an absolute food shortage—was thus transformed into a problem of 'malnutrition' which might be overcome by 'a general improvement of agriculture and animal husbandry'.[15] The authors of the report offered the Empire Marketing Board reassurance as to the value of these studies: although they had 'no immediate bearing on the increased production or better marketing of any particular product . . . information obtained in investigations of this kind is calculated to hasten the improvement of the physical condition of the native and to increase his importance as an economic factor'.[16]

Walter Fletcher and A. T. Stanton, Chief Medical Adviser to the Secretary of State for the Colonies, were both members of the Dietetics Committee of the Economic Advisory Council. Both men also sat on the Colonial MRC, which came to an end in 1930. The decline was fairly abrupt, for in April 1929 Fletcher was conveying great optimism to Richard M. Pearce, the Director of Medical Science at the Rockefeller Foundation:

I think the Colonial Medical Research Committee is a really good piece of machinery. We have made more headway with the Colonial Office in the last three years than in all the previous years put together. I am hoping that the Committee will not only increasingly assist work in the overseas Colonies but also bring to bear upon it at suitable points the whole strength of the work being done here at home, whether of a primary or secondary kind. It will help also, I hope, the better progress of what I am very keen about, namely, the interchange of men between one place and another, and the steady creation of a real 'research service' over the whole Empire.[17]

Fletcher was clearly at this point thinking most expansively about the possibilities of colonial medical research. However, a year later, matters were going seriously awry. In his history of the MRC, Landsborough Thomson attributes this largely to troubles over the medical secretaryship of the Colonial MRC. Both the confusingly named William Fletcher (ex-Malaya) and his successor in this post, H. H. Scott (ex-Hong Kong) were, in Thomson's view, over-loyal to the Colonial Office. Walter Fletcher was apparently dismayed when Scott was appointed by the Colonial Office as Assistant Director of the Bureau of Hygiene and Tropical Medicine.[18] This was mainly an abstracting

[14] The women of the two tribes, whose diet was said to be more mixed, with greater overlap between the two groups, nevertheless showed a notable difference in stature—Masai women were on average taller than Kikuyu women.
[15] MRC *SRS* 155, p. 64 (see note 13).
[16] Ibid. p. 65.
[17] MRC 1333 (Cooperation with Colonial Office) I: Fletcher to Pearce, 17 April 1929.
[18] Landsborough Thomson, A. (1975) *Half a century of medical research*, Vol. II, *The Programme of the Medical Research Council (UK)*, pp. 199, 201. HMSO, London.

service, a descendant from the Sleeping Sickness Bureau founded by the Colonial Office in 1908, to collect abstracts of papers on relevant subjects and distribute them in the form of a Bulletin. It was said that Scott's duties for the Bureau would be light and that he could continue as the Medical Secretary of the Colonial MRC; Fletcher, however, expressed himself 'much perturbed' over this development.[19] At about the same time, other moves were taking place that might be judged to be of greater significance in the history of relations between the Colonial Office and the MRC.

On 26 July 1929, a Colonial Development Act was passed. This allocated up to £1 million for grants and loans to colonial territories, for assisting the development of agriculture or industry in ways that would benefit commerce and industry in the UK. The Act was passed six weeks after the defeat of Baldwin's Conservative Government at the polls by the Labour Party. Constantine has shown how the thinking behind this Act was rooted in the search by the previous administration for means to reduce unemployment in the UK; he spotlights in particular the 'imperial preference' theories of L. S. Amery, Secretary of State for the Colonies under Baldwin.[20] Wrangles with the Treasury had held up Amery's scheme, but it was taken up with enthusiasm by the new Labour Government, and received strong backing from J. H. Thomas, who was Lord Privy Seal with special responsibilities for unemployment. The actual administration of the Act was conducted by the Colonial Development Advisory Committee, apparently a semi-autonomous body although its members were appointed by the Colonial Office. Its Chairman, Sir Basil Blackett, an ex-Treasury official and businessman with interests in De Beers and other companies with imperial links, was President of the British Social Hygiene Council and took an especial interest in the question of public health in the colonies.

When Fletcher heard that matters to do with medical research were being considered by this advisory committee, he became concerned that the Colonial MRC was being bypassed.[21] A further, temporary, body, the Colonial Development Public Health Committee, which had been set up without Fletcher's knowledge, made recommendations to strengthen the colonial input into both the Colonial MRC and the Colonial Office's own Colonial Advisory Medical and Sanitary Committee.[22] The Colonial Office decided instead to amalgamate the two committees, on the grounds that they involved duplication.[23] In fact, this meant dissolving the Colonial MRC;

[19] MRC 1333/II: Fletcher to Stanton, 7 May 1930.
[20] Constantine, S. (1984). *The making of British colonial development policy 1914–1940*, p. 165. Frank Cass, London.
[21] MRC 1333/II: Fletcher to Stanton, 11 July 1930.
[22] *Report of Colonial Development Public Health Committee*, Colonial Office Misc. 413 (July 1930), para. 17.
[23] MRC 1333/II: Stanton to Fletcher, 3 September 1930.

official Colonial Office notification was sent to the MRC in November 1930, with an assurance to Fletcher that 'the new arrangements will involve no interruption in this valuable co-operation in the field of medical research'.[24] However, there appears to have been an almost total breakdown in communication between the Colonial Office and the MRC for a period of many months. A correspondence between Fletcher and Stanton on this topic faltered as Fletcher's health failed.[25]

One specific piece of research which Fletcher and Stanton argued over was a study of the chemotherapy of yaws. Fletcher called this 'about the first and almost the only effective piece of organised research work to be credited to the Col. M.R.C.',[26] whereas Stanton thought it had originated from the Colonial Advisory Medical and Sanitary Committee. However, the scheme had been supervised by a subcommittee which was, in effect, almost entirely within the MRC orbit.[27] The governments of several British colonies in Africa were asked to assist in the testing of different bismuth compounds, provided by the Association of British Chemical Manufacturers.[28] The rapid cure of yaws, by injections of arsenic or bismuth compounds, made a deep impression on victims of this widespread and potentially very disfiguring disease (caused by a spirochaete closely related to that responsible for syphilis). This had a double effect: it drew more people to the clinics, but it also led to an expectation that other diseases would be cured as effectively by injection.[29]

By 1932, Fletcher was unwell, and the MRC apparently gave up any attempt to remain seriously involved with Colonial Office policy making. A last note from Fletcher to Stanton on these matters, written in the middle of 1932, referred to triple cuts in resources: direct MRC funding was reduced, the Colonial Fund was less, and help from the Empire Marketing Board was dwindling.[30] While not giving up all activity in this area, the MRC had to limit its participation yet further.

During the period of considerable financial limitations, when there was no committee on research in tropical medicine (1930–6), the MRC was involved in two main strands of research relating to tropical medicine. Firstly, there

[24] PRO CO/70408/30(1): D. V. Vernon, Under-Secretary of State for the Colonies, to Fletcher, 4 November 1930. Fletcher suggested, and the Colonial Office accepted, that the word 'sanitary' be dropped, thus renaming the Colonial Office committee (see note 5) as the Colonial Advisory Medical Committee; MRC 1333/II: Fletcher to Stanton, 6 November 1930.

[25] MRC 1333/II: correspondence between Fletcher and Stanton, 18 March 1931–23 April 1931 (5 letters).

[26] Ibid. Fletcher to Stanton, 14 April 1931.

[27] Membership of the subcommittee on yaws was: Fletcher, King, Scott, and Col. H. W. Harrison, a venereologist.

[28] MRC: *Annual report, 1928–29* (1930), pp. 125, 138; MRC: *Annual report 1929–30* (1931), pp. 92, 111.

[29] Worthington, *Science in Africa*, p. 554 (see note 2).

[30] MRC 1333/II: Fletcher to Stanton, 3 May 1932.

continued to be an interest at various centres in testing drugs which might be used to treat tropical diseases. To a large extent, these were not produced by commercial firms but by research chemists in university departments. Interest continued to focus on major epidemic diseases, notably sleeping sickness or trypanosomiasis. A very large number of quinoline and other compounds were tested for trypanocidal action. Professor G. T. Morgan published with J. G. Mitchell on the 'search for trypanocidal activity', and Professor Warrington Yorke of the Liverpool School of Tropical Medicine received MRC grants for assistance by Drs F. Murgatroyd and F. Hawking to investigate the efficacy of these drugs and the development of drug-resistance in trypanosomes. This latter problem had been demonstrated by Ehrlich in 1908; Warrington Yorke recognized it as a potentially serious problem, although its wider applicability to antimalarials and antibiotics was not appreciated until considerably later. The most promising of the many trypanocidal drugs tested were to be given clinical trial in Africa.[31] Warrington Yorke's team also worked on a new class of antimalarial drugs, not analogous with those previously tried; these were guanidine and amidine compounds.

Another development, representing a second strand of research effort, was the establishment in 1932 of a Malaria Research Unit at the LSHTM, headed by Sir Rickard Christophers who had been Director of the Central Research Institute in India and had done much work on malaria. In discussing the reasons for setting up this unit, and for making a concerted research effort to counter malaria from many different directions, Fletcher compared Britain's record unfavourably with that of Germany. Later discussions were to revert to the theme of German superiority, and the advantage given by the investment of time and manpower by German drugs companies, compared with the lack of any equivalent effort by the drugs industry in the UK. The new synthetic compounds 'plasmochin' and 'atebrin' produced by German pharmaceutical companies were referred to as field leaders. Although Keilin's work at Cambridge on bird malaria was felt to be outstanding, it was not enough:

The council have long been reluctant to leave work in this field to be developed upon so small a scale when such immense vital and financial issues are at stake . . . The expenditure which would be needed for a fully developed scheme would always be quite insignificant in relation to the enormous financial, trading and humanitarian interests which are being sacrificed now for want of attainable knowledge.[32]

Yet the MRC, with its vision of conquering malaria through co-ordinated research—or at least of increasing the British contribution to solving the problem—could not afford to fund the new Malaria Unit. It was frankly

---

[31] MRC, *Annual report 1931–32* (1933), p. 110.
[32] Ibid. pp. 16–17.

admitted that the scheme would have been dropped, had it not been for funding from the Leverhulme Trust, which agreed to pay Christophers' salary for five years. Shortly after the Unit began operating, the MRC gave a grant to Kenneth Mellanby to work under Professor Buxton, also at the LSHTM, on the physiology of biting insects including some species of mosquitoes which carry malaria.[33]

In the Malaria Unit, where Christophers worked with the able assistance of Dr J. D. Fulton (on a Beit Memorial Fellowship), the mechanism of action and effectiveness of antimalarial drugs was investigated, using in-vitro techniques as well as birds and monkeys. Among other compounds, tests were made on one of Warrington Yorke's new series (undeca-methylenediamidine); the German antimalarial drug atebrin was also investigated. The unit kept closely in touch with the Malaria Therapy Laboratory run by the Ministry of Health at Horton, where malaria was used therapeutically in an attempt to treat various kinds of mental illness.[34] Christophers' unit received visits from workers at Horton, though it appears that only one joint experiment was conducted with the Horton team in the initial five years. Some of the most suggestive work at the unit was concerned with respiratory mechanisms of malaria parasites, and trypanosomes were included in this study too. The aim was to see how far, and at what concentrations, various drugs exercised an inhibitory influence on respiration in the parasites. It was difficult and inconclusive work, but important in opening new lines of enquiry and in attempting to elucidate some aspects of the mode of operation of the drugs. This was in-vitro work on first principles, as opposed to the chemists' approach of synthesizing and testing thousands of variations on compounds known to be effective.

Both the fuller understanding of how the drugs worked, and the goal of finding a drug that would counter all forms of the malaria parasite, were still remote when Christophers came to the end of his term in 1937. Leverhulme agreed to continue to support the unit for another two years, under Fulton, and with the continued co-operation of the LSHTM.[35] Clinical trials and advances in British (and American) drug manufacture in this field were later induced by wartime contingencies.[36]

[33] MRC: *Annual report 1932–33* (1934), p. 130; see also pp. 34–5 on medical entomology.
[34] MRC, *Annual report 1934–35* (1936), p. 148: a strain of monkey malaria maintained in the Malaria Unit, transmissable to man, was 'useful for the malaria treatment of general paralysis of the insane and other diseases, where the patient had become immunized against the malarial parasites more frequently employed'.
[35] MRC: *Annual report 1937–38* (1939), pp. 175–7; this passage also gives a summary of research in the Malaria Unit during its first five years.
[36] MRC: *Annual report 1939–45* (1946), pp. 58, 62–3, gives details of the setting up of a Malaria Committee after the world supply of quinine was cut off by the fall of the Dutch East Indies in 1942; mepacrine was introduced among British troops in malarial areas, and paludrine was synthesized by British scientists. The latter remains one of the most important prophylactic antimalarials.

In view of the later discussion of nutrition in relation to tropical medicine, it is worth noting exchanges which took place around this time between Fletcher and Ludwik Rajchman, the dynamic and relatively progressive Director of the Health Organization of the League of Nations. During 1927, Rajchman was attempting to interest Fletcher in convening a conference of biochemists and others interested in comparative aspects of nutrition, with a view to instituting international dietary surveys. On Rajchman's insistence, Fletcher had enlisted the help of E. P. Cathcart at Glasgow University's Physiological Institute; the latter produced a lengthy memorandum on directions needed in nutritional research. All were agreed that a preliminary conference should attempt to standardize methods of conducting dietary surveys, but that national bodies rather than international ones should be responsible for the substantive research.[37]

The matter appeared to rest there, from the MRC point of view, until four years later. Then, in the spring of 1931, Fletcher heard that a representative of the League of Nations was visiting European countries to secure their co-operation in nutritional surveys, and was about to arrive in Britain. Fletcher felt it was an 'extraordinary position'[38] that the League of Nations should begin such work without consulting the MRC, and wrote to the British representative in the Health Section at Geneva, Sir George Buchanan: 'It seems hardly credible that the Health Section can have proposed to set up a nutritional investigation in this country without any previous reference to us.' He wanted to know if this was 'some stunt that Rajchman is attempting off his own bat?'[39] He then checked the files, found the previous correspondence with Rajchman on the subject, and noted that the MRC line then had been to oppose international supervision of research—that is, to discount a role for the League. Fletcher suspected that, because these were his views, Rajchman had deliberately avoided consulting him further.

Fletcher's dismay probably deepened when he found that W. R. Aykroyd, of the Lister Institute, who had broken the news of the proposed investigation, was already deeply implicated and had been offered a job at Geneva by Rajchman. He advised Aykroyd to be slow to commit himself, in case Rajchman had no proper sanction to make such an offer. However, Aykroyd sent Fletcher a copy of a 14-page typescript report he had written for the League Health Section, concerning the possibilities for nutritional research on an international basis.[40] In some embarrassment, apparently, over Fletcher's hostile reaction to the whole concept, Aykroyd commented

---

[37] MRC 1520/3: correspondence between Rajchman, Fletcher, and Cathcart, 7 February 1927–7 May 1927 (10 letters).

[38] Ibid. Fletcher to Aykroyd, 12 May 1931.

[39] Ibid. Fletcher to Buchanan, 12 May 1931.

[40] Ibid. Aykroyd, W. R. *Report to the League of Nations (Health Section) on the possibilities of nutritional research on an international basis* (typescript, no date).

that perhaps the League, if it wanted to initiate active research, 'would do best to confine itself to more out-of-the-way countries where a little money would go a long way'.[41] Ignoring Fletcher's advice on his career choices, Aykroyd did take the post in Geneva where he worked closely with Rajchman for many years.

Changes in the MRC position on nutrition became visible after the appointment of Edward Mellanby, following Fletcher's death in 1933. However, other changes of a more general nature occurred first. The considerable shift in MRC policy apparently represented by its appointment of a new Tropical Medical Research Committee in 1936, can be traced in part to discussions between Stanton of the Colonial Office and Mellanby. The latter had expressed a desire to learn more about the 'obviously very important' field of tropical medicine soon after taking over as Secretary of the MRC.[42] He came to recognize what he described as 'the difficulties which Fletcher had found insurmountable'[43] in attempting to channel scarce resources into suitable research projects which, in the nature of the existing funding, generally had to be proposed by colonial governments. In the face of a lack of appropriate suggestions from the colonies, the MRC had been left with little to contribute to tropical medicine beyond its sponsorship of chemotherapeutic research in the UK.

Then, in April 1935, Mellanby received a letter from Kenneth Mellanby, who had previously been working at the LSHTM with Buxton but was now at the Human Trypanosomiasis Institute at Entebbe, Uganda. Kenneth Mellanby suggested that the MRC should take over the Institute, which was to be reallocated when its head, H. Lyndhurst Duke, retired at the end of 1935. He included advice on how to economize by Africanization of the technical services: 'I should never employ a European lab. man here . . . you can get natives with a great deal more intelligence for about a tenth the sum!'[44] Initially, Stanton welcomed the Entebbe idea, reminding Edward Mellanby of a somewhat parallel situation in which the Liverpool School of Hygiene had taken over a hospital in West Africa. (The Liverpool School had itself established the Alfred Jones Laboratory in Sierra Leone in 1918.) Mellanby was enthusiastic, seeing this as a scheme which 'would allow the M.R.C. to obtain a real footing in Colonial Medical Research'.[45] However, Stanton soon warned Mellanby of the Uganda Government's intention of taking over the Entebbe Institute to be run as a Government Medical Laboratory pending the possible opening of one near Mulago. He indicated

[41] Ibid. Aykroyd to Fletcher, 18 May 1931.
[42] MRC 1333/II: Mellanby to T. Drummond Shiels, Under-Secretary of State for the Colonies, 26 February 1934.
[43] Ibid. Mellanby, memorandum on discussion with Stanton at Colonial Office, 20 May 1935.
[44] Ibid. Kenneth Mellanby to Edward Mellanby, 31 March 1935.
[45] Ibid. Mellanby, memorandum, 20 May 1935.

that the Colonial Office would welcome a policy of expansion overseas by the MRC, for instance by sending research workers from the UK to work in government laboratories in colonial territories.[46] It was primarily to organize such a programme that the new MRC committee was established in 1936.

The Tropical Medical Research Committee had 12 members including Landsborough Thomson as secretary. Sir John Ledingham was in the chair, and members represented the major interests in tropical medicine, including the Colonial Office and the London and Liverpool Schools.[47] Its historical importance lies not so much in its achievements, since its activities were halted by the outbreak of war when it had only been in existence for three years, but rather in the fact that it represented a new departure—for the first time the MRC was formulating a definite policy with regard to tropical medical research. The purely *ad hoc* approach which had been in operation up to this date, in spite of some rhetoric by Fletcher suggestive of grand schemes, was now slowly beginning to retreat before the notion of a definite responsibility to aid in the planning of research in this field. At this stage, the plan was a fairly limited and pragmatic one: to provide a small number of research fellowships each year, enabling promising individuals to progress from a year of postgraduate study at a British centre, through a year of research here, to a year of research in an institution in the tropics. Certain diseases were singled out as particularly urgent targets: malaria, yaws, and trypanosomiasis. There was, however, an intention of utilizing the Tropical Medical Research Committee for broader promotion of relevant research, expressed in the discussion of liaison with other MRC committees on nutrition, tuberculosis, bacteriology, and chemotherapy, as well as consultation with other expert sources outside the MRC.[48]

In the event, grants made by the MRC during this period led to research on trypanosomiasis, yaws, yellow fever, filariasis, leprosy, and pellagra, while work on malaria continued at the LSHTM, Cambridge, and Liverpool.[49] In some cases, tropical medicine research fellows moved into established units or departments in the UK for their third year. The number actually sent abroad during this period was very small indeed: F. Murgatroyd to the Gambia, C. Hackett to Uganda, F. Hawking to Tanganyika, P. Ellinger to Egypt, and E. M. Lourie to Sierra Leone.

In two prominent pieces in successive annual reports for 1936–7 and 1937–8, the Secretary of the MRC linked tropical medical research firmly with two of the key fields of research in which the MRC hoped to continue to expand its operations. The first of these, chemotherapy,[50] received an

[46] Ibid. Stanton to Mellanby, 23 May 1935.
[47] MRC: *Annual report 1935–36* (1937), p. 157.
[48] Ibid. pp. 34–7.
[49] See pp. 117–18.
[50] MRC: *Annual report 1936–37* (1938), pp. 9–12.

enormous boost during this period from the successful trials of prontosil and sulphanilamide, which demonstrated the possibility of fighting bacterial infection with specific drugs. This was an important turning point; up till then, stimulating the body's 'natural' immune responses in a variety of ways had seemed to offer the main avenue of advance. The implications of the new drug breakthrough for tropical medicine were spelled out: it had already been expected that chemotherapy would provide the major answer for a wide variety of tropical infections caused by protozoa and spirochaetae, and now it seemed this approach would extend to bacterial infections.

The fact that the development of several of the most promising drugs for the treatment of tropical diseases had been achieved by German companies was viewed, more than ever, as a cause for concern. British firms could not or would not put equivalent resources into the tedious research needed to develop such drugs; the state therefore had to support the MRC's role in this development. In a sense, the tropical element was brought into the discussion to support the call for greater state intervention. The economic effects of tropical diseases were cited—malaria still held 'the premier place as a cause of premature death and inefficiency in the Empire',[51] with millions of sufferers causing a financial loss of millions of pounds. British as opposed to foreign development and manufacture of drugs for tropical diseases would also make sound economic sense because the British Empire was the chief consumer of such drugs. On the one hand, this was an argument for a bigger slice of any development funds that might be available; on the other hand, it was seizing the rising crest of war fever produced in this country by the Spanish Civil War and Germany's rearmament. It was pointed out that Britain and its Empire had been deprived of German manufactured drugs such as salvarsan in the 1914–18 war, and that similar problems could arise again.

The second field of growing importance was nutrition.[52] Mellanby, with his record of nutritional research including work on rickets, was predisposed to recognize the importance of nutrition in relation to tropical medicine. In this he differed markedly from his predecessor, Fletcher, whose horizons in this respect seem to have been rather limited, as indicated above. It might seem obvious that, whereas chemotherapy was necessarily bound up with a curative and single-disease approach to the problems of health and disease in the tropics, nutrition would involve a preventive approach in which many causative factors and many health outcomes would be considered together. However, this was only the case to a limited extent. As indicated in Chapter 5, the burgeoning research into nutrition in Britain in the inter-war period concentrated on separating out the different food factors and on attempting to link a given clinical syndrome with a deficiency of a particular factor. The

[51] Ibid. p .11.
[52] MRC: *Annual report 1937–38* (1939), pp. 17–18.

realization that ill health could be caused by a lack of a certain input, rather than always by the addition of some harmful influence to the body, had been such an important conceptual breakthrough that it had shaped the direction of much nutrition research, often with the aim of identifying the function of a vitamin or other food factor by studying the effects of its lack. True, there had also been attempts to measure the effects of overall dietary insufficiency, in surveys of populations known to be suffering from malnutrition (such as post-First World War Vienna, Glasgow slums, and miners' families). But the implication that socio-economic deprivation led to physical stunting was circumvented by experiments showing the beneficial effects on children's growth of various dietary supplements, from watercress to milk. Medical researchers—and the medical profession—in the main failed to make the explicit link between poverty, poor nutrition, and ill health which John Boyd Orr spelled out in his 1936 publication, *Food, health and income.*[53]

If this was the case for the UK, it was notably also true of the British colonial empire. There was a growing interest in types of diet, with the more sophisticated investigators suspecting that the interaction of many elements in the diet led to a greater or lesser susceptibility to certain diseases. However, it was still possible for colonial mine owners to earn praise for their experiments in improving their workers' efficiency and resistance to tuberculosis by adding meat to a maize diet—or more maize to the inadequate ration previously given. Better wages and a free choice of diet were not advocated by the nutrition experts any more than by the mine owners. The extent of complexity admitted by a report on pellagra, which showed 34 per cent of a sample population in the Nile Delta to be suffering from the disease, may be gauged from the following:

. . . pellagra in Egypt results from two concomitant but independent factors. Malabsorption due to parasitic infection of the intestines, and malnutrition due to a diet insufficient in the vitamin B_2 complex, cause an increased formation, circulation, and excretion of porphyrins—a condition of latent pellagra. In such people the onset of active pellagra is precipitated by very hard physical work, especially in the open air, by intensive exposure to sunlight, or by febrile infectious diseases.[54]

In other words, the conditions of everyday life for the vast majority of the peasant population in that area often resulted in ill health. It is not the intention here to suggest that medical researchers were performing a useless function in identifying particular disposing factors—here, lack of vitamin B_2 and hookworm infestation—and a measurable indicator—porphyrin

---

[53] Orr, J. B. (1936). *Food, health and income.* Macmillan, London: for discussion of attempts by government to suppress his findings, see Orr, J. B. (1966). *As I recall*, pp. 116–17. Macgibbon and Kee, London.

[54] MRC: *Annual report 1936–37* (1938), p. 162; research was carried out by P. Ellinger of the Lister Institute on a grant from the MRC.

excretion—in relation to a particular disease, pellagra. It is not to be expected that a medical researcher in 1937 would analyse the relations of production in this semi-colonial setting, which resulted in one third of the population in a fertile area suffering from a preventable disease (and most of them probably suffered from more than one). However, it would have been exciting to learn of some of these researchers taking note of the views of writers such as Orr, who saw that peasants suffering from malnutrition needed help if they were to reach a level of health which would enable them to produce enough food for themselves, let alone a marketable surplus. An even greater conceptual leap would have been required to grasp the relativity of concepts such as 'surplus', and to see that problems such as perennial indebtedness were probably more fundamental causes of pellagra among peasants than were vitamin shortage and worms.

A major initiative in this field came from the Colonial Office in 1936, when the Secretary of State for the Colonies, J. H. Thomas, asked the governors of the colonies to turn their attention to nutrition.[55] The Secretary of State emphasized the growing recognition of the importance of nutritional problems in the economic and welfare spheres, and referred to a report on nutrition by Aykroyd and Burnett, published in the *Quarterly bulletin of the Health Organization of the League of Nations*.[56] He requested that information be gathered and presented on a range of questions relating to food and cash crops, diet, and certain health indicators among the indigenous populations. The material submitted in response to this request was collated by an Advisory Committee on Nutrition under the auspices of the Economic Advisory Council, resulting in a two part report, *Nutrition in the Colonial Empire*, published in 1939.[57] The MRC, although represented on the Advisory Committee, did not detail the drawing up and publication of its report in its own annual reports of 1937–8 and 1939–45, in both of which 'Nutritional problems in the colonies' had a special subheading. Instead, there was mention of a subcommittee of the Advisory Committee on Nutrition, with Mellanby in the chair; its role was to prepare a plan for co-ordinated field surveys and research on nutrition in the colonies.[58] Although the MRC presented this project in a rather proprietorial manner, it could be seen as a logical next step, refining and perhaps redefining the work of the survey prompted by the Colonial Office.

Only one stage was enacted before the outbreak of the Second World War. This was the appointment of B. S. Platt, who had worked at the Lester Institute of Medical Research at Shanghai on nutrition and deficiency

[55] J. H. Thomas, Secretary of State for the Colonies, Circular Despatch, 18 April 1936.

[56] Burnett, E. and Aykroyd, W. R. (1935). Nutrition and public health. *Quarterly bulletin of the Health Organization of the League of Nations*, **4**, 1–140.

[57] Economic Advisory Council: *Nutrition in the Colonial Empire*, Cmd. 6050, 6051 (1939).

[58] MRC: *Annual report 1937–38* (1939), p. 17.

disease, to head a small team to make an in-depth study of nutritional problems in Nyasaland (now Malawi). The reasons given for the choice of Nyasaland are interesting: social, anthropological, and linguistic work had already been undertaken there, partly sponsored by the American-based International Institute of African Languages, so that by grafting on agricultural and nutritional studies it would be possible to make an integrated whole. The aim was spelled out:

. . . not only to see in what way the diets of native populations are defective, and the conditions of malnutrition which are developed in consequence, but also to determine means of remedying these defects by native crops grown in best accord with the agricultural, economic and social conditions of each country.[59]

The possibilities of improving the economic position of the colonies were also mentioned. This approach was not new—a few anthropologists such as Audrey Richards and Raymond Firth were paying close attention to diet, the Economic Advisory Committee survey was considering diet in relation to food production, while the League of Nations had published *The relation of health, agriculture and economic policy* in 1937.[60] There was even talk of a World Food Plan, with the combined aim of improving nutritional standards among colonial peoples and dispersing the surpluses of agricultural produce which were causing so much distress in the developed countries, in Britain's white Dominions particularly.

How far was the MRC participating in this internationalist approach through its sponsorship of Platt? It would be quite curious in view of prior tensions between the MRC and the League of Nations on the one hand, and the Colonial Office on the other, to find the MRC unduly influenced by either at this stage. The heavy reliance on finding the right man for the job could arguably have allowed Platt, once selected, to lead the MRC in this direction. However, a more dominant role for Mellanby is indicated in a telling passage in the Council's report for 1939–45, which says that during the inter-war period he had been 'actively concerned in the pioneer work of the Mixed Committee on the Problem of Nutrition of the League of Nations, and in the nutrition work of the League's organisation'.[61] Although the tropical countries were not foremost in mind in the work of the League's committee, Mellanby's work with the League was later taken to validate a leading role for the MRC in nutritional investigations in colonial territories.

Given that the MRC was involved in the pre-war establishment of field

[59] Ibid. p. 18.

[60] Firth, R. (1934). The sociological study of native diet. *Africa*, **7**, 401–14; Richards, A. I. and Widdowson, E. M. (1936). A dietary study in North East Rhodesia. *Africa*, **9**, 166–96; Fortes, M. and Fortes, S. L. (1936). Food in the domestic economy of the Tallensi. *Africa*, **9**, 237–76; League of Nations: *The relation of health, agriculture and economic policy* (1937). League of Nations, Geneva.

[61] MRC: *Annual report 1939–45* (1946), p. 103.

surveys of nutrition in the colonies, can it be said to have taken a lead in sponsoring a new, more integrated approach to these problems? A closer look at subsequent work undertaken by Platt, and at MRC policy on medical research in relation to colonial development during and after the war, would suggest that the MRC's apparent advocacy of an integrated approach should be interpreted with caution. Far from supporting such ideas as a World Food Plan, the MRC adhered fairly closely to the view that a more scientific approach to nutritional research was needed if solutions to the health problems associated with poor diet were to be solved. The MRC would continue to lend its weight, not to the call for redistribution of resources and more food or clinics for the poor, but for more scientific enquriy.

Wartime and post-war trends: the place of medical research in colonial development

The reasons behind the introduction of the 1940 Colonial Development and Welfare Act are too complex to be explored in detail here. It was more than part of the general move towards welfare legislation engendered by expectations that the effort put into fighting fascism should lead to a better future for all. In the case of colonial development, Britain as an imperial power was still motivated by a paternalist desire to improve the lot of its subjects, a desire which coincided comfortably with the view of enlightened capitalism that a more developed colonial possession was a greater asset to the metropolitan centre.[62] However, the introduction of 'welfare' into the title of this Act is suggestive of an increase in the benevolent side of the formula. The scale of funds allocated under the Act also represents a break, rather than continuity with the 1929 Act.[63] Although the 1929 Colonial Development Act had allowed for up to £1 million per annum to be spent on development, only £5 million in total had been spent in 10 years. The 1940 Act allocated up to £5 million per annum, to be channelled through colonial governments as before, but not only for capital expenditure (which the previous measures had done, in order to relieve unemployment in the UK). Recurrent development-related expenditure on services—in agriculture, education, health, and housing—now became eligible for grants. Most significant for the MRC, a sum of £500 000 per annum was specifically allocated for research.

---

[62] For a brief discussion of changing views on Britain's 'Dual Mandate' in tropical Africa during the 1930s, see Worboys thesis, pp. 364–5.

[63] The break may be more apparent than real, however, according to Constantine, who shows that UK sources had to underwrite large amounts of colonial government expenditure in the inter-war period through grants in aid, bank loans and so on. See Constantine, *British colonial development policy* (note 20).

Mellanby was invited to sit on a committee established to advise the Colonial Office on the use of this new research money. The other original members of this small Colonial Research Committee, appointed in 1942, were Lord Hailey (Chairman), Sir Edward Appleton, secretary to the Department of Scientific and Industrial Research, and Professor A. V. Hill, secretary of the Royal Society.[64] Questions were asked in Parliament concerning the ability of these very busy men to devote sufficient time to issues of colonial research.[65] Christopher Eastwood was appointed as secretary to the committee and suggested that members might like to begin by looking at Lord Hailey's *African survey* and the companion volume on *Science in Africa* by E. B. Worthington.[66] He offered to lend Mellanby a copy of each volume if the MRC library did not have them, an offer which Mellanby accepted. It is not possible to tell which sections of these volumes most accorded with Mellanby's views, but it is worth recording that both books stressed the importance of public health and preventive medicine, as well as an increased living standard, in order to improve health in Africa. Worthington, in perhaps an over-sanguine passage, said that 'the study of the major tropical diseases has now advanced to a point where nearly all are curable, so that many authorities now urge that increasing attention should be devoted to the preventive aspects of medicine, and the development of social services.'[67]

The view of medical problems as related to wider social issues comes through strongly, also, in the Colonial Office report of May, 1942, on *Medical policy in the Colonial Empire*. The committee (the Colonial Advisory Medical Committee) which drew up this report, under the chairmanship of Harold Macmillan, then Parliamentary Under-Secretary of State for the Colonies, included Mellanby among its members. In the introduction, it was stated that:

Medical questions cannot be divorced from the social and economic questions with which they are linked up . . . It is now generally realised how intimately medical issues are related to the daily life and habits of the people, and to their social and economic

---

[64] MRC 1333/d: Draft first annual report of Colonial Research Committee, list of composition during first year. By the time the Colonial Research Committee was appointed (June 1942), the Secretary of State for the Colonies had made 10 grants, to the value of £56 658, the largest being for research into cocoa diseases in the Gold Coast—see Morgan, D. J. (1980). *The origins of British aid policy 1924–1945*, p. 100. Macmillan, London. Morgan further calculates that between 1941/2 and 1960/1 a total of £24 051 062 was allocated, and £17 529 189 issued, for colonial research, and one-sixth of this went to medicine; ibid. p. 104.

[65] *Parliamentary debates (official report) House of Commons*, 5th series 1942, 381 (16 July 1942), 1349–50; ibid., 385 (16 December 1942), 1914.

[66] Lord Hailey (1938). *An African survey: A study of problems arising in Africa south of the Sahara*. Oxford University Press, London; Worthington, *Science in Africa* (see note 2).

[67] Worthington, *Science in Africa*, p. 461 (see note 2).

outlook. The position of malnutrition in relation to a number of diseases illustrates the close association that exists between disease and social welfare.[68]

The report thus reinforced the notions of welfare embodied in the 1940 Act, applying them to medical policy; and it pointed towards the multiple factors to be considered in relation to improving the health of the people in the colonies.

Representatives of social and economic studies and business presently joined the Colonial Research Committee. Then in March 1943, Eastwood was replaced as secretary to the committee by the anthropologist Audrey Richards. She was largely responsible for drafting the Colonial Research Committee's first annual report, attempting a summary of research so far undertaken, looking mainly at the 1920s and '30s.[69] There was little reference to the MRC's role, which disturbed Mellanby, and in the event Richards agreed to circulate the report as a progress report. This came out early in 1944, with the first full Colonial Research Committee report following in June 1944. One of the points which Richards argued for was the need to extend the range of research, especially on social and economic questions. In spite of the desire for an integrated approach, it was decided that the best means for extending these branches of research would be a separate body, the Colonial Social Science Research Council.

An illustration of the division between social science and medical research arose from a preliminary meeting of this new body, held in June 1944.[70] One item discussed at that meeting was a report of a 'most distressing state of affairs' in the British Cameroons, where a very high infant mortality rate was attributed to the low economic and cultural status of women. To analyse the twin problems of underdevelopment and underpopulation in the region, it was suggested that research on women, by a woman social anthropologist, was needed, and the name of Phyllis Kaberry, known to Richards and Firth, who were both present, was proposed. Lord Hailey's agreement to bypass the Colonial Research Council was secured; Mellanby was asked for his opinion on 'a survey on the economic position of women in the Cameroons' and readily gave his acquiescence.[71] It is not possible to be sure whether Mellanby realized that this proposal arose from concern over maternal and infant mortality. But it does seem that an opportunity for integrated medical, social, and economic study of a problem was lost, since the Colonial

---

[68] CO Misc. 505: *Medical policy in the Colonial Empire*, memorandum submitted to Secretary of State for Colonies by Colonial Advisory Medical Committee, 19 May 1942, p. 1.

[69] MRC 1333/d: draft first annual report of Colonial Research Committee.

[70] MRC 1333/d: minutes of preliminary meeting of Colonial Social Science Research Council, 13 June 1944; present were Prof. A. M. Carr-Saunders, Sir Frederick Clarke, Prof. A. L. Goodhart, Dr Audrey Richards, Prof. G. Thomson, Prof. R. L. Turner, all members of the committee, and also Dr R. Firth, Mr C. Y. Carstairs, Miss M. F. Lehmann, Mr D. J. Parkinson.

[71] MRC 1333/d: Carstairs to Mellanby, 23 June 1944; Mellanby to Carstairs, 26 June 1944.

Research Council and the MRC did not follow up this research topic. The position of women remained a 'social' problem and it was to be many years before it would begin to be integrated into the medical models of the etiology of child survival. Person-oriented rather than problem-oriented research continued, in the sense that each committee looked for its own bright young researchers.

In 1945, following consultations with the Colonial Office, a new Colonial Medical Research Committee was set up within the MRC, with members appointed by both the Colonial Office and the MRC. This was to continue for the next 15 years, presiding over a period of expansion in tropical medical research. A glance at the list of MRC research establishments related to tropical medicine (Table 6.2) confirms the lack of input before the Second World War, with a rather remarkable flourishing after the war. Nutrition was at the forefront of this expansion. The MRC, much impressed with the calibre of Platt's work, set up the Human Nutrition Unit in 1944 with Platt as Director, with the 'primary object of assisting a resumption of co-ordinated field studies of nutritional problems in the Colonies'.[72] The Field Research Station at Fajara in the Gambia started in 1947 and became an MRC Unit in its own right in 1953; it still continues. Also in 1953, a group was established at Mulago Hospital, Kampala, Uganda, to look specifically at infantile malnutrition. There were also units or groups established on climate and metabolism, bilharzia, and trachoma, either located in the tropics or with most of their research done there. The history of a number of these institutions deserves a chapter each, but here only a brief mention of the Fajara project is possible.

The combination of approaches and length of the field study at Fajara gave it originality. It was still 'colonial' medical research, with an assumption that the European experts could show the local people better ways of doing things. But it did involve a more comprehensive attempt than before to make a systematic study of 'normal' health and nutritional status in the context of an African village; and it engaged in some attempt, however skewed and initially hurried, to find out how Africans in the locality dealt with problems of health, nutrition, and agricultural development. Although early reports reveal a blunderbuss approach on the part of the 'experts', who ambitiously tried to alter many variables in a short space of time, it seems that these researchers learned by observation and experience that the situation was far more complex than they had appreciated.[73] The Gambian project, intended

[72] MRC: *Annual report 1939–45* (1946), p. 103.

[73] MRC 1333/e/1: Nutrition Sub-Committee, Colonial Medical Research Committee, minutes of third meeting, 19 August 1946, Platt, B. S. A note on nutrition work in Colonial Territories; MRC 1333/E/2 (Nutrition in the Gambia) II: Platt, B. S. The Nutrition Field Working Party—its inception, development and place in the central organization for nutrition investigations in Colonial Territories, typescript paper, 5 January 1950.

to provide a model for development and public health for the whole of Africa, may not have succeeded in those grandiose terms. However, it evolved into a source of ideas and a testing ground, probably more significant for current thinking than the parasitology-chemotherapy approach to tropical medicine into which the MRC threw most of its efforts in the inter-war years.

In view of the flowering of MRC establishments with an interest in tropical medicine after the Second World War, it is necessary to look at the reasons behind this growth, and to assess how far it represented a new departure in MRC thinking.

Firstly, in spite of an increasing sophistication of techniques visible in reports from some of these units, such as the use of isotope-labelled proteins in the study of malnutrition,[74] there is little evidence that the sudden

Table 6.2   MRC research establishments related to tropical medicine*

Dates	Title and location
1921–1986	Molteno Institute of Parasitology, Cambridge
1926–	Dunn Nutritional Laboratory, Cambridge (later MRC Dunn Nutrition Unit)
1932–1939	Malaria Research Unit, London School of Hygiene and Tropical Medicine
1944–1967	Human Nutrition Research Unit, London, with Field Research Station, Fajara, the Gambia
1948–	Climate and Working Efficiency Research Unit, Oxford; from 1962 became Environmental Physiology Research Unit at London School of Hygiene and Tropical Medicine
1948–1953	Royal Naval Tropical Research Unit, Singapore
1950–1962	Group for Research in Bilharzia Disease, St Albans (later Bilharzia Research Unit)
1953–1973	Group for Research in Infantile Malnutrition (later Infantile Malnutrition Research Unit, then MRC Child Nutrition Unit), Mulago Hospital, Kampala, Uganda
1953–	Medical Research Council Laboratories, the Gambia (continuation from Field Research Station, see above)
1955–1970	Tropical Metabolism Research Unit, University College (later University) of the West Indies, Kingston, Jamaica
1956–1973	Trachoma Research Group (later Unit), Institute of Ophthalmology, London
1962–	Epidemiological Research Unit (later MRC Epidemiology Unit), University of the West Indies, Mona, Jamaica

* From: Landsborough Thomson, Vol. II, Appendix C.

[74] MRC: *Annual report 1952–53 (1954), p.* 87, summary of research at Human Nutrition Research Unit, Holly Hill, Hampstead.

expansion of interest and research in tropical medicine was discovery-driven. In so far as there had been a breakthrough in approaches to tropical medicine, it was a conceptual one: the recognition that health in tropical countries could not be secured by investigation and conquest of separate disease entities alone, and that a more rounded approach was needed which would take into account a host of environmental circumstances. This in turn was predicated on another important shift that had been taking place throughout this period: the growing interest in the health of the people of the tropics rather than just of the colonial visitors.

Secondly, there was, as the MRC remarked, a growing 'public interest' in colonial issues.[75] One of the forms this took was the allocation of further money to development following the 1945 Colonial Development and Welfare Act. Investment in colonial development was taking place at all levels, from the basic infrastructure of roads and harbours through to higher education and medical research. Although with hindsight this is seen as the run-up to decolonization, it was not recognized in that way by many contemporaries. In an effort to make up for time lost during the 1930s and the war, the Colonial Office decided to form a new Colonial Medical Research Service as a branch of the Colonial Medical Service. As in very many fields, there was an immediate post-war shortage of suitably trained skilled staff. Possibly this helped further to strengthen the MRC's high valuation of workers like Platt whose credentials were already well established—and who had a vision of the direction which research needed to take.

Unfortunately—and this is a third point—there was still only limited co-ordination at this stage, in spite of the lip service paid to contact with other disciplines by the Colonial Medical Research Committee. For example, in relation to the setting up of a nutrition subcommittee, Mellanby told Carr-Saunders that it was 'primarily a matter of health'[76] but thought that contact with experts on agriculture and social science was desirable, and suggested Audrey Richards for the latter. But when Richards asked if socio-economic investigators could usefully collect data on food consumption whilst working on their own investigations, there was a lukewarm response.[77] It was generally felt in the committee that only nutritional experts should collect such data. Later, when Himsworth had replaced Mellanby as Secretary of the MRC, there was an acrimonious and protracted struggle between Platt and R. A. Webb, a scientist sent to the Gambia to look at the biochemistry of food and soil. This drew in the Agricultural Research Council and the

[75] MRC: *Annual report 1945–48* (1949), p. 32.

[76] MRC 1333/e/1: Mellanby to Carr-Saunders, 6 May 1946.

[77] Ibid. Minutes of 3rd meeting of Nutrition Sub-Committee, Colonial Medical Research Committee, 19 August 1946.

Director of Agriculture for the Gambia, as accusations and counter-accusations flew concerning the lack of laboratory accommodation for Webb, his underhand connivance with the Gambian government, and so on. In spite of Himsworth's protestations that the MRC attached 'considerable importance to this scheme for co-operation between the ARC [Agricultural Research Council] and the MRC',[78] the affair led to a rift between the agricultural and medical sides in the Gambian scheme.[79]

Landsborough Thomson's assessment of the fifteen-year period of the second Colonial Medical Research Committee brings out, albeit unconsciously, the tension between a policy of expansion overseas and the continuing MRC emphasis on a free interchange between the tropics and 'home', and on the value of basic research.[80] Whilst the Colonial Medical Research Committee initially played a full part in co-ordinating the regional medical research bodies for East and West Africa and the Caribbean, the growth of local expertise (encouraged by the establishment of full medical schools at the University Colleges of Uganda, Nigeria and the West Indies) inevitably squeezed out the British interest. Similarly, co-operation with the Overseas Research Service under the Colonial Office gradually faltered as successive British colonies gained independence, starting with Ghana in 1957. Decolonization was clearly a major factor influencing MRC and Colonial Office policies on tropical medicine, leading to lengthy debates over funding as independent former colonies lost their eligibility to receive money from the Colonial Development and Welfare Fund.[81]

Another factor influencing policies on tropical medicine singled out by Landsborough Thomson has a more dubious status. He sees a shift in the major concern in this field from tropical diseases in primitive conditions to diseases of urbanization such as tuberculosis and cardiovascular diseases in the tropics and at home.[82] Apart from the fact that tuberculosis is rampant in rural areas in many tropical countries subjected to colonialism, it is difficult to see where the supposed shift took place. While it is true that the original three subcommittees of the Colonial Medical Research Committee, on malaria, helminthiasis, and nutrition, were supplemented by others of a more

---

[78] MRC 1333/E/2 IV: Himsworth to W. K. Slater, Agricultural Research Council, 24 July 1951.

[79] Ibid. MRC 52/207 : report of working party on 'Future of the Field Research Station in the Gambia' by J. S. K. Boyd, J. Taylor and Landsborough Thomson, 14 March 1952; subsequently Himsworth expressed the opinion that Fajara was well run, but not enough research was done there and at the Human Nutrition Research Unit at Hampstead—the solution would be to diversify and expand, and have a Director resident in the Gambia: Himsworth to Platt, 16 April 1952.

[80] Landsborough Thomson, *Medical Research*, Vol. II, p. 209 (see note 18).

[81] Ibid. pp. 210–11; after 1960 the renamed Tropical Medicine Research Board of the MRC continued with funding from various bodies, eventually from the Overseas Development Administration.

[82] Ibid. p. 211.

general nature (East African Survey and Personnel),[83] and that research topics in UK and overseas institutions broadened to include the 'urban diseases', it is doubtful if this represents a decisive alteration of policy. The MRC may have been influenced by workers who saw the tropics as another clinical laboratory for studies of diseases such as cancer and heart disease, which were of major concern to medicine in developed countries. However, there continued to be a massive concern—perhaps a growing one—for those conditions most prevalent among the poor in underdeveloped countries. Cardiovascular disease does not figure very largely in this context. The MRC may have been influenced, via the Colonial Office, by international opinion in the form of bodies such as the World Health Organization, whose aims included the promotion of international co-ordination. The growth of the nutritional investigations at Fajara and Mulago bears witness to this trend; doctors and others from many countries were to visit these centres, to gain from them, and to contribute to the growing world-wide concern with malnutrition. It is also true, however, that the MRC continued to sponsor much basic laboratory research in the UK in relation to the tropical diseases and nutritional problems in the tropics.

Finally, and of particular interest in the light of current debates on the primacy of nutritional v. medical v. environmental factors in the whole picture of ill-health in the 'Third World', there was considerable recognition of the complexity of interlinked problems, at least among some workers, in the 1940s. This is beautifully illustrated in a letter from Professor B. G. Maegraith (of Liverpool) to Platt, written from Accra in 1949. Touching on environmentally linked health problems such as schistosomiasis in the diamond mines and onchocerciasis in the inland villages, he continued:

I think you are probably right. If you could get rid of some of the undernourishment, disease control might be possible. Any lingering doubts I had about the importance of diet were dispelled in my recent trip to Tamale and Yenguma [in the Northern Territories of the then Gold Coast, now Ghana]. As you know, hookworm is everywhere . . . Treatment of the worms and feeding up and the farmer is back at work producing food.[84]

This passage captures the difficulty of separating out the nutritional and disease (parasites, in this case) factors; the writer seems to veer from one to the other, because in a sense he sees them as fundamentally all linked to nutrition. In any case, his observations ring with a recognition of the reciprocal importance of nutritional and medical interventions. There is recognition, in the same letter, of the tremendous problems of controlling

---

[83] MRC: *Annual report 1945–48* (1949), p. 32; MRC: *Annual report 1948–50* (1951), p. 224.
[84] MRC 1333/E/3 (Colonial Medical Research Committee, Research Projects 28 March 1945 to 5 October 1950): Prof. B. G. Maegraith to Platt, 21 July 1949.

malaria. It was worse than before in some areas, according to Maegraith, partly due to diet and partly to loss of immunity; in spite of good efforts 'the disease keeps breaking out through the barriers'. Both in relation to malaria and to other diseases that are the objects of modern mass immunization programmes, similar problems are the focus of concern today.

Conclusions

The financial stringency of the 1930s has been noted by Landsborough Thomson as one cause of the dearth of activity during that period, in tropical medical research as in other areas of MRC interest.[85] In this chapter it has been argued that it is worth going a little further, to look into the way colonial policy in general was changing and in particular how ideas about 'development' were evolving. Whereas colonial development was entirely a metropolitan-focused concept in the inter-war period, there was a decisive shift in the 1940s towards development for the benefit of the colonial peoples, as well as to further Britain's interests. During the 1930s, with the view that colonies should be self-supporting, the Colonial Office favoured development expenditure only if it could be shown to increase the colony's contribution to its solvency and its consumption of goods manufactured in Britain. After 1940, spending on development became much more generous and broader, and 'welfare' was added to express the concern for the well-being of individuals as well as the colonial economy as a whole. This was partly a response to the growing movement for colonial freedom, partly to international criticisms of Britain's performance as a colonial power, and partly to the growing mood of welfarism induced by the communal struggle of the war.

While the war has been taken as a major turning point in this narrative, some attention has also be given to the change within the MRC when Mellanby replaced Fletcher as Secretary in 1934. Given the different personalities and interests of the two men, and the different flavour of their pronouncements on tropical medical research, there is a temptation to see this change as more significant than was probably the case. In very general terms, it can be said that Mellanby was more sympathetic to the need to encourage research in tropical medicine than was Fletcher. While Fletcher responded to the imperial imperative, and enthused about the progress to be made in tropical medicine, he saw it primarily as something to be done in the laboratories of British universities. Mellanby, on the other hand, supported the idea of research in the colonies themselves, though by British personnel. Another, perhaps more important element, was Mellanby's own research

---

[85] Landsborough Thomson, *Medical research*, Vol. II, p. 201 (see note 18).

background, which made him more sensitive than his predecessor to the question of nutrition in relation to tropical disease. Looked at in relation to nutrition, tropical medicine could no longer be broken down into separate disease entities, each to be placed under a microscope and attacked in the test-tube. A more integrated approach became necessary. But it would be a mistake to stress the role of Mellanby too greatly, since the initiative for research into nutrition in relation to health in the tropics came mainly from other sources.

It has been argued that the major changes in research in tropical medicine instituted after the Second World War should not be attributed simply to the effects of the war, although this had resulted in an increased awareness of social welfare issues and hints of decolonization. The Colonial Development and Welfare Acts of 1940 and 1945, which provided much greater resources than before, had their roots partly in pre-war politics. The increased funding enabled the MRC for the first time to play a major role in establishing and co-ordinating research centres in Africa and the Caribbean (they even took over two Rockefeller Foundation Institutes, at Entebbe and Lagos). The MRC, however, saw co-ordination mainly in terms of different types, institutional bases, and geographical locations of *medical* research. It saw, in a sense maintaining a continuity with the inter-war period, an inner world of bugs and dietary deficiencies, rather than an outer world of critically altered social relations, unfavourable terms of trade, and land hunger. The MRC could not have been expected to take a broader view in the 1950s, given the history of its narrow involvement with tropical medicine. Clearly, the urgent message for medical and non-medical researchers concerned with issues of health and disease in the present climate of crisis in Africa and elsewhere, is to increase communications across disciplinary as well as national boundaries.

7

Industrial health research under the MRC

HELEN JONES

Introduction

Industrial health was one of the MRC's first areas of interest. In 1914 a Special Investigation Committee upon the Incidence of Phthisis in relation to Occupations was set up and the following year it produced the first of the MRC 'special reports'. The Factory Department of the Home Office commissioned research into dangerous dusts and gases, but it was really the research for the Ministry of Munitions' Health of Munition Workers' Committee (HMWC) during the First World War which lay the foundation of much future industrial health research. From these early beginnings the MRC sponsored research into an expanding range of industrial health problems. So, for instance, in the 1920s a committee on miners' nystagmus was set up; in 1930 a committee on industrial pulmonary disease was established; in 1943 a Department of Research in Industrial Medicine at the London Hospital under Sir Donald Hunter was founded, and in 1945 the MRC's industrial psychology work was brought together under the Unit for Applied Psychology at the University of Cambridge.

This chapter concentrates on the Industrial Fatigue Research Board (IFRB) [after 1929 Industrial Health Research Board (IHRB)], which was set up in July 1918 as a committee of the MRC. Medical experts, civil servants from both the Industrial Division of the Home Office and the Ministry of Labour, Factory Inspectors, businessmen and trade unionists all sat on the Board. Investigations were undertaken by teams of researchers, working in both the laboratory and factories. By the time the Second World War broke out, over 80 reports had been published on an expanding range of subjects. Indeed, it was this widening of research horizons that in 1929 led to the substitution of Health for Fatigue in the Board's title.[1] The work of the South Wales Pneumokoniosis Research Unit (PRU), set up in 1945, is also discussed. Its work and ethos is an interesting and illuminating contrast with that of the Board.

In 1944 the first volume of the *British Journal of Industrial Medicine*

---

[1] Industrial Fatigue Research Board (IFRB): *First annual report to 31 March 1920* (1920), p .4. HMSO, London; IFRB: *Third annual report to 31 December 1922* (1922), p .6.

carried an article on the Board's history and future prospects by its then
Secretary, Professor Richard Schilling. Schilling presented a clear description
of the Board's investigations, alluding in passing to the problem of persuading
both sides of industry to take up its recommendations. Recently, Arthur
McIvor in an article on the IHRB in *Medical History* rightly points to financial
constraints, workers' suspicion and managerial parochialism hindering the
take-up of the Board's poorly marketed findings.[2]

The Board was active throughout the period of this book and so provides
continuity for the present discussion while exemplifying the changing
attitudes and interests of the MRC in relation to industrial health. The Board
was a planning and policy committee; after 1921 a series of expert
subcommittees appointed by the MRC vetted the technical data. Members of
the Board commissioned research from the MRC's researchers. In 1942 the
MRC took over policy-making and the influence of the Board declined, while
at the same time it became far more common for research to be undertaken by
the MRC's specialist units; in 1959 the Board was wound up.

Although the Board was established at the end of the First World War, its
initial purpose was to investigate an essentially war-time problem, that of
fatigue from over-long hours of work, and related to this, high accident rates.
By the early 1920s, however, very long hours of work were no longer a
problem: after the collapse of the restocking boom in mid-1920 there was a
move towards shorter hours and most workers were employed well within
legal limits. Consequently, the work of the Board shifted away from fatigue
caused by over-long hours, but its interest in accidents remained. As its early
findings suggested that accidents were not 'fortuitous', research began into
'accident proneness'. This led to a concentration on personal or individualist
'problems', and hence to research into selection tests. While problems of
fatigue through work were becoming less apparent, similar symptoms were
found, due to under-stimulation. Investigations then began into boredom
and repetitive work, its relationship to uniformity and variety in work, and
incentives. With the expansion of mass-production in the 1930s, fatigue from
boredom and repetitive tasks was a growing problem.

By the early 1930s the Board was looking at four broad areas: industrial
surroundings, such as atmosphere, lighting, and noise, methods of work,
including both physiological and psychological aspects, industrial fitness,
such as general sickness and absenteeism, occupational sickness and
accidents, and finally, selection tests. During the Second World War,
research into absenteeism took priority.

[2] Schilling, R. S. F. (1944). Industrial Health Research: the work of the Industrial Health
Research Board, 1918–44. *British Journal of Industrial Medicine*, **I**, 146; McIvor A. J. (1987).
Manual work, technology and industrial health, 1918–39. *Medical History*, **31**, 160–89. See also,
Landsborough Thomson, A. *(1975). Half a century of medical research*, Vol. II, *The programme
of the Medical Research Council (UK)*, Chap. 9. HMSO, London.

At the end of the Second World War a Pneumokoniosis Research Unit (PRU) in South Wales was established with Dr Charles Fletcher, Sir Walter's son, as its Director. The Unit throws into relief the nature of the IHRB and provides an interesting contrast to the Board's approach. Fletcher conceived the work of the Unit as a part of 'social medicine' and although it involved a break with the past this did not inhibit Fletcher, but it did bring him into conflict with Sir Edward Mellanby, Secretary of the MRC.

The IHRB's research was self-consciously pioneer work. As its field of research was so new it was considered vital to undertake very detailed research and present full data with the Reports, which repeatedly pointed to the newness of the field of research and so cautioned against reading too much into the data. Attempts to break away from this practice of presenting very detailed evidence hedged with warnings about its shortcomings created tensions within the MRC which peaked during the Second World War. The limited impact of the Board's research on industrial practices in the 1920s and 1930s in part lies in its own disclaimers; far more significant was the perceived conflict of interests on the part of many employers. During the Second World War industrial health came to be regarded as far more important by employers and the state; the findings of industrial health research were, accordingly, more readily taken up. Moreover, an examination of the research undertaken by both the IHRB and the PRU questions the current conceptualization and categorization of industrial health.

The argument is developed under six headings: the origins of industrial health research in the First World War, the continuation of the work of the Health of Munition Workers' Committee under the MRC, the pioneer nature of the research and other constraints on the practical application of research findings, the impact of the Second World War, the labour movement's criticisms, and the work of the PRU.

The origins of industrial health research

Until the First World War, research into industrial health had hardly begun. Apart from research by a private engineering firm, Mather and Platt, no systematic experimental research, as opposed to surveys, had been undertaken. During the course of the First World War concern over the health of strategically placed workers gradually developed as the correlation between good working conditions and maximum production, the guiding economic tenet on the Home Front, was recognized. Initially, appallingly long hours under poor conditions were widespread. As the negative effect of such practices on production became blatant, attitudes gradually shifted.[3]

[3] Jones, H. (1983). The Home Office and working conditions, 1914–1940, p. 45. Unpublished Ph.D. thesis. University of London.

At the end of the war, the Chief Inspector of Factories reflected on the remarkable change in public opinion: in the early days of the War, prosecutions under the Factory Acts for illegal hours were strongly criticized and sometimes unsuccessful, but by 1918 they were regarded with sympathy by both magistrates and the press.[4]

The Home Office and Ministry of Munitions led the way in this change of heart. Much of their evidence on the relationship between maximum production and good working conditions came from the MRC. Indeed, in its origins the MRC was much concerned with industrial health. In 1914 a Special Investigation Committee upon the Incidence of Phthisis in relation to Occupations was appointed. A number of investigations relating to dust were undertaken for the Factory Department of the Home Office and the MRC's Department of Applied Physiology investigated ventilation, heating, lighting, general hygiene, and canteen diets for the HMWC. From 1915, the Ministry of Munitions, in order to boost production and reduce labour turnover, took up the cause of a healthy industrial environment. The Ministry enforced in all factories under its control, health and safety measures which the Factory Inspectorate under the Home Office had been urging firms to adopt for years. The Ministry's best remembered effort was the creation of the HMWC in 1915 to 'consider and advise on questions of industrial fatigue, hours of labour, and other matters affecting the personal health and physical efficiency of workers in munitions factories and workshops.'[5]

It is important to appreciate the close links between the HMWC and the MRC, for it underlines the influence of Sir Walter Fletcher on health issues during the war and the wartime roots of much of the MRC's later industrial health research. Christopher Addison, Under-secretary of State at the Ministry of Munitions, 1915–16, gave the impression in his memoirs that the idea behind the HMWC was his own.

Addison wrote that

As our minds began to turn more and more towards an active campaign on Dilution we began to recognise the responsibilities it would entail in prescribing the conditions of employment of the new workers, and the importance of establishing some machinery for making a sensible and proper use of so great an opportunity became obvious.

The first step was taken by myself on August 9. On that day I held a meeting with the following gentlemen—Sir Thomas Barlow, Bart., the physician; Mr. Bellhouse and Dr. Collis from the Home Office; Sir George Newman from the Board of Education; Sir Walter Fletcher from the Medical Research Council, and Professor Boycott. I see that I expressed our aim in the following somewhat modest terms—'That it might be

[4] Parliamentary Papers 1918 Vol. X: *Annual Report of the Chief Inspector of Factories for 1914*, p. 9.
[5] *History of the Ministry of Munitions*, Vol. V, Pt. III, *Welfare: the control of working conditions*, (1920), p. 1. London.

worth while in our endeavour to increase the output of munitions to see whether something could not be done to sustain and improve the physical efficiency of the workers, to examine the supply of food, facilities for meals, hours, fatigue, ventilation and kindred matters.'[6]

Addison at no point indicated in his account that Sir Walter Fletcher, Secretary of the MRC, had written to him three weeks beforehand, outlining the problem and suggesting a course of action. Addison merely mentioned that the problem had not struck him until July 1915, the time, in fact, of Fletcher's letter. On 14 July 1915 Fletcher had sent Addison a memorandum, which he had asked him to pass on to the Minister of Munitions, Lloyd George. In this memorandum, 'Industrial fatigue in relation to output', Fletcher pointed out that England lacked industrial fatigue studies, even though their value was recognized in 'well-managed' works in 'normal' times; on the outbreak of war, knowledge of industrial fatigue was disregarded as work was hastily organized in make-shift factories, for what was initially assumed to be a short period. Fletcher therefore suggested the appointment of a small committee to visit munition and armament factories, to offer advice on how to improve output 'by attention to physiological conditions'. This prompted Addison into action. He made enquiries, and on 2 September informed Fletcher that Lloyd George, with the approval of the Home Office, had agreed to appoint a committee.[7] Both Walter Fletcher and Leonard Hill were members of the HMWC.

The Committee duly considered the relationship between industrial health and industrial efficiency and advised the Minister in a series of reports; the establishment of a Welfare Section at the Ministry of Munitions provided the machinery for implementing the Committee's recommendations. The Committee's final report was published in 1918, although it had already been disbanded at the end of 1917. In this Report it was suggested that individual health research should be undertaken on a permanent basis and the subject should be accorded greater importance.[8]

The continuation of work of the Health
of Munition Workers Committee under the MRC

In view of Walter Fletcher's close association with the HMWC it is not

---

[6] Addison, C. (1924). *Politics from within 1911–1918: including some records of a great national effort*; Vol. 1 (1924), pp. 212–13. Herbert Jenkins, London.

[7] MRC PF18: memorandum on industrial fatigue in relation to output (Armament and Munition Factories) Walter Fletcher to Christopher Addison, 14 July 1915; Christopher Addison to Walter Fletcher, 2 September 1915.

[8] Ministry of Munitions: *Reports and memoranda of the Health of Munition Workers Committee: final report, 1918*, Cd. 9065.

surprising that within a few months of its disbandment the MRC and Department of Scientific and Industrial Research, with the approval of the Home Office, decided to set up a committee, 'to consider and investigate the relations of the hours of labour, and of other conditions of employment, including methods of work, to the production of fatigue, having regard both to industrial efficiency and to the preservation of health among the workers'. The IFRB, with Sir Charles Sherrington as Chairman and Duncan (later Sir Duncan) Wilson, seconded from the Home Office's Factory Department, as Secretary, immediately took over from the Welfare and Health Section of the Ministry of Munition's investigations, which had been initiated by the HMWC, into the effect of different systems of employment on output in shell-making, an enquiry into the incidence of multiple accidents, and a statistical examination of output sickness and accident records accumulated during the war.[9] The HMWC used MRC researchers who were later used by the Board. The establishment and work of the IFRB thus grew directly out of wartime concerns.

Industrial health research carried out under the auspices of the MRC was part of a growing interest in the subject, both in Britain and abroad. After the First World War a variety of bodies promoted industrial welfare, of which industrial health formed an important aspect. The Institute of Labour (now Personnel) Management (ILM), the Industrial (Welfare) Society (IWS) and the National Institute of Industrial Psychology (NIIP) all promoted good industrial health. Both the IWS and the NIIP reflected the interests of businessmen. Like the IFRB, the IWS had personal connections with the now defunct Ministry of Munitions. Founded by Robert Hyde in 1918, it began life as the Boys' Welfare Association. Hyde had been working for the Ministry of Munitions previously, but had quarrelled with his colleagues; a running battle with the Ministry of Munitions, and later the Ministry of Labour, lasted several years. While at the Ministry, Hyde had established contact with a number of leading industrialists. He later claimed that the main purpose in establishing the Association was to persuade employers to accept responsibility for setting their house in order before reforms were imposed on them; this was reflected in the IWS's original aims 'to encourage the study of questions affecting the welfare of male persons engaged in industry'. As a result of discussions between the Queen and Sir Allen Smith of the Engineering Employers' Federation in 1919, the scope of its work was expanded to include women.

The IWS's diverse activities included advising employers on medical and health plans; building up Works Committees and suggestion schemes;

[9] IFRB: *First annual report to 31 March 1920* (1920), pp. 5–6.

planning sound pension funds; modernizing works' dining rooms; and maintaining a panel of suitable persons as welfare workers, employing managers and nurses, what the Duke of York, the President of the IWS, referred to as the 'raw material of goodwill in industry'.[10]

It was also at this time that the NIIP, with Charles Myers as its first Director, was founded. In 1919 Henry Welch, a businessman with a particular interest in the placement of young people in industry, and Charles Myers, Director of the Experimental Psychology Laboratory at the University of Cambridge (who also sat on the IFRB in the 1920s) both wanted to set up a body to use psychology in industry and commerce. By the summer of 1920 they had obtained the backing of some industrialists and were able to open an office; the following year the constitution of the Institute was drawn up, to promote and encourage the practical application of psychology and physiology to commerce and industry by any practical means.

The motives for undertaking psychological research in industry were elaborated a few years later by Myers at an NIIP symposium, 'the very reason for the formation of this Institute lay in an intended approach to the problems of industrial inefficiency from a new aspect, that of Psychology'. Myers drew a distinction between the Institute's work and that of scientific management, although, in fact, the two were very close. The Institute, however, hoped to inject more flexibility into its recommendations and in so doing to take full account of the individual needs of workers. Myers wanted the industrial psychologist to time-study the workers' movement in order to indicate *where* they were unsatisfactory, and *how* they might be improved so as to avoid waste of effort, time and perhaps, materials.[11]

Meanwhile the Government continued to promote safety and health at work through the Home Office's Factory Inspectorate. Indeed, it was the Factory Inspectorate which proved the most consistent advocate of the Board's research. A close working relationship operated between the Inspectorate and the Board. The Home Office advised the Board on appropriate industries for its first investigations, joint investigations were undertaken and Inspectors sat on the Board.[12] Sir Duncan Wilson had been seconded from the Factory Inspectorate to act as the Board's first Secretary. The Annual Reports of the Chief Inspector of Factories reported on the Board's activities in glowing terms, for example, in 1920 and 1929, and in 1938 the Chief

---

[10] Sidney, E. (1968), *The industrial society 1918–1968*, pp. 13–17. Industrial Society, London; Hyde, R. (1968). *Industry was my Parish: being the autobiography of Robert Hyde*, p. 75. Industrial Society, London; Industrial Society Archives: 2nd General Meeting, 14 November 1929.

[11] Frisby, C. B. (1970). The development of industrial psychology at the NIIP. *Occupational Psychology*, **44**, 35; The attitude of the employees towards the Institute's investigations: a symposium. *Industrial Psychology* (1928), **4**, 99–102.

[12] MRC 2080/2 IHRB VIII: D. R. Wilson to Sir David Munro, 12 July 1938; IFRB: *First annual report to 31 March 1920* (1920), p. 6.

Inspector, D. R. (later Sir Duncan) Wilson, even gave Sir David Munro, the Secretary of the Board, a draft of his entry in the Annual Report for Munro's approval.[13]

On the Continent, industrial health research was already under way before the First World War. Well-known studies had been undertaken in Belgium by Zeiss Optical Works in 1901 and Engis Chemical Works in 1905. In the USA and Germany, research into industrial physiology had also begun.[14] In the USA in the post-war years a whole range of institutions were involved in the 'human factor', as contemporaries referred to it, but, as in Britain, most of the findings were not taken up by industry. Although America had no government-funded body such as the IFRB, a Personnel Research Federation acted as a 'clearing-house' and played a co-ordinating role from the mid-1920s. Transatlantic cross-fertilization was common, and involved visits from members of the Board to the USA and Canada.[15] Contacts also existed with South Africa; in 1930 an MRC representative attended a conference there on silicosis.[16]

Pioneer work

It has been asserted that private organizations can more easily pioneer new research methods, and services than government-sponsored bodies. They are less constrained by the weight by bureaucracy and limited resources.[17] By implication, therefore, government bodies are less likely to pioneer new fields of activity. While the financial constraints on the Board were very real, nevertheless, the early years of the IFRB show a government-sponsored body playing, what it quite explicitly perceived to be, a pioneer role; those involved with the IFRB saw themselves as pioneers in the field of industrial health research. For this reason it was regarded as inappropriate for the Board even to attempt to have an immediate or major impact on practices in industry.

The First Annual Report of the Board published in 1920 emphasized that very little research had previously been undertaken, so the Board was pioneering new ground. Industry was not asked to support the research

---

[13] Parliamentary Papers, 1921 Vol. XII: *Annual report of the Chief Inspector of Factories for 1920*, p. 8; Parliamentary Papers, 1929–30, Vol. XIII: *Annual report of the Chief Inspector of Factories for 1929*, p. 73.

[14] IFRB: *First annual report to 31 March 1920* (1920), p. 4.

[15] MRC 2080/a: H. Wilson, personal note on activities in America by D. R. Wilson, C. S. Myers and M. Tagg, pp. 3, 30.

[16] Parliamentary Papers, 1930–31 Vol. XIII: *Annual report of the Chief Inspector of Factories for 1930*.

[17] See for example, *Report of the Working Party on Social Workers in the Local Authority Health and Welfare Services* (Younghusband Report) (1959), p. 300. HMSO, London; Marshall, T. H. (1963). *Sociology at the Crossroads*, p. 339. Heinemann, London.

because industries under investigation were also seen as 'pioneers' in a little-known field, and as such were entitled to any benefits received through the work of the Board. When the subject was 'fully established' it was suggested that the financial basis might then change. The Report stressed that the Board's work was tentative and would remain so for a long time; research would involve investigations over a long period.[18]

Initially, the Board did not aim to produce evidence which would involve industry changing its practices. The Board saw its role 'primarily with the acquisition of scientific knowledge. In the practical application of such knowledge, industries are the best judges of their own needs.'[19] The Board consciously refrained from initiating research with the object of arriving at immediate practical results. Rather, it set out to study 'fundamental' issues, so that practical recommendations in the future could be placed on a firm foundation. Thus, while the Board's Reports did often contain practical suggestions, these were incidental.[20]

Although conscious of its methodological limitations, and with only 25 researchers, the Board did undertake a wide range of investigations. The first work of the Board was to finish off the investigations of the now disbanded Ministry of Munitions. The Board initiated investigations into long-established industries, not specifically wartime ones. The industries chosen were iron and steel, silk, boots and shoes, laundries, and tin-plate. As well as these general enquiries, research into certain specific problems connected with industrial fatigue, such as fatigue tests, vocational selection, and motion study were conducted irrespective of any particular industry.[21] In 1923 the Board claimed that the industry-specific nature of much of its early research made it inapplicable on a broad front, but the following year it maintained that it was continuing to concentrate on problems of general industrial interest which would be investigated in the laboratory.[22]

In an effort to establish the 'scientific' worth of its research, full data and detailed reasoning accompanied all the Board's Reports. A typical example can be found in *A study of telegraphists' cramp* published in 1927, which prefaced its study, 'The investigation, which has proved to be one of exceptional difficulty, has proceeded in several stages . . .' The Report concluded that telegraphists' cramp tended to affect those who were 'highly strung' or 'nervous' and that 'so far as these findings are correct, the conclusion would be that people who show psycho-neurotic symptoms or poor muscular co-ordination . . . should not be advised to take up

[18] IFRB: *First annual report to 31 March 1920*, (1920).
[19] IFRB: *Second annual report to 30 September 1921*, (1921), p. 14.
[20] Ibid. p. 6.
[21] IFRB: *First annual report to 31 March 1920*, (1920), pp. 6–7.
[22] IFRB: *Third annual report to 31 December 1922*, (1922), p. 20; IFRB: *4th annual report to 31 December 1923*, (1923), p. 4.

telegraphy'. But, the Report emphasized its research problems and therefore warned against reading too much into the conclusions, 'In an investigation like the present, conducted largely along untried lines, more definite results than those obtained could hardly be expected . . . they are unsuitable as a basis for any administrative changes . . .'[23] Before an investigation was undertaken, the Board drew up a plan for an enquiry, which was submitted to one of its committees of technical experts, for instance the Committee on Industrial Psychology, and to the IHRB's Statistical Committee. When the investigation had been completed a Report was submitted to both committees for their criticisms before publication.[24]

The Board's policy of careful 'scientific' research which avoided sweeping claims was not shared by other industrial health researchers and brought it into conflict with the NIIP, the body whose work was closest to that of the Board's. For instance, Julian Huxley in a BBC talk in December 1933 on the contribution of science to improving working conditions, referred to the work of a range of bodies, including the IHRB and the NIIP. A member of the Board wrote to Huxley, annoyed that the industrial psychology work of the Board (which had begun before the NIIP's investigations), was played down. He complained that 'The Institute, no doubt because of its need for funds, indulges in active publicity which keeps it constantly in the limelight . . . the Institute, in its practical application of industrial psychology, is apt to make claims which, in our view, outrun the advance of sound knowledge and which therefore tend to bring the subject into disrepute.'[25] The point this letter raised was the fundamental one of methodology, that is the criterion of validity to be applied to the methods and results of the research; the NIIP's methodology was a recurring criticism of the Board, and this was aggravated by personal friction. Work done for the Board by the NIIP during the 1920s was severely criticized by the committees, on grounds of both its methodology and its conclusions. Hardly surprisingly, such criticisms were not welcomed by the NIIP. Charles Myers, the NIIP's Director, who sat on the Board for most of the 1920s, did not appreciate challenges to his methodology.[26]

As well as the impact of the *pioneer* nature of the research on *presentation*, other methodological problems, in part a result of the newness of the field of research, also imposed constraints on the work of the Board. For instance, given the number of variables, how could cause and effect be proven? It was

[23] MRC, IFRB: *Report No. 43A A study of telegraphists' cramp* (1927), pp. III–IV, 34–36. HMSO, London.

[24] MRC 2080/2: IHRB (Reconstituted) III, Sir David Munro to Sir Arnold Wilson, 24 June 1930.

[25] *The Listener*, 6 December 1933, pp. 867–869; MRC 2080/2: IV I. Thomson to J. Huxley, 8 December 1933.

[26] MRC 2080/2: IHRB (Reconstituted) III, Sir David Munro to Sir Arnold Wilson, 24 June 1930.

difficult to isolate specific causes of ill health, especially as they frequently had to be deduced from secondary phenomena, such as output. The industrial health pathologist had to start with the symptoms, but as one symptom could be caused by a whole range of factors, variations in occurrence and intensity had to be measured, and not all variables could be controlled. Moreover, once a 'cause' and a 'symptom' had been identified, its treatment was beyond the scope of the investigator.[27]

The economic climate aggravated both the methodological problems and the adoption of new ideas. Changing conditions made it difficult to undertake long-term investigations. Short, irregular hours were being worked in the early 1920s and small orders, involving frequent changes, displaced making for stock, with its steady continuous work on articles of one type; the usual influences on fatigue and efficiency were greatly modified. This meant that the researchers had to be more finely attuned to work practices than during the war when excesses quite clearly showed negative effects. Moreover, industry was coping with the immediate problems that economic recession brought in its wake, rather than looking to the long term. Optimum conditions for maximum production were irrelevant to many firms. In 1923 the Board admitted that industry was uncooperative and the atmosphere of industry was unfavourable to the adoption of novel ideas and methods.[28]

The Board *chose* a low profile, presenting technical data with its Reports, and refraining from making great claims for its findings. This did perhaps make the Board's literature inaccessible to businessmen who were not scientists. However, Reports carried summaries of their findings, and some effort was made to guide the non-specialist through the technical minutia. For instance, an investigation into sickness, especially tuberculosis, among printers in 1929, provided a short and simple outline of the methods of the research and the results precisely because it was recognized that the report comprised a large number of statistical tables and an intricate and long analysis of them, which was inaccessible to the laymen.[29] Further, as mentioned above, the Annual Reports of the Chief Inspector of Factories extolled the Reports of the MRC to industry, and mentioned their findings so that the information was available to businessmen. It was then left to the businessmen to decide whether or not to act on the MRC's findings. The Central Council for Health Education's publication *Better Health* also carried articles on MRC Reports, written in a layman's language.

Bearing in mind the depression and pressure on profits, it is hardly

---

[27] IHRB: *11th annual report to 30 June 1931*, (1931), pp. 4–5.

[28] IFRB: *4th annual report to 31 December 1923*, (1923), p. 21; IFRB: *Third annual report to 31 December 1922*, (1922), p. 4.

[29] MRC, IFRB: *Report 54, an investigation into the sickness experience of printers (with special reference to the incidence of tuberculosis)*, (1929), iv-ix.

surprising that a massive gulf existed between knowledge of industrial health and its application in the inter-war years; this was not confined to the IHRB's work. Although industrial medicine was taken up by large, prosperous firms, most of industry was unaware of industrial health and medicine before the Second World War. The IHRB's findings were not widely studied and were rarely put into practice.[30]

Evidence about the impact of industrial health findings when they were applied to industry is patchy. Whatever workers' attitudes towards researchers, Factory Inspectors were struck by how inured workers were to health hazards at work and how little attitudes were changing.[31] Aspects of industrial health that trade unionists were interested in tended to be ignored by the Board.

Doctors employed by firms were the best placed to take up the Board's research findings, but they were employed in industry to only a limited extent before the Second World War. They were located primarily in London, but also in Birmingham and York, and were concentrated within particular firms. ICI employed more than any other single firm and all the Industrial Medical Officers working in York were employed by Rowntree's. Medical services developed in large firms such as ICI and Boots, and in firms with a tradition of welfare provision, such as Cadbury's of Birmingham.[32]

While the pioneer nature of the research, its methodological and presentational problems hampered the dissemination of information, it was the character of industry, not the research, which was by far the most important factor in the low take up of the research findings. Most firms in the 1920s and 1930s were not interested in spending part of their profits on improving health and safety, even if it would have improved production in the long run. Where industrial health and medicine was taken up, it was as a response to the demands of labour management, not developments within industrial medicine or industrial health research.[33] Even if the IHRB's findings had been better presented, there is no evidence that this would have made a great deal of difference in the economic climate of the 1920s and 1930s. 'Evidence' does not in itself lead to action.[34] Across the whole gamut of research related to industry and health there are problems of implementation.

[30] Political and Economic Planning: *Report on the British Health Services*, (1937), p. 313, London; Stewart D. (1941). Industrial medical services in Great Britain: a critical survey. *British Medical Journal*, i 763.

[31] Jones, H. (1985). An inspector calls: health and safety in inter-war Britain. In *The social history of occupational health*, (ed. P. Weindling), p. 233. Croom Helm, London.

[32] Archives of the Society of Occupational Medicine.

[33] Jones, H. (1989). *Politics, health and industry*, Chap. 4. Manchester University Press (in press).

[34] Witness the lack of action by present-day governments following the *Report of the Working Group on Inequalities in Health: Black Report*, (1980). HMSO, London; Townsend, P. (1979). *Poverty in the U.K.* (1979) Penguin, Harmondsworth or a whole range of Child Poverty Action Group and Shelter publications.

Suggestions by the Board in the early 1920s that joint committees should be formed in all the major industries to deal with the 'human factor' and to consult bodies like itself and the NIIP met with a poor response.[35] Similar efforts by the Factory Inspectorate to encourage joint safety committees in industry also faced an uphill struggle, and tended to be established only after the Home Office threatened to take statutory powers to enforce them.[36] Yet, a strong belief in voluntary rather than statutory committees continued to be voiced by politicians of all shades, as well as industry.

Industrial health and medicine gradually expanded from the 1930s as the medical experts and their knowledge came to be used by businessmen. Employers used industrial medicine as a means of exercising control over the labour process and to complement a 'scientific' approach to management. Workers who did not fit the methods of scientific management were to be 'treated' by industrial medicine. Hence, a concentration by those involved in industrial medicine practice and industrial research on problems such as absenteeism and accident-proneness. The definition of 'fit for work' shifted from an ability to perform a task, to how well that task could be performed. The medical profession was not only used as a symbolic expression of social concern on the part of some employers but also as part of the process of accumulation: industrial health and medicine was taken up when it was perceived as a means of achieving maximum production and profits. Both industry, and the state in wartime, used industrial medicine for these purposes.[37]

The Second World War

While welfare provisions expanded in the 1920s and 1930s it was not until the Second World War that industrial medicine made any widespread impact. The war intensified the hazards of industry. The introduction of workers new to a process increased the risks of a process, longer hours and nightwork meant greater fatigue, in addition to which transport difficulties lengthened the time spent away from home. As in the First World War, it was during the initial stages of war that the hazards of work were greatest, and industry operated in almost total ignorance of the research undertaken between the wars.[38] In 1941 research in Glasgow showed an increase in pulmonary tuberculosis, which the medical profession blamed on a combination of long hours, overtime, strain and ill-spent leisure.[39] Yet, good health was especially

[35] IFRB: *4th annual report to 31 December 1923*, (1923), p. 26.

[36] Jones, H. (1983). Unpublished Ph.D thesis (1983), pp. 264–266. University of London.

[37] Jones, H. *Politics, health and industry*, Chap. 4, (see note 33).

[38] Browne, R. C. (1947). A conception of industrial health. *British Medical Journal*, **1**, 839.

[39] *Parliamentary debates (official report) House of Commons*, 5th Series 1941, 374 (21 October 1941), 1693 Mj. Haden-Guest, quoting an article in the *BMJ*.

important in wartime because it could affect production. The lessons of the First World War may have been lost on many employers in the early stages of the war (aircraft production actually *fell* in the first month of the war) but the war nevertheless gave a spur to the advocates of industrial medicine.[40]

The key motive behind all the wartime activity was the effect absenteeism was thought to be having on production. Time and again ill-health, absenteeism, and production were linked together.[41] Fears about production were well founded. The British aircraft industry's output per man-day was well below both Germany and the USA. During 1942–3 absenteeism was double the American rate.[42] Various bodies investigated the problem of absenteeism. The Ministry of Labour encouraged employees to keep a record of absenteeism from September 1942. In January 1943 the Lord President's Committee instigated an official inquiry into the causes of absenteeism, for example, health, transport problems, or indifference. At its peak, 14 per cent of munition firms were involved in the survey, which lasted until the end of the war. The survey found women's absenteeism to be twice as high as men's and married women's was 'significantly' higher. The IHRB found married women's absenteeism to be three times higher. Sickness was the most common cause given for absenteeism. Both the Lord President's Committee and some employers questioned the genuineness of the plea of 'sickness' and the Lord President's Committee, whose primary concern was production, urged workers to go to work even when they were 'feeling seedy' and to visit the doctor or nurse at work.[43]

The IHRB was much concerned with absenteeism, especially of women. Any assessment of women's health and absenteeism was hindered by the lack of statistical evidence; most firms did not keep sickness records or they kept them in such a variety of ways that comparisons were not possible. In 1945 it was estimated that at least 10 per cent of total time lost was through illness. The reasons given for this illness rate were the strain of war, a gradual lowering of physical fitness of those accepted for employment, and a great increase in the numbers of older women and women with family responsibilities. Also, there was a strain caused by a shift from previous occupations. The three main causes of illness were respiratory, nervous and fatigue, and digestive. The Report went on to show the sickness rate of production workers was more than twice that of clerical workers. To some

[40] Collier, H. (1940). *Outlines of industrial medical practice*, preface. Edward Arnold, London; Burnett, J. (1943). *Outlines of industrial medicine, legislation and hygiene*, J. Wright, Bristol.

[41] For example see, *Parliamentary debates (official report) House of Commons* 5th Series 1941, 371 (15 May 1941), 1233; ibid. 1941, 371, (24 June 1941), 948; ibid. 1941, 373 (10 July 1941), 342; ibid. 1943, 392 (23 September 1943), 464; ibid. 1943, 392, (13 October 1943), 893.

[42] Barnett, C. (1986). *The audit of war*, pp. 146, 155. Macmillan, London.

[43] Summerfield, P. (1984). *Women workers in the Second World War*, pp. 124–6. Croom Helm, London.

extent the differences were seen as a reflection of disparities between the type of work and between working conditions. It was recognized that factors outside the factory, such as transport, housing, and nursery provision could also affect production rates, but the only advice given in the Report was to 'make sure that you observe the commonsense rules of hygiene. Cleanliness, well-balanced and, if possible, regular meals, enough sleep, and as much fresh air as you can get . . . .'[44]

As well as increasing its work on absenteeism, the scope of the Board's work expanded from 1942 to include industrial diseases. The MRC had previously undertaken research into industrial diseases, but not the Board, so the work of the two now became much closer.[45] At the same time the MRC rather than the Board, as previously, planned overall Board policy. Efforts were made from the late 1930s to present the findings in a more accessible form. In 1938 the Board's Annual Report carried a summary of past work. However, not all its findings, it was thought, were ready to be put into practice. It was still regarded as inappropriate for the Board to engage in any widespread or intensive propaganda, on the grounds that once a scientific body began pressing for particular reforms, it lost a 'detached attitude' towards scientific truth.[46]

As soon as war broke out it was suggested that the IHRB should put out advice on hours of work in order that employers would not repeat the mistakes they had made in the First World War. In 1940 a pamphlet, accessible to the layman, *Emergency Report No. 1: Industrial health in War* was produced, which various bodies, such as the Trades Union Congress (TUC), Industrial Welfare Society, Institute of Labour Management, and Joint Industrial Councils, helped to circulate.[47]

The work of the IHRB was part of a whole range of wartime industrial safety, health, and welfare activities. On its own it is unlikely that it could have had a major impact for there was no guarantee that its advice would be acted upon. However, improving physical well-being proved an attractive strategy to government and employers because it offered an apparently concrete and self-contained goal. The provision of medical services, canteens, and an improved physical environment was a natural extension of the activities already encouraged by Factory Inspectors and established in some firms. To encourage the burgeoning pre-war medical supervision, the Factories (Medical and Welfare Services) Order was made in July, 1940. This enabled the Chief Inspector of Factories to demand munitions or crown factories to provide medical supervision, nursing and first-aid services, and welfare supervision. The government encouraged all aspects of health and

[44] MRC, IHRB: *Why is she away? The problem of sickness among women in industry* (1945).
[45] MRC 2080/2 X: 20 February, 1942.
[46] MRC 2080/2 VIII: 26 July, 1942.
[47] MRC 2080/2 IX: minutes of 53rd meeting 28 March 1940.

safety during the war by making Orders, establishing an Industrial Health Advisory Council, and working with other bodies in organizing conferences, supporting the training of personnel, and campaigns to reduce the accident rate.[48]

The Labour Party, the TUC, and the medical profession all contributed to the mounting activity. The question of a state occupational health service came to the fore, a *British Journal of Industrial Medicine* was launched, and the Nuffield Foundation began its funding of university occupational health departments.[49] From 1940 the Central Council for Physical Recreation received a grant from the Ministry of Labour which helped provide physical recreation facilities out of work time for adults engaged on work of national importance. Later, when it was thought that suitable physical training could reduce accidents and absenteeism, the Ministry of Labour approved classes in work time.[50] Campaigns to promote health such as mass radiography and anti-influenza were carried out in industry. Health committees were established in some firms as subcommittees of works committees or joint production committees, usually comprising representatives of management, medical and personnel departments, safety committees, and workers from each floor or section, in order to promote health education, health supervision of working conditions, and preventive medicine.[51] The Central Council for Health Education (CCHE), which had previously worked through local authorities, now took its message directly to industry. In this way it was possible to target large numbers of people while studying the effectiveness of the CCHE's work. Posters, films, and leaflets were distributed on subjects such as food handling, rehabilitation of injured workers, spitting and tuberculosis, and victimization of venereal disease patients.[52]

With long hours of work and irregular meal-times it was thought necessary to provide hot meals at the place of work. Only a few canteens had survived from the hundreds provided during the First World War. Some large firms provided facilities, there were about 1500 canteens at the outbreak of war, as well as cafes around dock sites. From 1939 the Home Office, with the co-operation of the British Employers Confederation, encouraged firms to provide adequate facilities, and in November 1940 the Factories (Canteens) Order empowered the Chief Inspector of Factories to require a canteen at any factory employing over 250 persons and engaged in munition or other

[48] Jones, *Politics, health and industry* (see note 33).
[49] Ibid.
[50] MRC 2080/88: CCPR Industrial Subcommittee.
[51] McMichael, J. (1944). Health education in industry, *Health Education Journal*, April, 54–7.
[52] Ibid. MRC 2080/44: Health education for factory workers; MRC 2080/44/1: CCHE Factory Committee.

government work. Early in 1941 Orders were made under which canteens could be required at construction and dock sites.[53]

The time spent working in artificial light had increased owing to the amount of nightwork and overtime, and the complete or partial blacking-out of factory premises even in daytime. This aggravated the ill-effects of bad lighting on the vision, morale, and output of workers. Therefore, the Factories (Standards of Lighting) Regulations were made in 1941 which imposed a minimum standard of general illumination in factories where long hours were regularly worked. This tended to include factories in which the work was essential and involved substantial use of artificial light.[54]

This picture of expansion of industrial safety, health, and welfare, and of various institutions and government departments all pulling together hides many of the wartime tensions. In 1941 Wilson complained to Munro that after the outbreak of war an opportunity for doing valuable work in the industrial field was missed. For example, while the Emergency Report No. 1 was an excellent beginning, with the notice and publicity it deserved, it was not followed up.[55] Some staff were transferred to other work, such as pre-selection of men for special occupations in the Services, or heating and ventilation in air-raid shelters.[56]

The most serious problem concerned relations between the IHRB and government departments. When the Board began investigations into the relationship between output and long hours of work, it was hampered by the Ministry of Supply, which at first only gave permission for the Board's researchers to *visit* Royal Ordnance Factories. Later, when the Ministry wrote letters of introduction to contractors working for the Ministry, no right to demand information was conferred. The Ministry of Aircraft Production was unwilling to grant facilities at all. The investigation continued, but was less comprehensive than it might otherwise have been and related to only a limited range of war industries.[57]

The sensitive nature of industrial health research during war, the need to make criticisms and recommendations without offending too many interests, and indeed the number of interested parties in a report on absenteeism is demonstrated in a Report by Dr S. Wyatt on absenteeism, which caused dissension both between the Board and the Ministry of Supply, for whom the investigation was undertaken, and between Board members themselves. The Ministry disliked the criticisms made of it in the Report, and while some

[53] Jones, unpublished Ph.D. thesis, p. 292 (see note 36).
[54] Ibid. p. 293.
[55] MRC 2080/2 IX: D. Wilson to Munro, 14 July 1941.
[56] MRC 2080/2 IX: MRC: IHRB, 8 July 1941. Information desired by the subcommittee on Home Defence Services of the Select Committee on National Expenditure.
[57] MRC 2080/2 IX: 19 September 1941 for members. The Ministry of Labour also had a poor relationship with Ministry of Aircraft Production: Bullock, A. (1967). *The life and times of Ernest Bevin*, Vol. 2, pp. 157–8, 250–2. Heinemann, London.

members of the Board did support its publication, others opposed it on a range of grounds. Critics did not consider it to be 'scientific' research; there was too little detailed evidence on which the Report was based; it was too long and drawn out; hours of labour should not be raised by the Board at all as this cut across the Ministry of Labour's and Supply departments' work; it was a security risk and would undermine morale; it was undesirable to imply that the work incentive was sometimes weakened by the 'excess of earnings over needs'; and it was useless to recommend the provision of more nurseries. Added to this were problems within the Ministry of Labour over whether the Ministry should have been consulted about changes the Board was making in the scope of its work.[58] Difficult relations also existed between the MRC and IHRB after 1942 when the MRC took a closer hand in the direction of the Board; the Chairman, Lord de la Werr, never came to grips with this increased control by the MRC.[59]

The ever increasing range of activities, given a fillip by the war, also produced problems in the long term. The IHRB oversaw activities as diverse as toxicology; specific occupational illness; non-industrial illness in industrial communities; sickness absence; working environment; design of machines; the problems of skill, learning and capability; the handicapped and disabled; the integration of different age groups into society; general social factors bearing on health; and relationships in groups. All these areas, so far as they concerned health, were of interest to the Council. But, from the outset the IHRB was orientated towards industry, although the industrial aspect was but one facet of many of the problems with which it was dealing. As a result, as was suggested in a confidential memorandum in 1950, many problems which could only be successfully approached in a broad fundamental context, were being considered on a 'cramped ad hoc' basis, while the Board and its committees, by diffusing their efforts, failed to give some specific industrial problems the intensive consideration they required. An example of the frustration this caused was made apparent in two memoranda submitted by members of the Occupational Medicine Committee. One complained that too much time was devoted to broad problems of health and too little to specific industrial hazards, the other suggested that too much attention had been paid to specific industrial hazards and too little to the broader social factors affecting health. The author of the memorandum argued that the time had come to restructure research although keep the title IHRB. It was suggested that the Council's research be regrouped under 'Social and Environmental' Health and that industrial health be included under this category.[60]

[58] MRC 2080/2: 12 August 1942; 23 September 1941.
[59] MRC 2080/2: 23 May 1945.
[60] MRC 2080/2a/2: 7 July 1950.

The Labour movement's criticisms

This widening scope of Board activities should not detract us from the labour movement's serious criticisms of the MRC. Wilson and Levy, in their classic study of workmen's compensation, point to the IHRB's self congratulation that in 1938, after twenty years of research, 'some of the conclusions have already [!] been translated into practice'. Yet, the kind of changes made were short rest pauses and the use of spectacles for very fine work—obvious devices which cost virtually nothing and were directly recuperated in output. Wilson and Levy complained that research had thrown no light on diseases such as nystagmus or silicosis and had done nothing to encourage re-employment and light-work, while injured workers suffering from traumatic mental disorders owed nothing to the MRC. Wilson and Levy also criticized the MRC for having done nothing towards the development of disability schedules, even though they operated in most other countries, and the 1919 Holman Gregory Committee on Workmen's Compensation had suggested a detailed investigation.[61]

Ernest Bevin, a member of the IHRB in the 1930s, pressed the Board from 1928 to undertake an investigation into London bus drivers. He recalled in a speech to the British Medical Association (BMA) in 1937 that in the late 1920s he was conscious of a group of men with a high standard of health who were beginning to show signs of intensified gastritis, different from previous ones, and Bevin had called on the MRC to investigate the bus drivers. It took Bevin six years to persuade the IHRB to undertake the investigation and it was another three years before a Report was published.[62]

In 1933 the TUC unsuccessfully called on the Government to extend workmen's compensation to cover all lung diseases caused by industry. Miners engaged in haematite ore mining were not included in Silicosis Schemes, because the MRC had failed to recommend their inclusion, even though there was cumulative evidence that their work caused the disease. The MRC was roundly criticized, ' You have had many years; we have supplied you with x-ray photographs, we have allowed you to dissect our members, we have given you all the evidence you require, and we are not going to permit the lives of our men to be sacrificed', to the 'cold formula of professional etiquette'.[63]

In 1936, the Chief Medical Officer of the Silicosis Medical Board informed the MRC's Committee on Industrial Pulmonary Disease (CIPD), appointed in 1930, that claims for compensation made by South Wales coal-miners were

[61] Wilson, A. and Levy, H. (1941). *Workmen's compensation*, Vol. 2, pp. 179, 357. Oxford University Press, London.

[62] Bevin, E. (1942). *The job to be done*, p. 169. Heinemann, London. Speech to Medical Sociology Section of BMA, Belfast, 1937.

[63] TUC: *Annual report 1933* (1933), pp. 354–355.

increasing and the proportion refused by the Silicosis Medical Board was also going up.

	1933	1934	1935
Claims	234	316	398
No. refused	23%	39%	52%

These figures suggested that there was a disabling pulmonary disease which was not scheduled. During a debate in the House of Commons, Geoffrey Lloyd, Conservative Under Secretary at the Home Office, claimed the CIPD was already investigating the matter; after the debate the Home Office suggested to the MRC that it should in fact do so. So began a series of investigations by the CIPD, which published a number of Reports, and in 1942 pneumokoniosis was finally recognized as a mining industry disease.[64] In 1945 the MRC admitted that many questions remained unanswered and an extended research programme would be undertaken into chronic pulmonary disease among South Wales miners.[65]

In South Wales between 1931, when compensation for silicosis was first introduced, and the end of 1945, out of some 100 000 underground coalminers, just over 12 000 had been certified by the Silicosis Medical Boards to be suffering from silicosis or pneumokoniosis and had been suspended from working in the industry. No after-care service existed for these men and little was known about their requirements for medical treatment, rehabilitation, or special types of employment.

Pneumokoniosis Research Unit (PRU)

In the summer of 1945 a PRU was set up by the MRC after consultation with the Ministry of Fuel and Power with Charles Fletcher as its Director. The aim of the Unit was to investigate the cause, incidence, and prevention of pneumokoniosis in coal-mines, and to introduce possible rehabilitation schemes for miners who had been disabled by the disease so that they could work full time in alternative employment.[66]

The early years of the PRU were in stark contrast to those of the IFRB. The PRU was not set up to deal with what was quintessentially a wartime problem although its work was influenced in two important aspects by wartime

---

[64] MRC: *Chronic pulmonary disease in South Wales coalminers I. Medical studies* (1942), Preface, pp. V–VI HMSO, London; *Parliamentary Debates (Official Report) House of Commons*, 5th Series, 1936, 311 (7 May 1936), 1853–6.

[65] MRC *SRS* 250: *Chronic pulmonary disease in South Wales coalminers* (1945), Preface.

[66] MRC 800 Vol. III: MRC Pneumokoniosis Research Unit (South Wales) Brief account of researches carried out by the Pneumokoniosis Research Unit between 1 October 1945 and 30 September 1947, written by Charles Fletcher, 26 November 1947.

developments. First, the Unit was interested in the rehabilitation of workers. Although there had been some hesitant steps towards rehabilitation services in the earlier part of the century, it was the Second World War's insatiable demand for manpower that brought rehabilitation to the fore. Second, the Unit drew on the social survey technique developed during the Second World War, even though its use was regarded unsympathetically by Sir Edward Mellanby, Secretary of the MRC, who did not regard it as 'scientific' or 'objective'. Third, and related to the use of social surveys, Fletcher was greatly interested in the broad social context of medical research or 'social medicine'. Social medicine's roots lay in the 1930s, but it was given a fillip during the war. Moreover, unlike the IFRB, the Unit was concerned with the immediate practical application of its research, and Fletcher was not behind in making known the usefulness of his Unit's work. Indeed, he was even accused of seeking out the media limelight. The pioneering nature of Fletcher's work did not act as a constraint as it had on the IFRB's activities.

Fletcher wanted to use the wartime social survey, introduced in 1941 by the Ministry of Information, in order to investigate the social consequences of pneumokoniosis. The survey enquired into a host of subjects during the war, including attitudes towards rationing, conscription of women, and cinema going.[67] The use of the social survey was an important part of Fletcher's 'social medicine' approach. Social medicine looked at the influence of social, environmental, and genetic factors on the incidence of disease, and the identification and promotion of those factors which were favourable to good health. Social investigations into standards of health and determinants of these standards began in the 1930s, but the term 'social medicine' was not in circulation until the creation in 1942 of the first chair of Social Medicine at the University of Oxford.[68]

Fletcher's approach was, therefore, just as 'new' as the IFRB's had been in the early 1920s, but unlike the Board he did not operate his own self-denying ordinance, but rather put his case to Mellanby in order to combat the latter's scepticism.[69] Typical of Fletcher's attitude was a letter to Mellanby in January 1946:

I would not for one moment pretend that I think our investigation is likely to result in any fundamental scientific advance, but the problems of pneumokoniosis down here, so far as human suffering is concerned, are as much social as medical, and if social measures are to be taken to alleviate them they must be based on social investigations, just as any medical methods of treatment must be based on medical investigation.

---

[67] Calder, A. (1971). *The people's war: Britain 1939–1945*, pp. 467, 309, 424. Panther, London.

[68] Lewis, J. (1986). *What price community medicine? The philosophy, practice and politics of public health since 1919*, pp. 38–9. Wheatsheaf, Brighton.

[69] MRC 800 Vol 1: PRU, 1 November 1945, extract from Sir Edward Mellanby's note on C. Fletcher's visit.

It is quite true that the technique of social investigation is in a very early stage of development and our methods may be crude and inadequate, but I do not feel that we shall make any advance unless we are prepared to try with the best methods that are available.[70]

Mellanby continued to warn of the dangers of being led astray by using subjective answers to questions as if they had the same value as 'objective factual' answers.[71] Fletcher carried on his work, however, despite Mellanby's hostility to social medicine, which did not abate even after the MRC established its own Social Medicine Unit at the Central Middlesex Hospital in 1948.[72]

Whereas the IFRB had been concerned to establish its 'scientific' respectability and to avoid making claims for the practical application of its research, Fletcher made no such fallacious commitment to 'scientific objectivity' and employed the services of social scientists. Moreover, the research actually involved making practical changes and medical provision.

The purpose of his first investigation was to discover what types of employment men with certified pneumokoniosis managed to obtain and what types had been found suitable, to discover the difficulties involved in their getting employment, and to investigate the financial consequences of certification. The Social Survey undertook a personal visit to a random sample of one in ten of those certified as having pneumokoniosis up to the end of 1944, with a questionnaire designed to obtain full information about the employment and social circumstances of these men.[73]

A similar questionnaire to that used by the Social Survey was applied to all the certified men attending for clinical and radiological examination. From this it was hoped to get more detailed information about the relation of clinical conditions to social and employment circumstances.

An investigation was carried out into the performance of men with pneumokoniosis in light industry, in terms of absenteeism, sickness rates, and the employees' opinion of their ability. The main findings of these investigations were that when there was full employment, as in the war years, at least 60 per cent of men with pneumokoniosis found work, but that as unemployment reappeared they were the first to suffer. In 1946 only 40 per cent of the men were in work. The performance of the partially disabled man compared with the non-disabled in light industry, but the more seriously disabled required special provision.[74]

[70] MRC 800 Vol. 1: C. Fletcher to Sir Edward Mellanby, 26 January 1946.

[71] MRC 800 Vol. 1: interview with Sir Edward Mellanby, 1 February 1946.

[72] Lewis, *What price community medicine?*, p. 40 (see note 68).

[73] MRC 800 Vol. III: problems with which Pneumokoniosis Research Unit is concerned, unsigned, undated.

[74] MRC 800 Vol. III: MRC Pneumokoniosis Research Unit. South Wales C. Fletcher, 26 November 1947.

In the absence of any system of after-care or follow-up of men certified with pneumokoniosis or silicosis, little was known of the natural history of the disease after they avoided the dust hazard. Suspension from underground work was intended to take place at a stage at which further exposure to dust would result in serious deterioration, but it was not known whether suspension did in fact prevent such deterioration. In order to study this question and in order to provide a rational basis for a system of treatment, a sample of men certified between 1931 and the end of 1944 was asked to attend for examination at Cardiff. In this way it was possible to assess their state of health and also to determine the progression of the disease by comparing the X-ray taken at the time of certification with that taken on attendance at Cardiff. Men in various stages of the disease, selected from those already examined as out-patients, were admitted for trials of treatment to Llandough Hospital. In the absence of precise knowledge as to the cause of the progression that so often occurred it was not possible to attempt any strictly curative treatment; but considerable relief of symptoms in the more advanced cases was seen, particularly by the treatment of the asthmatic condition from which many of them suffered. It was also found possible to lessen the disability of many men at all stages of the disease by general and breathing exercises.

Once the frequent occurrence of progression in certified men after suspension from underground work had been shown, it was necessary to investigate the effect of continued exposure to dust in cases in the early stages of the disease. The X-rays of some 1600 miners in 1938–40 were available. Many of the men then X-rayed had remained at work underground, and among them were cases who might have been certified at the time of their first X-ray had they applied to the Board. A sample of these men was asked to attend for examination and X-ray, so that the progression of the disease, if any, could be assessed. It became apparent that it is possible for a man with a certifiable degree of disease to continue in underground work for a period of 7–8 years without detectable deterioration. Efforts were also made to measure the incidence of pneumokoniosis in relation to the working environment in a variety of ways such as X-raying two groups of miners, one who had worked mainly under dust-suppression conditions and the other group who had not done so.[75]

Conclusion

The industrial health research of the MRC covered a wide range of activities. However, until the PRU was set up, research into industrial health dealt

---

[75] Ibid.

solely with the impact of various aspects of the workplace on workers' health. Industrial health beyond the workplace was not considered (except by the HMWC in the First World War). So, for instance, no research was undertaken into the impact of unemployment on industrial workers' health, or the effect of industrial injuries on future job prospects. With the advent of the PRU these aspects were also included, and industrial health research under the MRC became a part of 'social medicine'. The distinction between Dr Charles Fletcher's work and that which had gone before is an important one, glossed over by Landsborough Thomson.

The range of industrial health research undertaken by the MRC defies neat categorization, and questions, therefore, the conceptualizations of the relationship between health and work which have been put forward by academics. Vicente Navarro has identified a number of ways in which the relationship between health and work have been analysed. First, work may be viewed as an environmental problem, exposing individual workers to physical, chemical, and environmental agents that may make them ill or cause them to have accidents. Second, work can be regarded as a source of resources (which lead to studies of peoples' diet, life-styles, utilization of health services etc.), health is part of the consumer society to be sold while disease and death are compensated. Third, work can be seen as one stressful factor among many determining death and disease in advanced capitalist societies. Navarro himself argues that health is determined by the nature of the capitalist labour process; the alienation of the labour process causes ill-health among workers.[76] This chapter has shown that those involved with industrial health research did not draw the conceptual distinctions which Navarro has catalogued. Rather, environmental health and the alienation of the labour process were viewed in tandem by the IHRB. Precisely because the environment of work is an alienating one, workers have to be 'educated' or 'treated' in order that they will find it less alienating. The idea that the labour process is alienating is not the property of Marxist academics, it was quite explicitly recognized by researchers, doctors, and capitalist employers. The difference lies in their prescriptions: for the Marxist academic the labour process should be altered, for industrial health researchers and practitioners of industrial medicine the worker must be won over by adapting both him/herself *and* the environment without altering power-relations in the labour process.

While government-sponsored research drew conclusions, albeit tentative in the early days, about the need for adapting both the worker and the working environment to the labour process, governments' lack of control over the labour process, meant that they did not have the power to

[76] Landsborough Thomson, A. (1975). *Half a century of medical research*, Vol. II, *The programme of the Medical Research Council UK*, p. 165. HMSO, London.

implement the findings. This was a fundamental weakness of the MRC's work.

The Board's findings were taken up only indirectly. It contributed, along with Factory Inspectors, the IWS, NIIP, ILM, and practices abroad, to changing opinion among employers. Governments did not respond directly to the Board's findings. The 1937 Factory Act was based largely on proposals from the mid-1920s and reflected current good practices in industry. If the Board had an influence on the Factory Act it was indirectly through influencing the views of Factory Inspectors and a few employers. Research into health at work that influenced government policy was directly commissioned and produced evidence which supported already formed governmental thinking. The PRU bypassed the formal governmental policy-making process and its research was linked with the immediate practical application of its findings. In part, the different approach of the IHRB and PRU is a reflection of the constraints of research by committee under which the Board laboured, and the fresh dynamism an individual such as Charles Fletcher can bring to the work of a well-established research institution.

8

The MRC and the pharmaceutical industry: the model of insulin

JONATHAN LIEBENAU

When the Medical Research Committee was formed there was little concern for commercial problems and no foresight about the role the MRC might need to have in the regulation of medical industry. Although precedents had already been set in Germany and the United States for the supervision and licensing of some kinds of drugs manufacturers, British attitudes towards non-intervention excluded any consideration of a regulatory role.

In this chapter the conditions under which this changed are considered. Initially, during the First World War, this occurred in response to a need for a co-ordinated strategy to replace key medicines previously imported from Germany; later it occurred in response to an offer by the developers of insulin to control UK rights.[1] It will be argued that insulin in particular set the model for the relationship between the MRC and the pharmaceutical industry. Later still, in relation to the efforts to mass produce penicillin, and more recently with cortisone, the MRC worked towards a regulatory and supportive role in relation to drug manufacturers.

In the early twentieth century British officials took a peculiarly ambivalent attitude toward commercial involvement in contrast to their German and US counterparts. For example, while the health departments in those two countries accepted public expectation that they would assure consumers of the safety, and in some cases even the efficacy, of new medicines, in Britain even the mechanism for contracting and negotiating with manufacturers was lacking prior to the MRC's involvement. Although the industry was not passive in Germany and the US, it needed to be particularly aggressive in Britain to assure that governmental actions would be of significant size and appropriately directed.

The background to German and American regulation, and the support the French government offered, helps to explain why manufacturers were so concerned to affect the government's role. During the late nineteenth century a new attitude towards public health coincided with the availability of new

---

[1] The best general history of the development of insulin in Toronto is Bliss, M. (1983). *The discovery of insulin*. New York.

ranges of therapeutic substances. The tangible products of the new sciences of bacteriology and immunology were serums, antitoxins and new vaccines, as well as antiseptics. With public health services concerned to apply advanced medical science to rapidly urbanizing areas such as Hamburg and Berlin, New York and Philadephia, these substances were seen as major contributions to co-ordinated, government-sponsored campaigns. Diphtheria antitoxin was the first such substance to galvanize these views. First developed in Berlin by Emil von Behring and at the Institute Pasteur by Emil Roux, diphtheria antitoxin was soon seen as a potentially major weapon for public health campaigns. Almost as quickly, however, its dangers and shortcomings were noticed. Its potency was difficult to test, and contamination in the production process was a constant danger.[2]

In Germany the response was to establish a government testing station to approve all batches made. In the United States a federal licensing procedure was enacted with powers to inspect manufacturers. Both countries made efforts to enlist the support of manufacturers, and in both cases the largest manufacturers, and those with significant investments in scientific staff and facilities, co-operated. That co-operation grew even closer as it became increasingly clear that governments needed the scientific expertise and production know-how of manufacturers in order to regulate effectively. Manufacturers, for their part, were divided on their response to potential regulation. Those producers who had invested in scientific staff and laboratories saw high standards as a means of differentiating themselves from less scientifically inclined competitors. A system of testing, certifying, and regulating developed in the years around the turn of the century, which had the side effect of identifying products and brands that were trusted in international trade, as well as by public health departments and other domestic buyers.

For the first few years of these developments overseas, British producers were unconcerned about these changes in business practice. They affected sectors which no British producer (with the exception of Burroughs Wellcome) was interested to compete in, and concerned markets which were outside their traditional trade. Before the outbreak of the First World War, however, some producers were taking note of foreign practices. That attitude began to change during the First World War when the shortage of certain key medicines from Germany changed the way people thought about the role of government. The response of the industry to salvarsan, the first effective chemotherapeutic agent against syphilis, was meant to be a turning point. Produced in Frankfurt in 1909 and tested amid enthusiastic publicity, salvarsan was only just beginning to be relied upon on a large scale at the

[2] Liebenau, J. (1987). Public health and the production and use of diphtheria antitoxin in Philadelphia. *Bulletin of the History of Medicine*, **61**, 216–36.

outbreak of war. Within a year the interrupted dependency on German supplies became a *cause célèbre*. By joining the list of key products that Britain relied on Germany for, such as dyestuffs, gyroscopes, and optics, salvarsan became a symbol of British industry's inability to hold its own. The patents covering salvarsan's production were available for abrogating but the technical ability was not in place. Only the Burroughs Wellcome company was capable of making salvarsan in 1914, but there were persistent problems of toxicity. May & Baker was able to produce salvarsan by 1916, but only with the help of Poulenc Frères of Paris, and even then there were quality problems.[3]

With the special need for salvarsan already identified by the conditions of wartime, the newly formed MRC envisaged an active role for itself in regulating it. Three reasons made intervention especially opportune. Salvarsan was only just becoming widely accepted for use in all cases of syphilis; experience had shown that freshly mustered troops were liable to high rates of venereal disease, and the conspicuous failure of British manufacturers to produce this new German product invited derision. In collaboration with the Board of Trade, which co-ordinated the seizure of enemy-held properties (including patents), licences were granted to Burroughs Wellcome and Poulenc Frères to produce salvarsan for the British market. The companies were held to the unique provision, however, that all samples 'be submitted to biological tests' by the MRC. Official certificates were granted by the MRC for each batch, but the cost of testing was charged to the manufacturers. The whole procedure was undertaken in a new government laboratory which maintained good contact with Burroughs Wellcome in particular. This arrangement seemed to function well for all parties involved, and within a year the MRC was petitioning the government to extend regulations to cover sera, vaccines, other biologicals, chemotherapeutics, and certain new medicines as they entered the market. Leading British medical scientists saw this as a move both to bring the UK into line with other countries whose products were regulated, and to put an end to a 'period of anarchy'.[4]

The earliest action the MRC took in relation to salvarsan, in 1916, concerned the employment of Dr A. J. Ewins, who later had a distinguished commercial career. Ewins was identified by E. Mellanby as being 'of special value to the department which tests salvarsan which is one of the important new functions of the Committee which may have widespread consequences hereafter'. Ewins was to be well paid for this work, but his income was more than made up for by the income generated for the MRC from salvarsan

[3] Slinn, J. (1986). *A history of May & Baker*. May & Baker, London.
[4] Liebenau, J. (1984). Industrial R&D in pharmaceutical firms in the early twentieth century. *Business History*, **26**, 331–46.

producers to test their product. This assured that testing work would at least be a self-financing activity.[5]

In conjunction with the War Office and the Local Government Board, the new Biochemical Department of the Medical Research Committee began testing salvarsan in 1917.[6] By early 1918 a special Salvarsan Committee was established 'to consider the methods of manufacture, of biological testing and of clinical administration of Salvarsan and its substitutes'. That committee consisted of Dr W. Bulloch, Dr Henry H. Dale, Lieut. Colonel Harrison of the Rochester Row Military Hospital, Surgeon General Rolleston, Major F. W. Andrews, FRS, RAMC, and the Medical Inspector of the Local Government Board, F. J. H. Coutts. Although announced to the press soon after formation, the Committee had nothing to report for 18 months, well after the end of the war, when the pamphlet *Effects of arsenical compounds in treatment of syphilis* by P. G. Fields and R. J. G. Parness was published.

Problems of quality and consistency continued to plague British manufacturers. Even as late as October 1921 Burroughs Wellcome and May & Baker were having trouble assuring that their neosalvarsan was equal to the German product.[7] In the meantime, pressures had been mounting to introduce a British 'Therapeutic Substances Act' which would provide assurances to the medical profession that medicines were being produced following some accountable standards, would provide government guidelines to follow for effective enforcement, and would allow producers to compete in international markets along with German and American companies who could boast that their products were 'certified' by their respective governments. In 1920 the British Medical Association spoke out to urge the Ministry of Health to provide a legal authority to enforce the testing 'of certain potent and dangerous chemical or biological products'. This stand was reiterated four years later, stressing the frustration of seeing so little happen in the meantime.[8] Changes in the law had to wait a bit longer, and it was not until 1925 that the Therapeutic Substances Act was passed. In the interim another case arose which was to set new precedents and procedures, and challenge the entire concept of a relationship between the MRC and the pharmaceutical industry.

The case of the response to insulin is particularly instructive of both official and commercial reactions to new products. Insulin was developed at the University of Toronto in 1921/2 and immediately attracted attention in

[5] Ewins started on £300 p.a. when he was hired on 1 October 1914 and received rises to £350 p.a. on 1 April 1916 and £400 p.a. from 1 April 1917. MRC General Correspondence 1914, 1915, 1916 PF 2/1 29 May 1916 letter from Mellanby (?) to Mr C. Roberts.
[6] MRC Board Minute Book, Vol. II, 1915–1926, 1 February 1918, p. 60.
[7] MRC 137/1103: salvarsan-testing, 18 October 1921, Dale to Fletcher.
[8] Editorial (1924). Therapeutic substances Bill. *British Medical Journal*, i , 677.

Canada and the United States. By the summer of 1922, officials at the MRC had taken intense interest in insulin, partly as a response to its general promise, but more particularly because there was an indication that Toronto wished to offer the MRC the British patent rights for insulin. The Toronto researchers, Frederick Banting, Best, and Macleod, already had arranged with the Eli Lilly Company to manufacture and distribute in North America, and there was the possibility that the MRC might have a comparable role in Europe.[9]

The first indication of the intentions of the University of Toronto was reported by Fletcher to the MRC before many details were known.

The Secretary reported that the University of Toronto had asked whether the Council would be willing to accept the patent rights in this country of a pancreatic extract known as 'Insulin'. The Council will be prepared to accept these if there be no express or implied restriction upon their complete freedom of subsequent action.[10]

The MRC was hesitant. Accepting responsibility for a patent under the best of circumstances was liable to be tricky. There were two additional issues which made these arrangements especially difficult: the possibility that the patents might be inadequate, and the unprecedented difficulties associated with supervising and controlling the production commercially. There was one other aspect which entered into consideration: the reluctance to accept foreign standards.

The possibilities that this opportunity presented were not overlooked, however. Apart from the opportunity to bring this important diabetes medication to Britain and to have some control over its production and use, the desirability of securing the MRC's role in any new legislation was foremost in the minds of the MRC's administrators.

The key attitudes were formed during mid- to late summer 1922 in preparation for a trip by H. W. Dudley and Henry Dale to visit the University of Toronto and other sites involved in the development, production, and testing of insulin. In a report by Fletcher to Dawson Williams,[11] the interests of the MRC were spelled out. The initial offer of control over the insulin patents by the University of Toronto were 'informal' and the MRC indicated that it would be prepared to accept these rights, if its complete independence and freedom of action thereafter be fully recognized. There was, already at that stage, a strong feeling of suspicion of the appropriateness of the venture, and Fletcher went on to specify that

If the claims made for insulin are justified, it will be important not only that confirmatory and additional work should be done here, but also that proper steps

---

[9] MRC 1092: A. Landsborough Thomson memo, 26 July 1922; ibid.: Dawson Williams to Fletcher, 28 August 1922; ibid.: Fletcher to Williams, 30 August 1922.
[10] MRC Minute Book, Vol. II, 1915–1926: Pancreatic extract, 2 July 1922, p. 256 (min. 316).
[11] MRC 1092: July 1922–February 1923: ibid.: 30 August 1922.

should be taken at the National Institute towards standardisation and towards the help and guidance of the profession in the therapeutic use of the substance.

The role mentioned for the National Institute for Medical Research (NIMR) would have followed activities in supervising and standardizing salvarsan carried out there during the war. The lack of any mention of the commercial sector in this context is conspicuous. Fletcher's attitudes toward other aspects of the logistics involved were equally explicit.

I am personally inclined to think that the patent rights which the University holds, and which seem likely soon to be vested in my Council for this country, have only an uncertain validity. Whatever the Council can do in this matter will be done, of course, with a view to getting the quickest availability of the drug for the profession and the public, preventing improper exploitation by commercial interests, and getting such increase of knowledge as we can.[12]

While this level of suspicion may appear to be extreme, it was no more than Fletcher expressed at other times, and it would not have surprised those in industry, who could not have expected much more respect.

The attitude of Dale and Dudley was quite different. First of all, they had fewer illusions about the possible 'increase of knowledge' which the MRC might be expected to provide, and they saw their roles more clearly as facilitators towards more effective production, should the opportunity present itself. They collected data on the costs and methods of production.[13] They were interested in particular in the arrangements of the University of Toronto–Eli Lilly Company agreement and in the difficulties the Eli Lilly laboratory had in replicating the level of efficiency of Toronto production and the potency of their insulin. They were led to the conclusion that,

In general the manufacture of the extract, both in Toronto and Indianapolis, is in a very unsatisfactory state. The yield is much below that obtained in small scale experiments and is very irregular, sometimes a potent and sometimes a very weak end product results, and the reasons for these frequent failures are not known. . . . Just before we left America both the Lilly Co. and the Toronto laboratory were in great difficulty owing to the fact that their products were proving to be unstable, the potency falling off to practically nothing in a week.[14]

This did not deter them from proposing areas of research that might help alleviate the problem: 'The lack of an accurate simple test for the substance, and the great clamour for material for clinical purposes have prevented investigation of points at which loss of activity occurs and the reasons for its occurrence'.[15] These proposals also followed a pattern recognizable from the

[12] MRC 1092: Fletcher to Williams, 30 August 1922.
[13] MRC 1092: Dudley's report, October 1922, Methods of preparation. p. 9.
[14] Ibid. p. 7.
[15] Ibid.

strategy of aiding in the commercialization of diphtheria antitoxin and salvarsan. The most appropriate aid a governmental laboratory could give to a commercial enterprise, and the first requirement of the regulating body were the same thing: find a means of standardizing the substance and thereby check its suitability for sale.[16]

Dale took further advantage of the American visit to stop at the Hygienic Laboratory of the US Marine Hospital Service (later the US Public Health Service) to discuss the similarities, differences, and special difficulties of standardizing salvarsan, the 'pituitary extract' [insulin] and antitoxic sera.[17]

These investigations only served to confirm many of the MRC's prejudices. As Dale put it,

We had serious doubts, before our visit to America, as to the efficacy of the patent, for which application has been made, in giving the desired protection and control. What we have seen of its working in America only makes these doubts stronger.[18]

The patent claim seemed weak, vague, and too general. Any attempt to specify the practices then in use for the purpose of a specific process patent would, on the other hand, bring about easy circumvention. Already there were numerous rival patents being filed in America. Eli Lilly had registered their trade name 'Iletin' and Fairchilds, a maker of ferment preparations, were advertising an extract of pancreas which they implied contained the active hormone, but which clearly had no insulin. Evidently even the most fundamental purposes of the patent were inadequately served. The Toronto inventors were unable to control the quality and price of the substance, and even the Hygienic Laboratory had difficulty legally adding insulin to its list of regulated substances because of the limited definition provided by the patent.

The implications for the MRC were clear. Although Dale believed that the MRC ought to accept the University of Toronto offer, it should do so only with the proviso that exempted the Council from any obligation to defend the patent. The inadequacies of the patent had implications for British producers as well. Not enough information was contained in the patent, Dale believed, for anyone satisfactorily to make or test insulin. This, however, would provide the MRC with an opportunity to

exercise a moral control over manufacturers, and would induce [them] to submit to a system of supervision, as regards this product, which the law does not enable the

---

[16] A number of patents were, nevertheless, granted to in Britain under the auspices of the MRC. These included: BP No. 203,778 (13 June 1922, expired 12 June 1931): University of Toronto, Banting, Best and Collip. A method for the preparation of insulin; BP 209,766 (12 January 1923, expired 11 January 1932): University of Toronto, Banting, Best and Collip. Improvements in the production of insulin; BP 212,238 (2 March 1923, expired 1 March 1932): University of Toronto, Waldon. Manufacture of a purified form of insulin; BP 216,979 (27 March 1923, expired 26 March 1932): H. W. Dudley and the MRC.

[17] MRC 1092: methods of preparation.

[18] Ibid. p. 12.

Council at present to enforce. The holding of the patent would simply regularize and define the Council's authority in relation to the insulin work. If the position were handled firmly and wisely, and with an obvious desire to help and not merely to restrict manufacture, it seems probable that the makers would submit to control willingly as they still do in the case of the Salvarsan products, in connexion with which the legal authority for the Council's control has become more nebulous as the control has become more effective.[19]

These advantages, however, did not work to everyone's favour. Unsurprisingly, problems arose about how to regulate supply and who would be willing to produce under the MRC's restrictions. Less predictably, there was a general outcry about the possibility that the MRC would sanction patenting.[20]

Initial approaches were made to the British Drug Houses (BDH), Burroughs Wellcome, and Allen & Hanbury and later arrangements reached with Boots and the Evans Medical company. The details of a proposed licensing agreement were sent to Burroughs Wellcome; BDH; Evans Sons, Lescher & Webb; Duncan Flockhart; and Boots. In general, the licences were not to be limited except as the supply of raw materials (sources of fresh pancreases were not as readily available in Britain as near the great slaughterhouse areas of Midwestern North America). The limits would be for only two producers in London and one each in three or four regions. All products would have to be submitted to the MRC for testing, and while no restrictions would be made on imports, some import conditions would apply, implying some advantage for domestic producers. Nine specific terms were attached:

1. Manufacturers had to demonstrate that they had appropriate equipment and staff for proper biological and other testing.
2. The NIMR would test every batch and issue certificates.
3. All initial sales would be handled by the MRC.
4. Costs to manufacturers had to be supplied, and although these data would be confidential, a fixed maximum selling price would be imposed.
5. 'Insulin' would be the only name the product could trade under.
6. The MRC reserved the right to review all published statements.
7. A standard MRC statement on the use of insulin was to be supplied to consumers by the producer.
8. Batch numbers and a measure of the level of activity would be included on all labels.
9. A nominal royalty was payable to the MRC.[21]

[19] ibid. p. 15.

[20] Armstrong, H. E. Medical research, changed scientific outlook, position of the Royal Society. Letter to *The Times*, 21 November 1922.

[21] MRC Minute Book, Vol. II, 1915–1926: 12 January 1923, p. 276, min. 3.

With these conditions in place, the MRC took on the parallel tasks of imposing controls on producers and of co-ordinating research. Initial results came quickly indeed. Fletcher reported to Charles Sherrington that Dale and Dudley had already increased the average yield of insulin from pancreases by more than eightfold, while reducing the amount of alcohol use by four-fifths. They had also shortened the production time and developed a means of heat-sterilization. 'If we had let the manufacturers begin two months ago, they would probably have made little progress and would now be scrapping their plant for changed methods. As it is, we hope to have five firms started very shortly, two are already beginning.'[22]

From that point the programme of production was well under way. In March 1923 the BDH–Allen & Hanbury partnership produced enough insulin to test, and they were eager to begin to distribute 'before the American preparation arrives'.[23] At about that time it also became clear that the MRC had to be 'rather innocent critics' of the costings submitted by manufacturers. 'I have no idea,' Dale wrote, 'whether they intend to act in competition, or in collusion.'[24]

The MRC took responsibility for licensing those manufacturers, testing batches, and protecting the industry from imported insulin. They also took on a considerable research project to standardize production and lower costs, which by 1924 succeeded in cutting prices by almost 75 per cent. Protection became a heated issue when it was claimed that the companies were in danger of being undersold by Danish suppliers.

By October 1924 the strategy for organizing a series of trials at selected clinics was chosen while large-scale production was explored. Samples were immediately sent to St Bartholomew's, Guy's, St Thomas's, The London, and University College Hospitals in London, and to major hospitals in Sheffield and Edinburgh. These led to a series of clinical trials all under the co-ordination of the NIMR.[25] This was all approached before any kind of arrangements had been made with manufacturers, and while Eli Lilly was clamouring to be allowed to export insulin to Britain through the MRC; a move resisted, with much forethought, on the ground that they could not 'contemplate any arrangement which, by popularizing a proprietary name, or in any other way, might compromise the possible development of manufacture of this remedy in Britain'.[26]

It was not long before a host of objections to this entire venture were raised. Henry E. Armstrong of the Royal Society, who was to become an increasingly

[22] MRC 1092: Fletcher to Sherrington, 8 January 1923.
[23] MRC 1092: Dale to Fletcher, 21 March 1923, ibid. 3 April 1923.
[24] MRC 1092: Dale to Fletcher, 3 April 1923.
[25] Ibid. p. 14; MRC Minute Book, Vol. II, 1915–1926: p. 268, 17 November 1922, min. 375 (insulin treatment of diabetes).
[26] MRC 1092, methods of preparation, p. 18.

vociferous critic of the MRC, wrote in *The Times* and *The Lancet* that the proposed patenting 'cannot be countenanced by public opinion'.

> In every direction, science to-day is being commercialized, if not directly, through the creation of a scientific bureaucracy and the multiplication of scholarship and prizes from the Nobel Prize downwards. The old conception that scientific discovery was its own great reward is all but lost to us, and we are forcing on the development of a class of a-moral scientific workers. The virus is already at work, not only in the Medical Research Council, but also in the Board of Scientific and Industrial Research; both bodies are interfering with and checking in the progress of discovery and invention by imposing rules and taking action to prevent what they are pleased to call overlapping—the attack of a problem by more than a single worker or at more than one centre. Patents are only one form of this interference . . . [27]

Fletcher responded immediately in a private letter scolding Armstrong and pointing out that the MRC had not patented anything; 'If you give us sympathy instead of abuse, I could have explained to you the diplomatic reasons against snubbing a Canadian University by refusing an offer made in a purely courteous and friendly spirit to the home country.'[28]

Had Armstrong known what actually occupied the time of Fletcher, Dale, and others who were trying to figure out how to proceed, he might have directed his criticisms elsewhere. A means for contacting appropriate companies and establishing procedures for collaboration was still being sought. They were disposed to accept a concept proposed by Noel Paton of Glasgow University, who supported the idea that a large manufacturer such as Burroughs Wellcome & Co. be engaged 'on the understanding that all the preparations are to be tested and standardised under our direction, e.g. at Hampstead, and to be made available only at selected cliniques'.[29]

Trying to control matters through hospital centres would not work because they had limited experience; such decentralization would be wasteful. Aside from that, proprietary information would certainly leak to competing businesses.

> The other method—by including one or more business firms—has the advantage that we will have at our disposal the vast experience of these people in making such preparations, e.g. adrenalin, idothyreoglobulin, pitcitrin, etc., and it is more likely that they will hit upon improvements in method.[30]

Within two weeks of this letter Dale had held discussions with ten chief firms' representatives.[31]   Burroughs   Wellcome's   response   was   particularly

[27] Armstrong, H. E. Letter to *The Times*, 21 November 1922; see also *The Times* (17 November 1922) and *Lancet* (1922) **ii**, 1086.
[28] MRC 1092: Fletcher to Armstrong, 21 November 1922.
[29] MRC 1092: Paton to Fletcher, 23 November 1922.
[30] Ibid.
[31] MRC 1092: Fletcher memo to MRC members only, 5 December 1922; MRC Minute Book, Vol. II, 1915–1926: 8 December 1922, pp. 272–3, min. 389.

gratified, as they offered 'unqualified acceptance' except for the suggestion that all sales should be limited to the medical profession.[32] Other interest was similarly forthcoming. BDH applied for a licence on behalf of themselves and Allen & Hanbury, prompting Dale to urge haste and 'go ahead as quickly as possible with the firms who have expressed their willingness to accept our conditions'. In light of a potential avalanche of unsanctioned activities, such as the case at the Wellcome Laboratories where Dr O'Brien prepared, 'without reference to us', some insulin which he had tentatively arranged to provide to Dr Graham at St Bartholomew's Hospital. 'I put my foot down on this very heavily,' Dale wrote, 'and had a very straight talk with O'Brien, who now realises that any such action will be regarded by us as a breach of confidence, and treated accordingly.'[33] BDH, in any case, wished to avoid unnecessary complications by proposing to regard the arrangement as 'something in the nature of a partnership agreement'.

Also in December 1922 the issue of how Britain should make use of insulin was being widely discussed. E. Sharpey Schafer sought to link the Toronto work with his own work ten years earlier, and C. S. Sherrington reported on 'The use of pancreatic extract in diabetes' to the Royal Society and in *Nature*.[34] By the start of the new year a detailed description of the insulin production process had been sent to seven centres of research by Henry Dale.[35]

Not all interested parties were granted permission to manufacture. Problems with the supply of suitably fresh pancreases was seen as the first stumbling block, but when R. Sumner & Co. asked for permission they were summarily refused on these and other grounds: 'You will realise that the manufacture of insulin is not a process which you could in any event undertake without some months of experimental work and a large outlay on plant.'[36] The Sumner company felt quite aggrieved. It seemed unfair for them to have to refer to their large list of customers (3000 physicians and 3000 pharmacists, they claimed in November 1923), and not to use their strong connection with the University of Liverpool Department of Pharmacology. They objected to the concept of the MRC granting what they claimed to be monopoly rights to a chosen few manufacturers.

The mechanisms for contacting suitable manufacturers was discussed at some length by Dale and Fletcher in November 1922. Dale pointed out that, following discussions with representatives of Burroughs Wellcome, Allen & Hanbury, BDH, and May & Baker, there was a great deal of interest among

---

[32] MRC 1092: Dale to Fletcher, 22 December 1922.

[33] Ibid.

[34] MRC 1092: E. Sharpey Schafer to Fletcher, 6 December 1922; Sherrington, C. S. (1922). Presidential address to the Royal Society, 30 November 1922. *Nature*, **110**, 774.

[35] MRC 1092: description of insulin production by Dale, 30 December 1922.

[36] MRC 1092/10F: R. Sumner & Co. correspondence, P. Overton to Thomson, 1923.

manufacturers concerning the prospect of making insulin. A private approach by the MRC to one or two firms, however, would cause 'dissatisfaction' among the others. 'On the other hand, a free announcement of willingness to license suitable makers would produce a deluge of applications from utterly unsuitable people.' This would imply a compromise strategy, to invite one representative of each of the six to eight firms 'whom we know as having, prima facie, a reasonable chance of making insulin if licensed . . .'.[37] At the subsequent meeting Dale pointed out 'the difficulties due to restricted supply of pancreas, excise limitations on duty-free alcohol, biological control, etc.'.[38] The outstanding problem clearly was, however, that if only one London firm were to receive a licence, it would be Burroughs Wellcome, the only one with elaborate enough laboratory facilities and a high quality scientific staff.

Interest from medical scientists throughout Britain was intense. Leading figures at St Thomas's Hospital, University College Hospital, St Bartholomew's Hospital and elsewhere wrote to Fletcher and Dale to ask for guidance and permission to commence research.[39] Clinical results were reported in British medical journals in April 1923 at the same time that commentary about costs began to appear in the popular press.[40] C. P. Crewe claimed in *The Times* that the British price was three times that in America, while G. F. McCleary, the Secretary to the new advisory body, the Insulin Committee of the Ministry of Health, weakly countered with the statement in *The Times* that prices had already been dropping substantially, and that American producers had advantages of both a longer period of experimentation and manufacture, as well as large-scale factors. The price did continue to drop (see Table 8.1); by the end of 1923 significant reductions were reported, and by February 1924 the UK prices were at or below US levels. American imports continued, however, to have their supporters, who claimed that the Eli Lilly product was in some way superior, and in any case was better packaged than the A-B Brand (for Allenbury–BDH).[41]

The matter of the MRC holding patents cropped up again when the Council agreed to take out at least one new patent for a method of concentration devised by Dr Dudley. At the same time they recognized that they were unable to remain responsible for methods of distribution, neither with regard to meeting priorities nor where restrictions might be imposed.[42]

[37] MRC 1092/10: Trade questions, Dale to Fletcher, 27 November 1922.
[38] Ibid.
[39] MRC 1092/3: H. MacLean, St Thomas's Hospital, to MRC; MRC 1092/2: T. R. Elliot, University College Hospital, to MRC; MRC 1092/4: Francis R. Fraser, St. Bartholomew's Hospital, to MRC.
[40] Lancet (1923). i, 814, 824, 905; *British Medical Journal* (1923). i, 341, 690–1, 695, 733, 737; Crewe, C. P. Letter to *The Times*, 10 July 1923; McCleary, G. F. Letter to *The Times*, 11 July 1923.
[41] Dr Shoetee Sack, Letter to *The Times*, 20 July 1923.

Table 8.1 British insulin prices in the UK: retail prices of 5 cm^3 (20 units per cm^3, 1923–1934)

Date	A.B.	Burroughs Wellcome	Boots
1923 (Apr)	25/0	25/0	25/0
(July)	17/6	—	12/6
1924 (Jan)	12/6	12/6	—
(Feb)	—	6/8	6/8
(Apr)	6/8	—	—
(May)	—	4/8	4/8
(June)	—	—	3/0
(July)	—	2/8	2/8
(Oct)	2/8	—	—
1929 (May)	2/0	1/8	—
1934 (Jan)	1/10	1/10	1/5

These powers were, in effect, transferred to the Ministry of Health, which later in 1923 took on responsibility for conditions covering the distribution of insulin through the Insulin Committee.[43]

With the testing system in place for only one year, Dale already began expressing doubts about the appropriateness of the MRC continuing to take those responsibilities. Finding sufficient merit in the majority of what he tested, he proposed to drop all testing of US imports and transferring all routine testing to the manufacturers.[44]

A new issue arose mid-1924 which was to hound the MRC for 10 years: the Danish licencee, Leo Company, applied for a British import licence to sell and re-export insulin. Leo had the rights from Toronto University to produce and sell to the Danish market, and it had been successful in conducting an export trade to most of the world, other than the British Isles. Fletcher's response was to reject the request on the grounds that it would overburden the testing mechanism.[45]

By 1926 the dimensions of the insulin business began to change. Over one-third of regular production was being exported as opposed to negligible imports, despite persistent requests by the Leo Company and later Bayer Products Ltd. (a British I. G. Farben company).[46]

---

[42] MRC Board Minute Book, Vol. II, 1915–1926: 23 March 1923, p. 284, min. 26.

[43] MRC Minute Book, Vol. II, 1915–1926: 4 May 1923, p. 288, min. 53.

[44] MRC 1092 v/4: memo, Fletcher, recommendations made by the Insulin Committee, 15 July 1924.

[45] Ibid.

[46] MRC 1092, VI: 18 September 1929.

These issues came to a head in 1933 when Parliament announced hearings by the Tribunal appointed under the Safeguarding of Industries Act to consider the cases of insulin. BDH produced an elaborate statement for the Parliamentary Medical Committee. In pleading for a continuation of the tariff on Danish insulin, BDH stressed the importance of the product and reminded the committee of the conditions under which the Act was passed in 1921. Ignoring the irony of the passing of thirteen years, BDH admitted that the protection which was intended to allow British companies quickly to catch up with their German counterparts had failed to stimulate companies to do much in the way of catching up, and stated that 'It is no less true today than it was then that for the retention of British initiative in research in furthering the manufacture of fine chemicals the industry as a whole needs to be safeguarded.'[47] The statement further pleaded that British manufacturers had 'led the world in reducing the price of insulin' and only Denmark, Norway, and Sweden had such low prices. Allowing imports, which were in any case unnecessary as the supply of A-B Insulin could be increased at any time to meet higher demand, would just weaken the domestic producers, losing the assurance that the British public then had for a constant, local supply.

When the predicted decision was made to abolish the tariff anomaly, in May 1934, F. H. Carr, on behalf of BDH, complained bitterly to Mellanby:

In taking this step, the Government are denying to an industry which makes very small profits and at the same time calls for the use of science and skill in a greater degree than most other industries, the principle of protection which is extended to practically every other industry in the country. . . . Since British insulin manufacturers set up the manufacture with great assistance and sympathy from the Medical Research Council, I cannot help feeling that this is a matter in which they must take some interest.[48]

Directly and indirectly, BDH pressed their two main points: that protection was due to them, and that the medicine was of particular importance and its supply should not be threatened. 'In order that there may be assured to the British diabetic a constant supply of reliable, high quality insulin prepared under accurate scientific control,' BDH argued in their formal statement, 'it is absolutely necessary that the industry should be protected from unregulated price competition.'[49]

Another foreign producer, N. V. Organon of the Netherlands, pressed their claim alongside the Leo company. N. V. Organon had started their plans to be allowed to export from the Netherlands to Britain as early as October 1923. They argued for the following years that as the Netherlands and Britain were both countries devoted to free trade, they should not be

[47] MRC 1092, VIII: BDH statement, January 1934.
[48] Ibid.
[49] Ibid.

stopped from exporting. Through their UK agents, British Colloids Ltd., they expected better treatment. It was only after the parliamentary hearings of 1931, however, that a licence to import was granted.[50] Other foreign interests had expressed the desire to market insulin in the UK just as plans were getting underway. Enquiries from Copenhagen, Amsterdam, and Strasbourg all offered to bring foreign-produced insulin to Britain for testing and trade.[51] The greatest such concern, as might be expected, came from Eli Lilly, the large American producer. Early in 1923 Lilly recognized that the British market was just about ready for insulin, while British producers were well behind.[52] Lilly were already well along in their export drive, and their American prices had begun to fall dramatically. These pressures could not long be ignored, and by May 1923 Dale had to report to Fletcher that Lilly:

desire to sell in competition with British manufacturers, and I expect that they think that they could drive them out of the market. I think it not unlikely that with the advantage of nearly a year's start, and an almost unlimited supply of accessible raw material, they could beat our manufacturers in price, and make it impossible to produce Insulin here on a remunerative basis. The question is obviously one of high policy rather than science, and I must leave it to you whether the matter should be decided by the Insulin Committee of the Medical Research Council or referred to the Ministry of Health Committee in conjunction with the Board of Trade.[53]

They resolved to allow regular shipments to the British Isles of limited quantity, and to grant no UK licence to Lilly directly, but only for the purpose of sending specified shipments. This continued until December 1923, when Landsborough Thomson could report to Lilly that UK firms were producing enough for the domestic market, and that Lilly would have to deal through British firms directly.

Links with Copenhagen continued as Professor August Krough kept up the pressure through his interests in Nordisk Insulinlaboratorium to export to Britain. A large, well organized producer, Nordisk had originally been founded to supply the Scandinavian market with insulin, but it was not long before a rather considerable export market developed. They used guidelines and methods prescribed by the Health Organization of the League of Nations and felt that compliance with these standards, as well as an export market

[50] MRC 1092/35: N. V. Organon.
[51] MRC 1092/1A: insulin: special inquiries, F. L. Blum of Strasbourg to Fletcher, 5 May 1923; Prof. August Krough of Copenhagen to MRC, May 1923; E. Laqueur of Amsterdam to MRC, May 1923.
[52] MRC 1092/19: Eli Lilly, 1922–1924, correspondence of G. H. A. Clowes, Director of Research, to Dale, 16 March 1923, 2 April 1923.
[53] MRC 1092/19: Lilly, Dale to Fletcher, 28 May 1923.

already consisting of 28 nations outside the five Scandinavian countries, were good enough arguments.[54]

Similar arrangements were entered into by Squibb of New York, which acquired special permission from the University of Toronto to sell to the MRC. They approached the MRC in autumn 1925 with a commercial proposal, but were told that there was no further need for imported insulin in Britain, as domestic producers were by then able to keep up.[55]

Problems with pricing continued well after all arrangements seemed to be settled. In one case, in 1925, Allen & Hanbury Ltd. was accused by Landsborough Thomson of dealing in Eli Lilly American insulin at a retail price of about 50 per cent higher than the price at which it was available in the United States.[56]

Similar irritations continued with the timing and wording of various announcements, which were supposed to be controlled by the MRC, but which participating companies had difficulty complying with, given their normally competitive behaviour. Boots announced a price decrease before the end of one information embargo, getting their name in first, and were constantly having to be reminded of agreements, explained to about arrangements and proceedings, and generally creating bureaucratic problems.[57] The use of any reference to the MRC's involvement was at best controversial.

The role of Burroughs Wellcome & Co. in exposing problems was invaluable to the MRC, but at the same time irksome to Dale, who had himself worked in those laboratories and was well aware of their procedures. Dale wrote to Landsborough Thomson,

It cannot have escaped your attention, that complaints of this kind almost invariably originate with Burroughs Wellcome & Co. It is very difficult to snub them, when there is a genuine basis for their complaint. I have been rather annoyed, however, by their tendency to use their own laboratories for detective purposes, with regard to competitive products. If they report to the Ministry that some therapeutic substance from another source has been found by them to be deficient in activity, we cannot refuse to investigate the matter, and do so with the knowledge that their statement will

[54] League of Nations 1926 III 7. Coc. CH 398; MRC 1092/34: Leo Ltd; see pamphlet 'Nordisk Insulinlaboratorium' Copenhagen 1930; correspondence with A. Krough and Fletcher, 31 May 1924, 12 June 1924.

[55] MRC 1092/38A: Squibb, John F. Anderson to MRC, 12 October 1925, Thomson to Anderson, 12 November 1925.

[56] MRC 1092/10B: BDH July 1924–February 1927, correspondence between Allen & Hanbury Ltd. and A. Landsborough Thomson, January–September 1925.

[57] MRC 1092/10C: Boots Pure Drug Co., November 1922–January 1933, see correspondence in May 1923.

probably be substantially correct. At the same time, I find their assumption of this function as private spies and detectives for the Authority under the Act, or the MRC, an annoyance which I would willingly discourage.[58]

The facilities provided by the major producers were significant by the scale of drugs production at that time. Boots boasted that they were the largest officially authorized makers and devoted a 'huge establishment' to its preparation, with an 'unrivalled analytical department' within their plant of over 14 acres and more than one million feet of floor space.[59] Evans Sons, Lescher & Webb Ltd. similarly claimed 'exceptional' facilities, including 'a completely equipped Organo-Therapeutic Department' in which insulin was being made along with a large number of other products. They also maintained a physiological laboratory and 'expert chemical workers to deal with any chemical investigations which may be necessary'.[60]

The question of how the MRC could work in conjunction with drug companies arose again during the drive to develop penicillin. In 1941 five companies, Boots, May & Baker, Glaxo, BDH, and the Wellcome Foundation incorporated a consortium, the Therapeutic Research Corporation (TRC), to collaborate in certain limited areas of research. By early 1942, given the wartime conditions and the supposed opportunities that earlier penicillin research promised, the TRC concentrated on means of large-scale antibiotics production.[61] Although the TRC was in good contact with the MRC, no formal links were established until 1943 when the MRC Penicillin Clinical Trials Committee was established. Their supervisory function was limited to reviewing clinical work and they never tried to take on any regulatory or supervisory role with regard to the commercial production of penicillin.[62]

The attitude of the companies was one of some frustration. Although they could not have expected the MRC to have intervened where it might have been really necessary, such as with the allocation of construction materials controlled by the Ministry of Supply, a more aggressive stance by the MRC might have helped some aspects of penicillin development. It seems that the difficulties experienced with trying to co-ordinate things for insulin production had an effect on the MRC's attitude toward penicillin. Without the championing attitudes of Dale and Fletcher (Mellanby showed no special enthusiasm), and without the added incentive such as the push for the Therapeutic Substances Act, the MRC kept its distance from manufacturers.

[58] MRC 1092/34: Leo Ltd., Dale to Thomson, 4 November 1930.
[59] MRC 1092/10C: Boots Pure Drug Co., November 1922–January 1933, see clipping 'Boots Pure Drug Co. Ltd., *The Graphic*, 16 January 1926, pp. 148–9.
[60] MRC 1092/10E: Evans Sons, Lescher & Webb Ltd., 1 December 1922–July 1928.
[61] See Liebenau, J. (1987). The British success with penicillin. *Social Studies of Science*, **17**, 69–86.
[62] Ibid. p. 79,

The relationship forged between the MRC and the four main companies involved with insulin production came to set the standard by which the Council dealt with businesses. The debates that were argued, the precedents that were set, and the awareness of the sensitive nature of government/industry relations, stayed with the MRC throughout its future dealings with the industry. Fletcher's style of leadership and Dale's personal involvement were not found in the relations regarding penicillin, but the sensitivity was very much present. As with insulin, there was great uncertainty about what to do with the companies when there was a potential public risk but where government involvement could look to nothing other than wartime controls as a model.

9

The MRC's support for experimental radiology during the inter-war years

DAVID CANTOR

This chapter examines the MRC's policy towards experimental laboratory studies of the biological effects of radiation (hereafter experimental radiology[1]) between 1920 and 1939. It is a story of the relationship between laboratory research and medicine, for the Council's experimental radiology was always justified in terms of its ultimate benefit to clinical practice. Moreover, it is a study of the allocation of scarce resources. The Council's forerunner, the Medical Research Committee, entered experimental radiology for the first time during the First World War, when it financed research at the Middlesex Hospital, London, into the physiological effects of small doses of X-rays.[2] However, it was the Committee's acquisition of 5 grams of hydrated radium bromide in 1919 from surplus government stock that provided the basis of the Council's programme of radiological research, supplemented in 1924 by an additional 800 milligrams of the salt. Radium was in limited supply, and its scarcity fostered tensions over its distribution, tensions enhanced by post-First World War concern over rising cancer mortality figures. If radium

---

[1] Today the term radiology is generally reserved for the diagnostic use of radiations. However, this is a relatively recent innovation. The Committee which supervised the Council's inter-war programme of research into the medical use of radium and other sources of radiation was named the Radiology Committee. This Radiology Committee predominantly looked after research into radium therapy. Consequently, the phrase 'experimental radiology' should not be taken to refer to experimental work on imaging, neither should the adjective 'radiological' be taken to refer only to diagnostic radiology.

For the purposes of this essay, experimental radiology will refer simply to any experimental laboratory research studying the biological effects of radiation. This term was used by contemporaries, though at times they also used it to refer to physicists' studies of the distribution of radiation in the body.

The term 'radiological' will refer to any work using radiations. However, 'radiologist' will refer *only* to medical users of X-rays. X-Ray radiotherapy was closely linked to the diagnostic uses of radiation, and was often carried out by physicians. Some radiologists used radium. However, most radium therapy was carried out by surgeons, gynaecologists and laryngologists (hereafter referred to collectively as 'surgeons').

[2] Middlesex Hospital Cancer and General Research Committee minutes: Fletcher to Russ, 22 November 1917, and minutes of meetings for 14 December 1917 and 15 January 1918. The results of this study were published in Russ, S., Chambers, H., Scott, G. M., and Mottram, J. C. (1919). Experimental studies with small doses of x-rays. *Lancet*, i, 692–5.

181

was to be supplied for laboratory research, then laboratory research had to be seen to provide benefits to medicine.

Many medical practitioners were highly dubious of the value of experimental laboratory research. Yet during the inter-war years the Council's radiological research policy moved more and more towards this form of research. In 1920 experimental radiology was more or less ancillary to clinical studies of the use of radium in therapy. But by 1939, new allocations of radium went predominantly to laboratory studies, which did not promise immediate return to clinicians.

The shift in the Council's policy towards experimental radiology is well illustrated by periodic policy statements made during the course of the inter-war years. In 1920 the secretary of the Radiology Committee of the MRC, Sidney Russ, noted that, 'the main object of ... [the MRC] ... in this matter was to make it a clinical investigation, backed up, where facilities exist by laboratory investigations.'[3] The corollary of this policy was, as the Council noted elsewhere, a focus on clinical as opposed to laboratory or basic research: 'the great bulk of it will consist in studies of the clinical results obtained by the use of rays accurately recorded, and of the optimum methods and doses to be employed'.[4]

In 1924 came the first hints of a change in this policy, as the Council informed the Ministry of Health that biological (rather than medical) research did in fact form a significant part of its programme:

Our Radiology Committee, while they can serve all the radiological needs of cancer research, is not limited to cancer research, and has very valuable work in hand upon the actions of rays on living tissues as such from a general biological point of view.[5]

In 1931 the Council noted in its annual report on the medical uses of radium that,

not only is there an increasing amount of purely experimental work being done on radiological lines, but . . . studies are at last being undertaken of a fundamental physiological character. These may not quickly provide the answers to the problems of the clinic, but they must inevitably broaden the basis on which the general principles of radiotherapy are being laid.[6]

In fact, not only did the Council recognize that its policy would not 'quickly provide the answers to the problems of the clinic', it also used its support of experimental research to distance its radiological research from the routine

---

[3] MRC 1074/A: Russ to Fletcher, 7 December 1920.
[4] MRC 1082 I: MRC to Murray, 8 December 1921.
[5] MRC 1383 IV: Fletcher to Newman, 22 October 1924.
[6] MRC *SRS* 174: *Medical uses of radium. Summary of reports from research centres for 1931.* (1932), p. 6.

assessment of practice. Landsborough Thomson, the Council's assistant secretary, noted this point in a 1937 review of policy:

The suggestion is that the Radium Commission (and presumably the King's Fund for London) should become wholly responsible for the promotion of all *clinical research work* which consists merely in recording the results of different methods of treatment. This responsibility would apply both to the supply of radium and the collation of results. The M.R.C., aided by their Radiology Committee, would then be free to use their radium solely for *fundamental experimental work* and for short-term loans for clinical work of a truly experimental character.[7]

So sensitive was the Council about distinguishing its research from routine radium work that the words 'clinical research work' in the above quotation were replaced with 'clinical inquiries'. This chapter examines the reasons why the Council financed experimental radiological research during the inter-war years, and why the Council wanted to use this policy to distinguish its research work from routine medical practice.

The MRC's early support for research into the medical uses of radium, 1920 – 9

The quotations at the start of this chapter suggest that between 1920 and 1924 the role of experimental research in the Council's programme of studies into the medical uses of radium was unclear. On the one hand, according to Sidney Russ, the secretary of the Radiology Committee, laboratory research would only back up a clinical investigation into the use of radium in the treatment of cancer. On the other hand, the Ministry of Health was informed that biological research would not be limited to studies of cancer. In fact, the bulk of radium was used for clinical research. Thus when the first of the MRC Radiology Committee's annual reports was published for 1923, only 221.4 milligrams of radium bromide were allocated for purely experimental research.[8] Other loans of radium for experimental research had to be shared with clinicians. Often radium could only be used outside of clinical hours, and in quantities and forms compatible with clinical usage. What is more, if accepted by the Radiology Committee, projects were almost always under the

---

[7] MRC 1070: A. Landsborough Thomson, Arrangements for research in radium-therapy, 9 February 1937 (my emphasis).

[8] MRC: *Medical uses of radium. Summary of report from research centres for 1923* (1924). The Council noted that experimental research was also carried out at the Cavendish Laboratory at Cambridge. This radium was, however, something of an exception, being supplied as an attempt to appease the DSIR which was miffed at the MRC's securing the entire quantity of government surplus radium.

aegis of local, medically-dominated radium committees.[9] These local committees oversaw the running of the project, and cared for the radium. In consequence, the bulk of problems tackled by experimentalists were of clinical relevance.[10] Indeed, at least one experimental project was rejected on the ground that it did not form a part of a combined clinical/experimental programme.[11]

At first the Council loaned the entire 5 grams of radium to the Middlesex Hospital for a combined clinical and experimental research project.[12] Hitherto no one had had access to such a large quantity of radium either for experimental or clinical purposes. However, it was impossible to keep all the radium in one place,[13] and after 18 months the unit was broken up and the 5 grams redistributed in fractions to several centres throughout the country, mainly for clinical research.[14] Clinical reasons could not justify maintaining all the radium in one place—perhaps 9 per cent of the entire radium available for medical purposes in the country[15] —and with no clinical reason to keep the 5 grams together the experimental programme ended. Nevertheless, the *Lancet* had noted that the unit provided a sufficiently intense source of radiation to tackle, 'matters of fundamental importance in the field of radio-biology'.[16] Experimental reasons alone could not keep the radium together.

What gave clinicians such a hold over the Council's radium was the enormous cost of the element. The 5 grams cost £72 500 (ie. £14 500 per gram), a huge sum when set against the £76 000 the Council received in its 1919/20 recurrent grant from the Treasury intended to cover all its other research.[17] While prices were coming down—from £36 per milligram in 1914 to £22 per milligram in 1922[18] —the huge cost of radium ensured supplies were limited. Indeed, so scarce was radium that no other comparable quantity of it was available for purely research purposes.

[9] The membership of these local committees is listed in the MRC's annual reports on *The medical uses of radium*, 1924–39.

[10] Experimental radiology funded by the MRC can be found in the MRC *Annual reports*, and the *Medical uses of radium* series.

[11] See MRC 1074/A: discussion on St George's Hospital's application.

[12] The results of this initial research were published in MRC *SRS* 62: *Medical uses of radium. Studies of the effects of gamma rays from a large quantity of radium* (1922).

[13] MRC 1776 I: Russ, memorandum on bomb therapy, 15 March 1933, noted that 'economic pressure and the limited quantities of radium available in the country, led to the splitting up' of the 5 grams allocated to the Middlesex Hospital.

[14] For details of the centres to which radium was allocated see the MRC's annual radium reports *The medical uses of radium*. The original proposals for some of the projects are still available in the MRC's radium files, however their preservation has been somewhat unsystematic.

[15] Supply and distribution of radium, the subcommittee's report (1929). *British Medical Journal*, i, 722–4.

[16] Investigations with a large quantity of radium (1920). *Lancet*, i, 164.

[17] Landsborough Thomson, A. (1973). *Half a century of medical research*, Vol. I, *The origins and policy of the Medical Research Council (UK)*, p 205. HMSO, London.

[18] Commerce in radium (1928). *British Medical Journal*, i, 19–20.

Clinicians also maintained control over radium because of rising post-war public concern about cancer. The Ministry of Health noted in 1923 that in the 20-year period between 1901 to 1921 the mortality rate from cancer had risen 20 per cent. In contrast the general death rate had fallen by 32 per cent, and that of infants by 45 per cent. Even the tuberculosis death rate had fallen by 38 per cent. The Ministry stated that allowing for the ageing of the population, the mortality rate from cancer in England and Wales had trebled in the space of two generations from 0.33 in 1851–60, to 0.97 in 1911–20, to 1.01 in 1921.[19] Such statements prompted widespread anxiety about cancer. This concern was evident in parliamentary questions on the rise in cancer mortality,[20] in newspaper offers of a reward for the cure of cancer,[21] and in renewed philanthropic and state interest in the disease. The Ministry of Health set up a Cancer Advisory Committee in 1922/3, the philanthropic research organization, the British Empire Cancer Campaign, was founded in 1923, and the MRC's own Radiology Committee was set up in 1921.

Rising cancer mortality figures stimulated interest in radium as an alternative and supplement to the mainstay of the medical response to cancer—surgery. Surgery had failed to stem the rise in mortality from the disease. Indeed, some practitioners even blamed it in part for the rise. 'Fresh surgical "triumphs"', wrote one critic, 'had been attended by rapid rises in the death rates of the organs concerned.'[22] To the patient, surgery offered the prospect of a long and painful operation that could leave him/her physically scarred and which would in all probability only extend his/her life for a limited period. Small wonder then if cancer treatment itself raised considerable fear among the public, despite the fact that the prognosis for untreated cancers was very poor. Indeed, advocates of radium therapy regularly claimed that radium entailed less mutilation than surgery. 'The appeal which radium makes to both surgeon and patient is the hope of a cure without disfigurement', said the

[19] Ministry of Health, *On the state of the public health. Annual report of the Chief Medical Officer of Health of the Ministry of Health for the year 1922* (1923). Cancer. Ministry of Health memorandum (Circular 426) (1923). *British Medical Journal*, ii, 421–3.

[20] Medical notes in Parliament. The increase in cancer (1922). *British Medical Journal*, ii, 102; Medical notes in Parliament. Mortality from cancer (1923). *British Medical Journal*, i, 605; Medical notes in Parliament. Cancer mortality (1923). *British Medical Journal*, ii, 39.

[21] Medical news (1922). *British Medical Journal*, i, 171; Prizes for research (1922). *British Medical Journal*, i, 200; Cancer research (1922). *British Medical Journal*, i, 238; Dr Sopie A. Nordhoff-Jung (USA) . . . (1923). *British Medical Journal*, i, 370; Bequests for cancer research (1923). *British Medical Journal*, i, 533; *The Yorkshire Evening News* . . . (1923). *British Medical Journal*, ii, 616; Cancer, its cause and cure (1922). *Lancet*, i, 236–7; Another £10,000 for cancer research (1922). *Lancet*, i, 1111; Prizes for cancer research (1923). *Lancet*, ii, 1214.

[22] Shaw, J. (1923). In, The need for public education in the control of cancer. *British Medical Journal*, i, 509–10, quotation at p. 510.

prominent St Bartholomew's Hospital surgeon C. Gordon-Watson in 1930.[23]

Rising cancer mortality and a scarcity of radium led to an emphasis on clinical research in the MRC's programme for three reasons. First, the Council's radium offered a means of overcoming surgical resistance to radium therapy. Second, and subsequently, increased interest by surgeons in such therapy promoted clinical research to counteract over-eager and incompetent use of radiations. Third, the Council's focus on clinical research was reinforced by the traditional resistance of leading medical practitioners to experimental research. The Council could not justify the allocation of significant quantities of radium to purely experimental work while clinical members of its Radiology Committee were primarily concerned with radium therapy. Indeed, the 1920s were characterized on the one hand by attempts by members of the Radiology Committee to popularize radium therapy among surgeons,[24] and on the other hand by attempts to discourage the entry of inexpert surgeons into radium therapy.

Resistance to radium therapy

First, the Radiology Committee's response to surgical resistance to radium therapy is examined. The 1920s were characterized by a reluctance among a number of surgeons to take up radium therapy. The high cost of radium probably inhibited some local purchases but, in addition, surgeons remained dubious of the value of the therapy. Referring to radiotherapeutic techniques, Victor Bonney, a surgeon at the Middlesex Hospital, claimed in 1925 that, 'it is nonsense blinding ourselves to the hard fact that as methods of cure they are disappointments, and even as means of palliation they leave much to be desired'.[25] When challenged a year later that he placed too much

---

[23] Gordon-Watson, C. (1930). The treatment of cancer of the rectum with radium. *British Medical Journal*, **ii**, 941–4, quotation at p. 941. Of course some mutilation of the tissue occurred in the course of implantation of the radium needles. However, when larger quantities of radium became available in the 1930s, enabling radium to be used at a distance from the body, mutilation was further reduced. Thus the surgeon George Gask noted in a review of the use of a 5-gram unit of radium in 1936, the treatment from this unit would prove to be no better than surgery except from the point of view of mutilation. MRC 1776 II: Note by Edward Mellanby (Secretary of the Council) of a discussion with Gask, 15 October 1936. See also Gordon-Watson, C. (1929). The new importance of radium. *Lancet*, **i**, 1005.

[24] For example the gynaecologist Malcolm Donaldson organized trips to the Paris Radium Institute for interested surgeons. MRC 1082 IV: Donaldson to Fletcher, 22 May 1926. MRC 1082 V: Donaldson to Fletcher, 12 June 1926 and 16 June 1926, and Fletcher to Donaldson 14 June 1926.

[25] Soper, G. A. (1926). *Recent English opinion on cancer. A review of a series of lectures delivered under the auspices of the Fellowship of Medicine, London, 1925*, quotation at p. 32. ASCC, New York.

emphasis on surgery in the treatment of carcinoma of the cervix, Bonney qualified these remarks stating he 'could not make head or tail out of the foreign radium figures and preferred to disregard them until British figures were published in corroboration'.[26] This point about the lack of British figures on the result of radium therapy was echoed in 1927 by another radium-doubter, the Manchester surgeon, William Fletcher Shaw. 'It is', he stated, 'surely not asking very much of British radiology to publish statistics on, at any rate, a five-year basis.'[27] Such figures, he claimed were already available for surgery.[28]

Against this resistance some advocates of radium therapy turned to the MRC, and were appointed to its Radiology Committee.[29] At first they appear to have hoped that by allocating radium to general hospitals the MRC would overcome local problems in purchasing radium. With radium readily available surgeons might have been willing to give up their doubts about the therapy. Indeed, there was much to suggest that radium would be amenable to surgeons. Its application often involved surgical manipulation: a surgery-of-access to open the tumour to the radium; the surgical implantation of tubes or needles containing the radium salt in or near the tumour; and the application of radium to the lymphatic areas draining the tumour which often could not be excised (at least not without massive mutilation).[30] Moreover, few radium enthusiasts advocated the complete replacement of surgery with radiotherapy. Most felt that in operable conditions surgery was the treatment of choice even in cancers where surgery had been least successful, such as cancers of the tongue, oesophagus, and rectum.[31] Radium was generally used in inoperable cases, or in conjunction with

[26] Bonney, V. (1926). Carcinoma of the cervix. *Lancet*, ii, 855–6, quotation at p. 856.

[27] Shaw, W. F. (1927). Treatment of cancer by radium. *British Medical Journal*, ii, 1244.

[28] Fletcher Shaw's comments sparked a controversy in the medical press about the value of surgery (Wertheim's hysterectomy) and radium in the treatment of carcinoma of the cervix. See the correspondence under the heading of 'Treatment of cancer by radium' in *British Medical Journal* (1927), ii, 1054, 1163, 1244, and *British Medical Journal* (1928), i, 75, 159, 197, 286.

[29] During the 1920s the membership of the Committee was the surgeon Cuthbert Wallace (Chairman), Humphrey Rolleston (Physician), S. G. Shattock (Pathologist) (1921–2), C. Thurstan Holland (Radiologist), Robert Knox (Radiologist) (1921–1926), Sidney Russ (Physicist, secretary), A. Burrows (Radiologist) (joined 1923), Malcolm Donaldson (Gynaecologist) (joined 1923), E. Kettle (Pathologist) (joined 1923), F. L. Hopwood (Physicist) (joined 1924), T. Horder (Physician) (joined 1924), A. E. Barclay (Radiologist) (joined 1927) and J. C. Mottram (Pathologist) (joined 1927). Those names without dates were members throughout the 1920s.

[30] For a description of the techniques of using needles or tubes see Cade, S. (1940). *Malignant disease and its treatment by radium*, chap. 2. John Wright & Sons, Bristol, Simpkin Marshall, London. See also Smith, A. B. and Smith, S. M. (1927). Radium and the 'surgery of access'. *British Medical Journal*, ii, 1053.

[31] Radium in cancer of the tongue, oesophagus and rectum (1923). *British Medical Journal*, i, 297–8; Radiotherapy in cancer (1924). *British Medical Journal*, i, 676–7; Radium, cancer, and the public (1928). *British Medical Journal*, ii, 999–1000; Birkett, G. E. (1929). The new importance of radium. *Lancet*, i, 898.

surgery and/or X-rays where the cancer was operable. It could be used to reduce inoperable cancers to operable size, and to diminish the tendency to recurrence (perhaps by stimulating an immune response, aiding the patient's own recuperative powers). Finally, even the most enthusiastic advocates of radium therapy were cautious as to its eventual place in cancer therapy. During the discussion of the radium therapy of carcinoma of the cervix in 1923, the St Bartholomew's gynaecologist, Malcolm Donaldson, thought 'it was much too early to discuss the ultimate value of the treatment'.[32]

As resistance to radium therapy persisted during the 1920s, public criticism mounted against die-hard surgeons' determination to maintain what one critic termed their 'ghastly monopoly' of cancer therapy.[33] Advocates of radium therapy who had turned to the Council were more cautious in their public attacks, distancing themselves from what they felt were excessive claims that radium should take over completely from surgery.[34] Nevertheless, they too felt uneasy with what they saw as surgeons' prejudice against radiotherapy. Thus, the Radiology Committee claimed that although most surgeons stated they did not believe in radiotherapy:

> If they [surgeons] are a little more cautious they would say that in their experience it does no good. The latter is quite a correct statement, because hardly any of them have had any experience of this line of treatment.[35]

As a consequence of this resistance, the Radiology Committee's advocates of radium therapy became disillusioned with providing general hospitals with radium. Thus in 1928 the Radiology Committee recommended the formation of a specialist centre where radium and other promising methods of treating cancer could be explored free from the constraints imposed by surgeons. Surgeons' resistance compounded the difficulties of carrying out research in general hospitals where a paucity of beds for cancer research, a shortage of really keen workers, and poor record keeping and follow-up hindered systematic research. It seemed clear to advocates of radium therapy that a specialist centre was needed especially in radiotherapy where the cost of

---

[32] Donaldson, M. (1923). Radium in carcinoma of the cervix. *British Medical Journal*, i, 151–2, quotation at p. 151.

[33] Radium, cancer, and the public (1928). *British Medical Journal*, ii, 999–1000, quotation at p. 999.

[34] Donaldson, M. (1928). Radium and cancer. *British Medical Journal*, ii, 1008.

[35] MRC 1210 II: proposals for creating a more intensive and efficient research in radiotherapy, 1928 [?]. MRC 1210 is Donaldson's MRC file, and the inclusion of copies of this memorandum in the file suggests that Donaldson was closely involved in its drafting. For other versions of the memorandum see: MRC 1210 II: scheme for promoting more efficient clinical research in cancer, 1927/8 [?]. MRC 1082 VI: suggested outline for a Radiological Centre, 1928.

apparatus was high. If radium were to be distributed over a large number of hospitals it would often remain unused, as many institutions did not receive sufficient cancer patients to justify its continuous use.

A growth of surgical interest in radium therapy

The second impetus to the Council's emphasis upon clinical research that derived from the post-war cancer scare was a product of growing surgical interest in radium therapy. In the late 1920s surgeons began to give up their doubts about radium therapy, and to adopt it in increasing numbers. One radiologist, A. E. Barclay, called this period the 'radium boom',[36] and yet this boom was greeted somewhat sceptically by Radiology Committee advocates of radium therapy. Malcolm Donaldson, one of the prime movers for a specialist cancer centre, complemented his complaints about surgical resistance to radium therapy with attacks on 'die-hard surgeons who are only taking up radium in self-defence'.[37] Those surgeons who now adopted radium therapy, their critics claimed, lacked experience and risked the health of patients and operators. Thus, Fletcher noted in a letter disparaging local attempts to raise money for a gram of radium for use by doctors in Totnes:

Radium used ignorantly is at best useless and at worst may actually stimulate cancerous growth instead of checking it. No doctor, however earnest, has nowadays any right to embark on the use of radium without careful study at first hand of the best methods as these have been worked out during the past years at one or two centres, chiefly abroad.[38]

Fletcher wrote this comment at the beginning of the 1930s, although if anything, concern had been greater when the Council set up its programme. Daniel Serwer has pointed out that the early 1920s were characterized by considerable public worry about the harmful effects of radiation. The deaths of certain prominent radiologists, and concern about the use of radiation in inexperienced hands, prompted the creation of the British X-ray and Radium Protection Committee. This committee was founded by the major radiological and physics professional organizations and the London Radium Institute. It aimed to set out recommendations for the safe use of

---

[36] MRC 2038: Barclay to Fletcher, 5 April 1930.
[37] MRC 84a V: Donaldson to Fletcher, 15 July 1932.
[38] MRC 1074/A: Fletcher to Elmhurst, 12 June 1930.

radiation.[39] While it had no respresentatives on the Protection Committee, the Council appointed the chairman of the protection committee to its Radiology Committee to facilitate liaison between the two.[40]

In the mid-to-late 1920s, advocates of radium therapy who turned to the MRC increasingly used the rhetoric of science to distinguish themselves from the growing numbers of surgeons who took up radium therapy. Barclay, a member of the Radiology Committee, commented cynically:

We see surgeons and gynaecologists rushing across to Brussels and elsewhere and, after a week of observation, returning as experts, writing up a few cases, and imagining they are advancing scientific progress.[41]

Then again, according to Donaldson (another Committee member), surgeons were not only handicapping the advancement of radium therapy by their ignorant resistance to it, but also by their lack of interest in research.

I am not going to suggest for one moment that the work done at Bart's is not extremely good, but I do say that a good deal of the material that goes into a general hospital is wasted, because it is distributed among various members of the staff who are not really interested in research. Again, there are not nearly enough beds. For instance, I could keep all my beds full of malignant disease, which I now send to Mount Vernon; but that would not be fair on the students. Clinical research needs a great number of beds and a special organisation, which I maintain is not possible in any general hospital.[42]

To Donaldson, specialist centres served to circumvent both surgeons who resisted radium therapy, and those who took it up with little interest in research.

Appeals to science became the key response to both surgical resistance and over-enthusiasm to radium therapy. In the first place it formed a response to those surgeons who rejected radium therapy, by suggesting that any failures they experienced in the use of radium were because the laws of its use were not

---

[39] The Membership of the British X-ray and Radium Protection Committee when it was appointed in 1921 was: Humphrey Rolleston, Archibald Reid and Robert Knox (appointed by the British Association of Radiology and Physiotherapy); S. G. Scott and S. Melville (appointed by the Electrotherapeutic Section of the Royal Society of Medicine); Harrison Orton and Cuthbert Andrews (appointed by the Rontgen Society); Sidney Russ (appointed by the Institute of Physics); G. W. C. Kaye (appointed by the National Physical Laboratory); and J. C. Mottram (appointed by the London Radium Institute). For further details of the founding of the Protection Committee see Serwer, D. (1976). *The rise of radiation protection: science, medicine and technology in society, 1896–1935*, Informal Report BNL 22279, Brookhaven National Laboratory.

[40] MRC 1082 I: MRC to Rolleston, 26 November 1921. Sidney Russ, Robert Knox, and J. C. Mottram were also members of both the Radiology Committee and British X-ray and Radium Protection Committee during the inter-war years.

[41] Barclay, A. E. (1929). The new importance of radium. *Lancet*, i, 1061–2, quotation at p. 1061.

[42] MRC 84a V: Donaldson to Fletcher, 15 July 1932.

fully understood. Thus the Radiology Committee noted while presenting the case for a specialized cancer centre that:

Those people who consider radiotherapy useless have not realised that it is not merely an empirical treatment, the dose and duration of application of which are only a matter of taste, but is in reality a vast science, the laws governing which are at present little known, and needing for their elucidation the combined efforts of physicists, biologists, chemists and clinicians.[43]

Secondly, science also served to distinguish Radiology Committee advocates of radium therapy from those who 'imagined' they were advancing science. Increasingly in the late 1920s and 1930s empiricism in radiotherapy was castigated as unscientific and, by implication, the bulk of surgeons who took it up became the butt of such criticism.

There is still an uncomfortable amount of truth in the gibe that the whole of radiology in its radiotherapeutic aspect lacks scientific basis and rests largely on an empirical footing.[44]

Those advocates of radium therapy who turned to the Council responded to this gibe, first by encouraging more systematic descriptions of clinical practice. For example, Donaldson claimed that clinicians seldom realized the importance of accurate descriptions of dosage in radium therapy. Because of differences in the size of tumours and the methods of application, radium dosage could only be calculated by a complicated estimation based on:

the number of hours for which application lasts, the number of mgr. of radium element employed, the number of containers, the thickness of their walls, the nature of the metal of which they are composed, their exact dimensions, and, as far as possible, the disposition of such applicators in relation to the tumour.[45]

Without such descriptions the 'laws' of radium therapy would remain hidden.

Those advocates of radium therapy who turned to the Council also claimed that experimental science would elucidate the laws governing the action of radiation. By the 1930s there were few sites in the body liable to the incidence of malignant disease that the Council felt it had not researched in its radium programme.[46] Its programme had 'helped towards the stabilisation of methods of treatment'[47] while, in contrast,

---

[43] MRC 1210 II: proposals for creating a more intensive and efficient research in radiotherapy 1928 [?].

[44] Radium and research (1931). *Lancet*, **i**, 140–1, quotation at p. 141.

[45] Donaldson, M. (1927). The radium treatment of carcinoma of the cervix since 1921. *St Bartholomew's Hospital Reports*, **60**, 97–111, quotation at p. 100. For a similar earlier comment on the difficulty of measuring dosage by another Radiology Committee member see Burrows, A. (1922). The problem of the radium therapy of cancer. *British Medical Journal*, **ii**, 33–4.

[46] MRC *SRS* 186: *Medical uses of radium* (1933), p. 5.

[47] MRC *SRS* 197: *Medical uses of radium* (1934), quotation at p. 5.

the reaction of tissues to irradiation remained a complex and bewildering topic.

The main problem in radiotherapy was to impose maximal damage to the tumour tissues, with minimal damage to the surrounding normal tissues. While clinical research had led to some understanding of the sensitivities of normal and pathological tissues to radiation, experimental research promised answers to a whole variety of related problems. How might radiation procure immunity to cancer, alter the radiosensitivity of tumours, affect different types of tissues, or stimulate cancer growth? What was the effect of variations in the wavelength, intensity, doses and combinations of the three on the biological effect? What stage in the life of a cell was its most radiosensitive? What was the latent period in a cell following irradiation before a biological effect became apparent?[48] For many experimentalists, however, the only way they could hope to answer these questions was to distance themselves from clinical work. Thus in 1933 the experimental radiologist, F. G. Spear, then a member of the Radiology Committee, noted in a prize-winning essay that,

we must not be afraid, for the time being, of losing sight of the patient in his bed in order that, armed with a scientific basis for our methods we may return to him with ultimate hope of his deliverance.[49]

Unfortunately for those who wanted to distinguish science from routine day-to-day practice the relationship between science and medicine was then the subject of heated dispute.

Experimental research and medicine

The third reason why the Council favoured clinical research in its 1920s radium programme resulted from the traditional resistance of leading medical practitioners to experimental research. Historians have charted the

---

[48] For contemporary British overviews of experimental radiology see Colwell, H. A. and Russ, S. (1924). *Radium X-rays and the living cell* (2nd edn). G. Bell and Sons, London; Colwell, H. A. and Wakeley, C. P. G. (1926). *An introduction to the study of X-rays and radium*. Humphrey Milford/Oxford University Press, London and Oxford; Colwell, H. A. (1935). *The method of action of radium and X-rays on living cells*. Oxford University Press/Humphrey Milford, Oxford and London; Scott, C. M. (1937). *Some quantitative aspects of the biological action of X-rays and gamma rays*. HMSO, London.

[49] Spear, F. G., Canti, R. G., Grimmett, L. G., Holmes, B., Cox, S. F., and Love, W. H. [?] (1933). *The biological effects and mode of action of radiations upon malignant and other cells*. Unpublished manuscript. This essay was submitted for the British Empire Cancer Campaign's Garton Prize in 1933. A note pasted into the cover states that although the prize itself was awarded to the King's College Hospital radiologist, H. A. Colwell, Spear and his colleagues were given an additional award for their essay. I am grateful to Mrs G. M. Carpenter for the loan of a copy of this manuscript.

difficult entry of experimental physiology into nineteenth-century English medicine. Anti-vivisection, the natural theology tradition, a long established preference for anatomy over physiology, and the low regard in which the life sciences were held all served to hinder the introduction of experimental research into medicine.[50] Among senior physicians and surgeons this hostility persisted until well into the twentieth century,[51] and the creation of the Medical Research Committee in 1913 gave it a new focus.

The Medical Research Committee, and its reconstituted successor, the MRC, represented the success of pre-clinical scientists and their clinical allies in advancing their control of State funding for medical research. The powerful secretary of the Committee/Council, Walter Fletcher, was an intellectual child of Foster's Physiology Laboratory, and both experimental and clinical scientists were strongly represented in the membership on both.[52] Under its original constitution the Medical Research Committee had nominally been responsible to a much larger body (the Advisory Council for Research) representative of different lay and medical interests. In fact the Committee maintained considerable autonomy from the Advisory Council, and this was recognized officially when the Committee was reconstituted in 1920 as the MRC. The new Council was responsible only to the Privy Council, an arrangement which ensured the Council's independence from the leaders of medical practice.[53] Unfortunately for the Council its leaning towards the experimental sciences sparked controversy with leaders of medical practice, especially the Royal College of Physicians and Surgeons.[54]

---

[50] French, R. D. (1971). Some problems in the foundations of modern physiology in Great Britain. *History of Science*, **10**, 28–55; French, R. D. (1975). *Anti-vivisection and medical science in Victorian society*. Princeton University Press, NJ; Lansbury, C. (1985). *The old brown dog: women, workers and vivisection in Edwardian England*. University of Wisconsin Press, Madison; Lansbury, C. (1985). Gynaecology, pornography, and the anti-vivisection movement. *Victorian Studies*, **28**, 413–37; Rupke, N. (ed.) (1987). *Vivisection in historical perspective*. Croom Helm, London; Geison, G. (1972). Social and institutional factors in the stagnation of English physiology, 1850–1870. *Bulletin of the History of Medicine*, **46**, 30–58; Geison, G. (1975). *Michael Foster and the Cambridge School of Physiology: the scientific enterprise in late Victorian society*. Princeton University Press, NJ; Cannon, S. F. (1978). *Science in culture: the early Victorian period*, pp. 272, 274. Dawson and Science History Publications, New York.

[51] Lawrence, C. (1985). Incommunicable knowledge: science, technology and the clinical art in Britain 1850–1914. *Journal of Contemporary History*, **20**, 503–20, quotation at p. 505; Lawrence, C. (1985). Moderns and ancients: the 'new cardiology' in Britain 1880–1930. In *The Emergence of modern cardiology, Medical History supplement No 5* (ed. W. F. Bynum, C. Lawrence, and V. Nutton). Wellcome Institute for the History of Medicine, London.

[52] For a list of the members of the MRC and its forerunner see, Landsborough Thomson, *Medical research*, Vol. I, Appendix H (see note 17).

[53] Landsborough Thomson, *Medical research*, Vol. I, Chaps. 2 and 5 (see note 17).

[54] I refer here to the English Colleges, as led by their presidents Lord Dawson of Penn (Physicians) and Lord Moynihan (Surgeons). Before becoming President of the Royal College of Physicians in 1931, Dawson was also President of the Royal Society of Medicine. In addition, he was President of the BMA in 1932. In these capacities Dawson also came into conflict with the MRC, and especially its secretary Walter Fletcher.

In view of the shortage of radium in the country, this controversy perhaps encouraged an emphasis on clinical research in the 1920s as the MRC sought to legitimate its acquisition of radium.

To the Royal Colleges the MRC seemed the institutional embodiment of the divide between practitioners and researchers. Lord Dawson, President of the Royal College of Physicians, complained to Fletcher that the Council tended to look down on men in practice as 'high-brows' looking down on 'low-brows'.[55] Similarly, Lord Moynihan, President of the Royal College of Surgeons, argued that the MRC tended to divorce medical research from practice to the detriment of both.[56] Moynihan argued that the advance of medicine was impeded by what he termed the 'truancy of physiology'.[57] Both rounded on Fletcher, blaming his prejudice against clinical practice for much of the problem.[58]

Underlying Dawson's and Moynihan's differences with Fletcher was a radically different concept of science. On the one hand, Fletcher tended to differentiate science from clinical practice, especially when discussing experimental and clinical science and the patronage of medical research. Fletcher believed that both clinical and experimental science had been hindered by their close association with clinical medicine, and that, consequently, medical research should be taken out of the hands of clinicians. In contrast, for both Moynihan and Dawson, science was very much a part of routine everyday practice. Indeed, to Moynihan the MRC was marked by its weakness in routine practice. He informed Fletcher that he could, 'see no hope for the advance of medicine until the M.R.C. is reconstituted'.[59] Of its twelve members:

only one, and he the most recent appointment (the very best possible) possesses any adequate knowledge of scientific clinical surgery; one only practises medicine, and his very able mind sways rather to the laboratory than to the wards.[60]

To both Moynihan and Dawson routine practitioners could engage in science, and consequently they opposed attempts to distance medical

---

[55] MRC PF100/18: Dawson to Fletcher, 15 December 1932 and 13 February 1933, Fletcher to Dawson, 21 November 1932 and 9 January 1933. At this time Dawson was also a member of the MRC. Fletcher was thus working against a member of the Council of which he was secretary.

[56] The hospital for tropical diseases (1930). *British Medical Journal*, ii, 927–8; Lord Moynihan (1930). The work of laboratories. *British Medical Journal*, ii, 979, 1103–4; Fletcher, W. (1930). The work of laboratories. *British Medical Journal*, ii, 1022–3. Fletcher and Moynihan also carried out a private battle over their correspondence in the medical journals, see MRC PF100/C.

[57] Lord Moynihan (1930). The science of medicine. An address delivered at the opening of the Banting Research Institute of the University of Toronto. *Lancet*, ii , 779–85, quotation at p. 783.

[58] MRC PF100/18: Dawson to Fletcher, 15 December 1932; MRC PF100/C: Moynihan to Fletcher, 6 January 1931.

[59] MRC PF100/C: Moynihan to Fletcher, 6 January 1931.

[60] Lord Moynihan (1930). Surgery in the immediate future. *British Medical Journal*, ii, 612–4, quotation at p. 614.

research from clinical practice. Thus they were uneasy about demands to liberate clinical research from practice and found this MRC advocacy problematic.

MRC proposals to create specialist centres of clinical research were not limited to radium therapy. One of the leading lights of clinical science, Thomas Lewis, noted that 'the almost constant association between clinical research work and the opportunistic atmosphere of practical or curative medicine'[61] was responsible for an endemic low standard of thought and work in clinical research. He persuaded the MRC to announce in its 1928/9 annual report that it intended to improve the career structure in clinical research by creating several new posts.[62] However, to the Colleges such statements seemed to confirm the MRC's disdain for the clinical practitioner. What is more, the Colleges' worries were reinforced by the simultaneous creation of the Medical Research Society (MRS) by Lewis. While the MRS aimed to promote clinical research and to facilitate closer co-operation between clinicians and experimental scientists, the Colleges feared that this co-operation would be at the expense of routine practitioners.[63]

Finally, the Colleges were alarmed by what they felt was an increasing willingness on the part of the State to ignore them in major policy decisions. Dawson was annoyed that the Ministry of Health had, in his view, largely ignored the medical profession in the Local Government Act of 1929. The upshot of these concerns was that the Colleges attempted to re-assert their leadership in medicine. Thus, Dawson and Moynihan persuaded the Ministry to appoint a Medical Advisory Committee in 1929 to ensure regular consultation between it and medical profession.[64] In addition, both tried to bring the Council into line. For example, angered by what seemed to him the hijacking by clinical and experimental science of State funding for medical research, Dawson noted in 1932 that medical science—by which he meant the basic sciences, medicine, surgery, obstetrics, education, and administration—should be co-ordinated by the Colleges. This co-ordination would, he hoped, bring the profession into the sphere of national policy-making.[65]

---

[61] CMAC GC/42/9: Lewis to Fletcher, 31 May 1929.

[62] MRC: *Annual report 1928–9* (1930). For Lewis and his associates attempts to persuade the MRC and the Rockefeller Foundation to establish departments of clinical medical and surgery see CMAC GC/41/9, GC/42/10, PP/LEW/D1/7, PP/LEW/D1/8, PP/LEW/D1/9, and PP/LEW/D2/1.

[63] The opposition of the physicians Sir John Rose Bradford and Lord Dawson of Penn (Presidents of the Royal College of Physicians 1926–31 and 1931 onwards respectively) to the formation of the Medical Research Society is noted in CMAC PP/LEW/D1/7: T. Lewis, 'Discussion and correspondence relating to clinical research. Part III. Article to *British Medical Journal* and events leading to the formation of the Medical Research Society'.

[64] PRO MH71/4, MH71/5, and MH71/6. These files on the Ministry of Health's Medical Advisory Committee provide details of Dawson and Moynihan's worries.

[65] Lord Dawson (1932). One hundred years and after. *British Medical Journal*, ii, 183–9.

Such a view was anathema to Fletcher and, at the turn of the 1920s, he and the Royal Colleges came into conflict. Fletcher fought back by suggesting that the Royal Colleges represented only a limited section of the medical profession—leading medical practitioners—and thus a limited view of medicine. They were alienated from scientists and unfit to co-ordinate research. Indeed, he argued, only the MRC could assume a co-ordinating role. He explained his position to Dawson:

I think you err (perhaps unconsciously) in thinking of the 'profession' as represented only by leaders in practice, whereas it truly includes all practitioners and hygienists as well as all the investigators in all the numerous fields of curative and preventive medicine, of scientific work in genetics, laboratory biology, statistics, sociology, and psychology, not yet brought into practical life. The M.R.C. covers the whole of these fields, and, while primarily aiding investigators as such, must be in close relation to the practitioners, whether doctors or officers of health and others, who bring results of investigation into practical value. You give me the impression that you have no vision of this width. The M.R.C. is the only instrument by which all the strength of the medical workers of every kind can be focussed in a common aim. . . . You are tending to make a cleavage in the unity of 'medicine' by claiming a dominance over it instead of a partnership—senior partnership if you like—in it.[66]

One of the examples with which Fletcher chose to illustrate his point was Dawson and Moynihan's recent involvement in an 'expert committee' set up by them to evaluate the use of radium 'bombs'—the use of large quantities of radium at a distance from the body. First, Fletcher asked why Dawson and Moynihan were members of the committee at all—'Neither of you would claim any expert knowledge of radium or has any first-hand knowledge of its uses and dangers'.[67] Secondly, he asked why their names were listed above that of the chairman, the cancer surgeon H. S. Souttar, a leading expert in the use of radium. It seemed to Fletcher that this incident illustrated both Dawson's and Moynihan's divisive effect on medicine and science, and their unwillingness to allow experts to develop radium therapy. In contrast, to Dawson and Moynihan radium represented part of the Council's threat to their leadership in medicine, and its encroachment on medical practice.

An expansion in experimental research, 1929–39

Just as the debate with the Colleges reached its climax, the Council announced it was expanding its experimental research into the medical uses of radium.[68] This was a curious pronouncement for not only did it appear to exacerbate its difficulties with the Colleges—Dawson and Moynihan had

---

[66] MRC PF100/18: Fletcher to Dawson, 9 January 1933.
[67] Ibid.
[68] MRC *SRS* 174 (see note 6).

complained that the Council was too committed to experimental research—but it also seemed that it might cause conflict with the growing numbers of surgeons who were taking up radium therapy. As demand for radium grew it might have been expected that the Council would come under increased pressure to allocate more radium for clinical purposes. But it did not. First, radium supplies increased dramatically in 1929–30 and, second, control of State-owned radium was divided between two organizations, the Council, which controlled that allocated for research, and the newly formed Radium Trust and Commission, which controlled that allocated for routine purposes. These developments fostered an expansion of experimental research in the 1930s.

In fact the division in control of radium developed out of the Dawson/Moynihan/Fletcher controversy. Realizing the demand for radium was growing rapidly, the Government had appointed a subcommittee of the Committee of Civil Research in 1928 to determine the radium needs of the nation.[69] The Committee reported in 1929, recommending the immediate purchase of 20 grams of radium for medical purposes, and the creation of a National Radium Commission to distribute the element.[70] However, the Royal Colleges had not been present at the early negotiations, and their exclusion heightened fears of a State challenge to their leadership in medicine. Dawson informed Fletcher that, 'The only reasonable conclusion was that you wished this report to go through without the prior knowledge of, or a consultation with, the leaders of the profession.'[71] Immediately, comments appeared in the medical press warning of the dire consequences for the future of the Commission of this lack of consultation.[72]

Once the report was out, the Colleges acted quickly to secure control of the Commission. Prompted by news that the Government was to announce its intention shortly, Dawson collected signatures from prominent members of the medical profession pointing out the need for consultation. *The Times*, through which the Government was to raise half the money by appeal, supported Dawson and refused to launch the campaign without the Colleges' co-operation.[73] Faced with this opposition, the Minister of Health agreed to call an informal conference at which he accepted, in the words of the President of the Royal College of Physicians, a majority of clinicians 'cognisant of the problems daily met with in the practical treatment of

[69] On the Committee for Civil Research see Macleod, R. M. and Andrews, E. K. (1969). The Committee of Civil Research: scientific advice for economic development 1925–1930. *Minerva*, **7**, 680–705; Howson, S. and Winch, D. (1977). *The Economic Advisory Council 1930–1939*, Cambridge University Press.
[70] Supply and distribution of radium. The sub-committee's report (1929). *British Medical Journal*, **i**, 722–4.
[71] MRC 2110/8: Dawson to Fletcher, 11 April 1929.
[72] *British Medical Journal* (1929), **i**, 695; *Lancet* (1929), **i**, 834–5.
[73] MRC 2110/8: Dawson (Editor of *The Times*) to Robinson, 15 April 1929.

disease' on the Commission.[74] With some justification a Ministry official later complained that the medical profession deprived the Ministry of any control over the use of radium, ensuring an absolute majority of six of their appointees on the Commission.[75]

The MRC in fact came off somewhat better than the Ministry. The Commission handed over its research function to the Council, and made an immediate loan of 1 gram of the element for this purpose.[76] This allocation suggests that it was not the nuts and bolts of radiological practice that divided the practitioner-dominated Commission and the research-orientated MRC. Rather, differences reflected fears about the domination of research, and its consequent political implications.

To the Colleges, the MRC had symbolized the encroachment of the State on their leadership in medicine. Fletcher had been on the Radium Committee when the medical profession had been excluded, and had been in the Minister's team when the profession met the Minister to complain about lack of consultation. What is more, the Council had embodied a threat to their leadership in radium therapy. Fletcher had informed Dawson before the report came out that at 'this state of knowledge the estimates of the "research needs" [for radium] are practically identical with those of "treatment needs" '.[77] To Fletcher, the experts who should develop radium therapy in the future were those who, throughout the 1920s, had been supported by the Council. Outside the Continental centres, these experts alone had carried out systematic research into radium therapy, and it seemed as if the Commission would ignore them. Thus, soon after the Minister met the representatives of the practitioner organizations, the prominent radiologist A. E. Barclay complained that it now seemed that 'those who have done the spade work, those who are experts in these methods, are hardly represented'[78] on the Commission.

---

[74] MRC 2110/8 includes the minutes of the meeting between the Minister and the representatives of the medical profession. The medical profession was represented by Lord Moynihan (President of the Royal College of Surgeons), Lord Dawson (President of the Royal Society of Medicine), Sir John Rose Bradford (President of the Royal College of Physicians), Sir Ewen Maclean (President of the BMA), Sir Farquhar Buzzard (Regius Professor of Medicine, Oxford), Sir Humphrey Rolleston (Regius Professor of Medicine, Cambridge), Sir Alexander Miles (President of the Royal College of Surgeons, Edinburgh), and R. A. Fleming (President of the Royal College of Physicians, Edinburgh). The Minister was accompanied by the Permanent Secretary (Sir Arthur Robinson), the Chief Medical Officer (George Newman), an assistant secretary (Michael Heseltine) and Walter Fletcher.

[75] PRO MH58/151: Robinson to Rucker, 26 January 1932.

[76] For an outline of the Radium Commission's programme see: Spear, F. G. and Griffiths, K. (1951). *The Radium Commission. A short history of its origin and work, 1929–1948.* HMSO, London. The Radium Commission offered to loan the MRC the radium in 1930, and the MRC finally accepted it the following year. MRC 1585 I: Russ to Fletcher, 9 December 1930, and Extract of Medical Research Council Meeting, 17 July 1931.

[77] MRC 2110/8: Fletcher to Dawson, 13 April 1929.

[78] Barclay A. E. (1929). The new importance of radium. *Lancet*, i, 1061–2, quotation at p. 1062.

With the threat to the Colleges' leadership in radium therapy out of the way, the Commission could loan the MRC radium without compromising the leadership of medicine. Indeed, with the bulk of radium in the country under its control, the Radium Commission soon became the focus for the new specialty of radiotherapy. It allocated radium to various centres throughout the country (except London which was covered by the King Edward's Hospital Fund for London) under similar conditions to those imposed by the MRC on its centres. At these centres it required 'radium officers' to be appointed, trained in radium therapy and responsible for the work of the centres. Initially under the supervision of consultant surgeons and gynaecologists, these radium officers developed from the status of house officers to that of consultant staff, and eventually formed the backbone of radiotherapeutic practitioners.[79] Each centre, moreover, was required to establish a records and follow-up department and eventually to appoint a full-time physicist. The physicist gradually took over the care and custody of the radium from the radium officer.[80] Finally, the Commission also promoted radiotherapy by instituting postgraduate radiotherapy training at the Mount Vernon Hospital and Radium Institute in 1930, and by encouraging the unification of radium and X-ray therapy under a radiotherapist familiar with both, separate from diagnostic radiology.

In fact, Barclay probably overemphasized the extent to which the Commission ignored those who had done the spadework of British radium therapy. Many members of the Radiology Committee were also members of the Commission. Indeed, the surgeon Cuthbert Wallace who chaired the Committee also organized the Commission's training course in radiotherapy. The formation of the Commission in 1929 simply marked the division already extant between radium research and radium practice, and the Council was left free to expand its experimental research programme.

Indeed to the Council, experimental research became a crucial way of distinguishing its work from the systematic monitoring of practice adopted by the Commission. It was a moot point whether systematic record keeping constituted research or practice. Until the creation of the Commission, clinical research and routine record keeping had been largely co-extensive under the Council's radium research programme. However, immediately on its formation, the Commission, in collaboration with the Council, the British Empire Cancer Campaign (BECC) and the King's Fund, drew up a standardized radium record form for use at all its centres. Subsequently in 1932, the Commission appointed a registrar under whose direction annual statistics were compiled from the summary cards received from its centres. By July 1937 some 40 000 follow-up cards were in the Commission's files, and

[79] Spear, F. G. and Griffiths, K. *The Radium Commission* (see note 76).
[80] Ibid.

the total was increasing at the rate of 10 000 a year.[81] The Council could not compete with statistical research on this scale and, as noted at the start of this chapter, in the same year (1937) Landsborough Thomson suggested that the Council should abandon such 'inquiries' to the Commission and turn instead to experimental research.

Now that clinical resources had shifted to the Commission, experimental scientists felt somewhat freer to flex their muscles within the Council. Thus, between 1930 and 1933 representatives of physiology, biochemistry, and of tissue culture research joined the Radiology Committee.[82] Pathology alone had represented the laboratory sciences on the Radiology Committee before then,[83] and the inclusion of the three additional pre-clinical sciences represented the culmination of a long struggle to expand such research. The result was that in 1931 the Radiology Committee recommended that the Commission's radium should be allocated for experimental research. Muriel Robertson at the Lister Institute was allocated 400 milligrams for work on the protozoon *Bodo caudatus*. The Surgical Research Department at Edinburgh University got 70 milligrams for research into the effects of radium radiation on the normal tissues of rabbits. Three hundred and fifty milligrams were also allocated to the Strangeways Research Laboratory for studies into the effects of radiation on cell division in tissue cultures. At the same time the Committee recommended that 30 milligrams of the Council's own radium should go to the Department of Physiology at Edinburgh for experiments on the calcium and inorganic phosphorus concentrations in the blood. Four hundred and twenty-five milligrams of the Council's radium was to be held in reserve for experimental purposes.[84]

The basis for an expansion of experimental research

During the 1920s the Council had laid the foundations for the expansion of experimental research by adopting three main strategies to fend off practitioner control of scientific research. In the first place it had challenged practitioner attempts to tap philanthropists for funds for medical research. This was most evident in the case of the BECC which had been started by a

---

[81] Ibid.

[82] The physiologists A. V. Hill and B. McSwiney, and the biochemist E. K. Rideal joined the Radiology Committee in 1931. The experimental radiologist, F. G. Spear, who specialized in research on the effects of radiations on cells grown in tissue culture, joined the Committee in 1933. For letters of invitation see MRC 1082 VIII: Landsborough Thomson to Russ, 16 March 1931; MRC 1082 IX: Landsborough Thomson to Spear, 3 April 1933.

[83] op. cit. note 29. The pathologist J. C. Mottram had been the recipient of the 221.4 milligrams of radium bromide allocated for experimental research alone.

[84] MRC 1082 VIII: radium: proposed allocations, 5 March 1931. For details of the projects see MRC 1074/R (Robertson), MRC 1074/T (Surgical Research Dept.), MRC 1074/Q (Sharpey Schafer) and MRC 1074/U (Strangeways).

small group of London doctors. To Fletcher, the BECC embodied the way in which leading medical practitioners could tap their patients for resources in a way that laboratory scientists could not.

It does not have to be fought so much in other countries, but in England, the Court and the Ministries and the newspaper proprietors are apt to get their ideas of medical science from the successful practitioners with whom they come in personal contact, and to whom they may feel indebted for personal services.[85]

In contrast, Fletcher felt the Campaign showed how such medical practitioners misrepresented science. The founders of the BECC wanted to develop a frontal assault on cancer, aimed at finding the cause of the disease as a prelude to finding a cure. To Fletcher this statement showed a fundamental misunderstanding of science, for laboratory scientists could not at this time find the cause—in the BECC's scheme a cure would be years away.[86] In contrast, Fletcher argued that, first, research should not be limited to cancer but should involve basic research in all the fields that looked as if they might give clues as to problems of cancer.[87] Second, he also suggested that the cure for cancer might come through radiotherapy before the cause was found. In this way he legitimated the Council's existing policy of funding clinical research in radium therapy—at a time when surgeons still questioned its efficacy—and laid out the reasons for future expansion of basic radiological research.

Through some deft political manoeuvring, Fletcher persuaded the BECC to accept what amounted to a scientific (MRC/Royal Society) veto on the BECC's Scientific Advisory Committee (SAC)—the SAC was to advise the BECC on its research policy, and all questions relating to research were to be submitted to it. The SAC had a membership of ten, of whom eight could be scientists. Of the eight, five were appointed by the MRC and the Royal Society, and a maximum of three by the Campaign itself. However, the MRC persuaded the Campaign that its three appointees should be selected in consultation with the Council and the Royal Society which, as guarantors of scientific credibility, could block any members they disagreed with. In this way Fletcher hoped that the Council would be able to control the Campaign's scientific policy by keeping anyone it opposed off the SAC. The Campaign could not even register a protest by appointing whom it liked into the minority.[88]

---

[85] MRC 1383 Vol II: Fletcher to Robinson, 28 July 1923.

[86] In 1923 the MRC complained that the clinicians who created the British Empire Cancer Campaign wanted laboratory scientists to mount what it felt was an inappropriate 'frontal assault' on the disorder. It felt that the time was not ripe for a direct assault on the cause of cancer. Laboratory work in biochemistry, immunology, cytology and virology could not, the Council felt, mount such an attack. MRC 1383 I: the proposed British Empire Cancer Campaign, 25 May 1923.

[87] MRC 1383 IV (see note 5).

[88] Fletcher lauded his triumph in the issue of the membership of the SAC in a letter to Lord Goschen, 19 January 1924 (MRC 1383/1b Vol. I).

What is more, Fletcher also persuaded the BECC to devote most of the income it received in its first year to radiotherapy, and to accept the MRC's Radiology Committee as its advisory committee on radiological matters. The BECC provided the Council with an extra 800 milligrams of radium. It also agreed to finance the building and running of the Council's Radon Centre at the Middlesex Hospital, and the salary of a radiologist to run a deep X-ray therapy centre at St Bartholomew's Hospital. While at the time this agreement enabled the Council to expand its clinical programme of research, it also laid the basis for the future expansion of experimental research. In persuading the BECC to accept the Radiology Committee as its advisory Committee, Fletcher made it clear that the Committee was not to be limited to cancer research. Rather it should support fundamental research into the biological action of radiation.

The second strategy which enabled the MRC to fend off practitioner control was to move major centres of laboratory research away from the London hospitals to the universities, independent research institutes, and to its own research centre, the National Institute for Medical Research. In those fields that impinged on radiology—physiology, pathology, biochemistry, and tissue culture work—the MRC attempted to secure an independent academic base for each to counter clinician influence. Physiology had been established in Cambridge since the nineteenth century, and Fletcher saw that department as the model to follow in the other pre-clinical sciences. Robert Kohler has indicated how Fletcher tried to free biochemistry from physiology, helping Hopkins to set up a biochemistry department in Cambridge with the aid of money from the Dunn Trustees.[89] Similarly, Fletcher also secured Dunn monies for pathology, believing it to be hindered by its close association with routine diagnosis. Thus he persuaded the Dunn Trustees to provide £100 000 for a new School of Pathology (and Pharmacology) in Oxford; £10 000 to build and equip a laboratory for the University Clinic at St Thomas's Hospital, London; £10 000 for the same object at St Bartholomew's Hospital, London; and £5000 for the enlargement of the existing laboratory at the London Hospital.[90]

In tissue culture research the MRC supported the Cambridge Research Hospital (after 1929 the Strangeways Research laboratory) with a block grant intended primarily for exploring the effects of radiations on cells grown in tissue cultures. In addition, in 1929 it provided a special grant to the Strangeways to build a new radiological laboratory, and in the following 2 years was instrumental in facilitating a joint Cambridge Radiotherapy Scheme. This scheme comprised a co-ordinated programme of research

[89] Kohler, R. (1978). Walter Fletcher, F. G. Hopkins and the Dunn Institute of Biochemistry: a case study of patronage in science. *Isis*, **69**, 331–55.
[90] MRC PF250/1A: Fletcher to Pearce, 25 October 1923.

between the Strangeways and a number of university departments—physiology, pathology, biochemistry, physics, medical radiology, and the Cold Temperature Station. Essentially, this scheme aimed to apply the results of the tissue culture research carried out in the 1920s to animals and to patients undergoing radiotherapy.[91]

The third strategy the Council adopted to fend off practitioner control of medical research was to use clinical scientists as a buffer between medical practitioners and laboratory scientists. In this strategy, it tried to encourage close co-operation between experimental scientists and clinicians with an interest in research. Elsewhere, it has been shown that the Council facilitated such co-operation between Malcolm Donaldson and the Strangeways Research Laboratory, enabling Donaldson to incorporate ideas and techniques from the Strangeways tissue culture research into clinical practice. Similar co-operation occurred at other major centres, notably the Middlesex Hospital and King's College Hospital. Indeed, at these centres and at St Bartholomew's, clinicians themselves often carried out some of the experimental research. Nevertheless, some clinicians felt that the Council placed too much emphasis on experimental research, and it is noticeable that once the Commission was formed, proposals for a specialist cancer centre sponsored by the Council were dropped.

Conclusion

It was the loan of the Radium Commission's 1 gram of radium that enabled the MRC to expand its experimental research. Its original radium was mostly tied up in existing projects. This was the largest amount of radium allocated for purely experimental purposes by the MRC. Hitherto, what radium had been distributed for experimental research had also been used largely for clinical studies. Ironically, however, the expansion of experimental research was still largely determined by clinical considerations. First, the Council had only expanded its experimental radiology programme once supplies of radium for clinical practice had increased. While radium had been limited, clinicians had had first claim over research supplies. Experimental research had been swamped by clinical desires to encourage interest in radium therapy and to improve standards of practice, and by the traditional hostility to experimental radiology. It had been clinical demand for radium that had improved supplies for experimental research.

Second, in the final instance clinicians still determined the physical conditions of radiation available to experimentalists. Just as research on the

[91] The Strangeways research programme and its relationship with clinical practice is discussed in Cantor, D. (1988). From research to routine: tissue culture radiobiology and experimental medicine in inter-war Britain. A paper given at the Annual Meeting of the American Association for the History of Medicine, New Orleans, 4–7 May 1988. Manuscript available from the author.

intensity factor had ended in 1920 when the Middlesex 5 grams was broken up, so too it ended abruptly when a 4 gram unit at the Westminster Hospital was broken up in 1931. Clinical reasons alone determined whether large quantities of radium could be held together in one place. Whether in 1920 or 1930, experimental reasons alone could not justify the maintenance of several grams together in one place.[92]

Third, experimental research had expanded because of the split in control of radium for research and radium for practice. While the Council had tried to develop the institutional foundations of experimental research during the 1920s, it was only the creation of the Radium Commission that enabled experimental work to develop. The Commission had been the product of a resurgence of practitioner attempts to assert their leadership in medicine, and the expansion of experimental research depended on these doctors. Clinicians had not (as experimentalists claimed) been opposed to experimental research *per se*, rather they had feared its political implications. Under the wing of the Council, experimentalists seemed to be defining medical research in ways that doctors feared would facilitate research of little value to clinical practice. They also feared that it would enable advocates of radium therapy to determine standards of medical practice independent of the leading professional organizations.

Finally, the Council still relied on sympathetic clinicians to support its experimental research. Research at the major centres of experimental research—the Middlesex Hospital, the Radium Institute, King's College Hospital and the Strangeways—was still largely carried out by clinicians or with their close co-operation. Elsewhere I have shown that these clinicians incorporated techniques and ideas developed in the laboratory into clinical practice. To these clinicians, laboratory practices symbolized claims to expertise that distanced them from the routine medical practitioner.[93]

Acknowledgements

I would like to thank the archivists at the CMAC, the MRC, the Middlesex Hospital, and the PRO for their help in this paper. The thesis from which this paper was derived was supported financially by a University of Lancaster Senate Studentship, and by a studentship from the (then) Science Research Council (No. 80302610). For help and encouragement I am also indebted to Mary Fissell.

---

[92] Cantor, D. (1987). The definition of radiobiology: the Medical Research Council's support for research into the biological effects of radiation in Britain, 1919–1939. Unpublished PhD thesis, Lancaster University.

[93] Cantor, From research to routine (see note 91).

10

Clinical research

CHRISTOPHER C. BOOTH

From its earliest days, the Medical Research Committee sought to encourage not only disinterested or 'pure' science, but also clinical research and experimental medicine. The Committee acknowledged in 1918 'the urgent importance of using the resources of the Medical Research Fund to forward the science of experimental medicine and its study at the bedside, in close conjunction with all the resources of the modern laboratory'.[1] Its endeavours to foster clinical research, however, were to be constrained from the outset by the lack of an effective university base in experimental medicine. For this reason, in describing the efforts of the MRC in the clinical field it is necessary to consider not only the activities of the Council but also to examine what steps were being taken to develop clinical academic departments in the medical schools at the time.

In 1913, there were only a few individuals, for example Sir Archibald Garrod and Thomas (later Sir Thomas) Lewis, whose scientific work in the clinical field was of outstanding merit. There were no full-time professors in clinical subjects in the medical schools and, in striking contrast to the situation in Germany, no traditions of clinical experimental work in the universities. Since his arrival in Oxford from Johns Hopkins Hospital in 1907, Sir William Osler, Regius Professor of Medicine in the University of Oxford, had been scathing in his condemnation of the state of affairs in British medical schools. Like others of his colleagues who had founded the Johns Hopkins School of Medicine in 1889, he had been deeply impressed by the medical academic scene in Germany. It had been this German influence that had played so important a role in the development of the hugely successful Johns Hopkins Medical School, where with William Welch, William Halsted, Kelly and Franklin Mall, he had had the opportunity 'to blaze a perfectly new road, untrammelled by tradition, vested interest or medical dead wood'.[2] In 1911 Osler gave evidence to the Royal Commission on University Education in London. Like the eminent American Abraham Flexner, who had given his evidence earlier, Osler had no hesitation in condemning the London Medical Schools, which had no clinical laboratory

---

[1] MRC: *Annual report 1918–19* (1919), p. 28.
[2] Cushing, H. (1925). *The life of Sir William Osler*, Vol. 2, p. 314. Clarendon Press, Oxford.

base, little or no link with the university, and no paid staff. In Oxford he bewailed the fact that there was no clinical school whatever. He concluded that the only solution was 'an active invasion of the hospitals by the Universities'. It was this evidence together with the testimony of Flexner and that of the distinguished University College physiologist, E. H. Starling, that led to the Commission's recommendation in 1913 to develop academic professorial units in the London Medical Schools.[3] In helping to promote these units, the work of the Medical Research Committee in clinical research, and of its successor the MRC, was to be complementary to that of the universities and medical schools.

Clinical research received serious consideration by the Medical Research Committee at its earliest meetings. Its original members included the distinguished Regius Professor of Physic from the University of Cambridge, Sir Clifford Allbutt, and C. T. Bond, a Leicester surgeon of wide interests. In October 1913, when the question of a central research institute under the control of the Committee was raised, it was recognized that hospital beds might be required and that they could be provided at Mount Vernon Hospital in Hampstead, which had now been purchased by the Committee to house its central institute. At the same time, it was realized that staff might be available in other institutions. At the meeting of the Committee held on 5 March 1914, two names were mentioned as possible recruits in the clinical field. They were T. R. Elliott, future Professor of Medicine at University College, and Thomas Lewis, who had been much influenced by the pioneering work of Sir James McKenzie and who had introduced the electrocardiograph with which he established the nature of the heart beat.[4]

With the outbreak of the First World War in August of that year, however, all immediate plans had to be set aside. As was discussed in Chapter 1, the Mount Vernon Hospital was handed over to the War Office and the Committee turned its attention to the problems of war. It was the war that was to give the new Committee its initial opportunity. The Secretary of the Medical Research Committee, Sir Walter Fletcher, in his reports on behalf of the Committee, drew attention to the way in which, 'the conditions of war [had] provided not only insistent demands for the application of the scientific method, but many exceptional opportunities at the same time for its easy and fruitful use'.[5] Studies of infection, both bacterial and parasitic, the treatment of wounds, the problems of poison gas, renal disease among men in the trenches, and the introduction of effective statistical methods into military practice were all supported by the Medical Research Committee.

[3] *Report of the Royal Commission on university education in London* (Chairman Viscount Haldane) (1913). HMSO, London.

[4] Landsborough Thomson, A. (1973). *Half a century of medical research*, Vol. 1, *The origins and policy of the Medical Research Council (UK)*, p. 27. HMSO, London.

[5] MRC: *Annual report 1916–17* (1917), p. 6.

There was also another problem of the First World War that was to be of great importance in the development of clinical research under the auspices of the MRC. This was the condition of 'soldier's heart' which was leading to increasing disability among military personnel condemned to the trenches. In 1915, when the disaster of gas hit the Western front, the Committee became deeply involved with the medical effects of mustard and other gases, and in 1916, when it became apparent that a curious ailment of the heart was afflicting soldiers suffering the horror and misery of trench warfare, Sir William Osler and his colleagues proposed that a special hospital should be set aside for the study of diseases of the heart. The War Office, however, initially opposed such special facilities and it was not until Osler, with Clifford Allbutt, McKenzie, and Fletcher, made a direct approach to Sir Alfred Keogh, Director General of Medical Services, that the War Office relented and Mount Vernon Hospital, now taken over for military use, was designated for cardiological studies. Osler was a friend, admirer, and enthusiastic supporter of Fletcher, and their mutual interest in medical history and in historical texts was an important bond between them.[6] Osler had written earlier in the year to Fletcher expressing the hope that Lewis could be induced to join in the work. Osler, together with Allbutt and McKenzie, was appointed to select the staff for the Mount Vernon venture, and they succeeded in having Lewis appointed to the full-time service of what was later to be the MRC.[7] It was also an important decision for Lewis personally. He had just got married and as his widow later recorded:

He never forgot that it was through the Medical Research Committee that he was enabled to follow his star and I well remember how delighted he was to receive his first appointment under the Committee, which made his research work possible in consequence with the increased expenditure of married life.[8]

By the end of the First World War the Medical Research Committee had established a commendable reputation for its handling of research into wartime medical problems, and Fletcher had become one of the most powerful figures in the developing world of medical research in Britain. A number of important monographs and reports had been published and Fletcher was able to point particularly to the practical and financial value of the work on 'soldier's heart'. Lewis and his colleagues had clearly shown that there was no organic abnormality of the heart in this condition, which was in fact a neurosis caused by a not unnatural reaction to the horrors of war. But Fletcher was able to calculate that the Medical Research Committee's work on soldier's heart alone was saving the Ministry of

[6] Cushing, *Osler*, Vol. 2, pp. 511–2 (see note 2).
[7] Ibid. p. 523.
[8] MRC PF 136 (2) : Lady Lewis to Landsborough Thomson, 3 May 1945.

Pensions as much as the entire grant to the Medical Research Committee.[9]

Fletcher was a strong supporter of the basic sciences throughout his years as Secretary to the MRC. It is clear, however, that in addition he sought to encourage clinical studies. He also believed in the ultimate applicability of science to practical problems. In a later report he referred to the field of muscle function in which he and Frederick Gowland Hopkins had been such important pioneers in Cambridge, and wrote: 'The studies of muscle function, which are almost notorious for their supposed uselessness to the student or physician, have laid down basic knowledge and are beginning to remove empiricism from practical studies of physical training and industrial labour'.[10]

The Committee had originally considered that it would establish hospital beds for clinical research as part of the central institute, following the plan that had been adopted with conspicuous success at the Rockefeller Institute in New York. The decision not to develop a research hospital at Mount Vernon was dictated by two considerations: first, that of cost, the Committee not being able to provide the very large expenditure necessary, and second, that 'it is undesirable on every ground to divorce research work from higher teaching'.[11] It was decided instead that it would support a Department of Clinical Research and Experimental Medicine at University College Hospital (UCH). There Thomas Lewis, on the permanent staff of the Committee since February 1916, would have beds available for 'research work and higher teaching ' and his clinical work would be in close relationship to the cardiographic department of the medical school. In addition T. R. Elliot was appointed to the permanent research staff of the Committee and was to work with Lewis. It was stressed, however, that although the clinical research activities of the Committee were to take place away from the Institute at Hampstead, the Department of Clinical Research was to be regarded as part of the Central Institute and its staff was to enjoy 'the fullest scientific intercourse with the others working there'.[12] Even though the major commitment at Hampstead at that time was to basic science, the Medical Research Committee, in establishing Lewis's department at UCH, had taken the first step towards developing clinical work as an integral part of its programme in the broader field of medical research.

In addition to directly supporting clinical research, Fletcher was also concerned with the development of other university departments carrying out research in the clinical field. In 1919, he drew attention to the unsatisfactory state of academic medicine in London, Oxford, and Cambridge.[13] The

[9] MRC: *Annual report 1917–18* (1918), p. 53.
[10] MRC: *Annual report 1923–24*, (1924), p. 13.
[11] MRC: *Annual report 1918–19* (1919), p. 29.
[12] Ibid. p. 29.
[13] Ibid. p. 10.

following year, he warmly welcomed the first steps then made by the London medical schools, in association with the University of London, to develop academic teaching units in medical and surgical hospital wards.[14]

The recommendations of the Haldane Commission on university education in London, made in 1913, had been shelved during the 1914–18 war, which provided the reluctant London teaching hospitals with an excuse for inactivity. The medical schools were in general not enthusiastic supporters of the Haldane proposals, but in 1919 St Bartholomew's Hospital appointed its first Professor of Medicine, Archibald Garrod, the pioneer of biochemical genetics and an outstanding clinical scientist who had brought biochemistry to the bedside. Garrod, however, never took up his post, for he left St Bartholomew's the next year to succeed Sir William Osler who had died in Oxford that same year.

By 1925 there were five chairs of medicine established at different schools at the University of London. Several of the appointees had sought training in the United States. Sir Arthur Ellis, first Professor of Medicine at the London Hospital, was a contemporary at the Rockefeller Institute in 1910 with Francis Fraser, who was to succeed to Garrod's chair at St Bartholomew's in 1920. Ellis later wrote to an American friend, 'I have often thought what a remarkable act of faith it was, that we should all have been consciously attempting to fit ourselves for full-time posts in medicine when no such posts existed anywhere.'[15]

Between 1920 and 1930 the MRC not only took note of clinical research in Thomas Lewis's Department, but also interested itself in the work of the new academic units which had been set up in the teaching hospitals. During that decade, the MRC annual reports included a section devoted to 'Experimental medicine and the research work of the clinical units'. In the Report for 1920–1, the paragraphs devoted to UCH start with 'The Council's Department of Clinical Research and the Cardiographic Department' and then describe the work of 'The Medical Unit of the Hospital', which was directed by the newly appointed Professor of Medicine T. R. Elliott who was therefore now working alongside Thomas Lewis.[16] There are then accounts of the work of the London, St Bartholomew's and St Thomas's Hospitals. All these units were receiving grants for research from the Council at that time. There is also a reference to the work at the Research Institute set up at St Andrews by Sir James McKenzie, who was particularly concerned to encourage research in general practice. The following year, the Royal Infirmary in Edinburgh joined the list, grants being made to the Department of Therapeutics. In 1923, the

[14] MRC: *Annual report 1919–20* (1920), p. 29.
[15] Corner, G. W. (1964). *A history of the Rockefeller Institute, 1901–1953*, p. 106. Rockefeller Press, New York.
[16] MRC: *Annual report 1920–1* (1921), pp. 23–38.

Council referred to the provision of special expenses for research work by Edward Mellanby in Sheffield on rickets and exophthalmic goitre.[17]

A year later, the tenth year of the work of the Council and its predecessor Committee, the Council thought it appropriate to conduct a broad review of its work since the war.[18] By now, the Council was pointing to the profound and far-reaching influence upon medical work arising from the new knowledge of nutrition derived from work carried out in laboratories of physiology and biochemistry (for detailed discussion, see Chapter 5). Insulin had been discovered, physiology was making special contributions, but in bacteriology and pathology 'relatively small progress has been made in recent years'. On experimental medicine and clinical research, the Council regarded the previous 5 years as of great significance in the progress of teaching and research in clinical medicine. 'The Council are of the opinion', it was recorded, 'that during the past five years these University clinics have wholly justified their foundation by their success.' Their establishment, however, had brought sharply to notice the virtual absence of proper laboratory accommodation in close association with the wards of the great teaching hospitals. The Sir William Dunn Trustees, guided by Fletcher, had provided the necessary funds to build and equip laboratories at St Bartholomew's, St Thomas's and the London Hospitals, and the Rockefeller Foundation had done the same for Edinburgh and Cardiff. The Council's firm interest in, and commitment to, the development of the academic 'units' in the medical schools was clearly stated: 'Their direct service to medical education as such and their many valuable but less obvious indirect services, are primarily for others to appraise. The Council, however, may estimate their work of investigation and they must regard these clinics as a quite indispensable part of the national system of medical research.'[19]

The Council continued to keep its directly supported work and the work of the teaching units under review. In 1927, it pointed out that in first supporting Thomas Lewis eleven years previously, it could justly claim to have established 'the first medical "unit" for research and higher postgraduate teaching in this country'. Its review of Lewis's Department of Clinical Research at that time was prompted by the publication of Lewis's monograph, 'Blood vessels of the human skin and their responses'. Fletcher noted, 'It is not an exaggeration to say that the output of valuable work from this Centre has constituted the central stream of progress made in this subject anywhere.'[20]

Lewis, however, was far from satisfied with the MRC's commitment to clinical research at that time. He considered that the Council could do more

[17] MRC: *Annual report 1922–3* (1923), p. 46.
[18] MRC: *Annual report 1923–4* (1924), p. 9.
[19] Ibid. p. 18.
[20] MRC: *Annual report 1926–7* (1928), pp. 12, 13.

by establishing a central institute for clinical research and that he himself should be provided with better facilities for training researchers. In a remarkable letter to Fletcher in 1929 he commented on the lack of progress on the clinical side of medicine (and surgery) which he thought was due chiefly 'not to inherent difficulties presented by the subject, but to what has become a traditionally low standard of work and thought from a scientific standpoint'. To remedy this, he thought that the MRC should 'develop a department or departments of clinical and experimental work on a broader and sounder basis than at present exists'. He had in mind an institute 'within which the workers may be free from the distractions presented by the petty and mainly diagnostic problems of diverse and obscure cases, and in which they can settle down to a more profound and uninterrupted study of the natural history of selected diseases'. He recommended that the Council authorize him to devote more time to the search for and training of suitable researchers, starting with two or three short-term contracts (6 to 12 months) at the rates of £200 to 400 a year.[21]

It was almost certainly the state of his health that prompted Lewis to send this letter at that particular time, for he had by now had his first coronary attack. Fletcher, in referring Lewis's letter to the Council, recognized that the Council members might well wonder why Lewis should be 'uneasy in regard to the stability' of his department. But he explained that Lewis felt that if a sudden accident removed him, his whole department would collapse and that there was no one to succeed him. Fletcher further explained: 'Former assistants, all able and picked men [*sic*], have either gone, like Dr. Cotton, to professional practice, or, like Dr. Verney and Dr. Drury, to experimental work in fields of pharmacology or physiology.'[22]

The Council appointed a subcommittee to consider Lewis's suggestions. Clearly, one of the questions before the Council was whether it should increase its support for the teaching units, or work towards establishing more full-time positions for clinical research workers, comparable to that held by Lewis himself. Fletcher consulted the clinical professors in the London teaching hospitals, who were asked in addition to provide information on the subsequent careers of individuals who had worked in their respective units. Francis Fraser replied from St Bartholomew's that two of the three asssistant directors were engaged in research and six of ten assistants were still involved in research work.[23] Among them were E. A. Carmichael, future director of a Research Unit at the National Hospital in Queen's Square, and C. H. Andrewes, later to found the Common Cold Unit at Salisbury. The assistants

[21] MRC 2011 (2): Lewis to Fletcher, 31 May 1929.
[22] MRC 2011 (2): memorandum by Fletcher to MRC, enclosing letter by Sir Thomas Lewis, 1929.
[23] MRC 1617: F. R. Fraser: enclosure to letter to Fletcher, 9 December 1929.

who had worked in T. R. Elliott's unit at University College included J. W. McNee (later Professor of Medicine in Glasgow), the neurologist F. M. R. Walshe, C. H. Kellaway from Australia, E. B. Verney (future Professor of Pharmacology at University College), A. E. Blake Pritchard, K. E. Harris and C. L. Cope (later to be Reader in Endocrinology at the Royal Postgraduate Medical School).[24] There were also responses from St Thomas's, St Mary's and the London Hospital. Hugh MacLean replied to Fletcher from St Thomas's:

You state that nobody of the various people doing research work in the units for the last 10 years has gone on to a life devoted entirely to clinical research [Fletcher wrote 'didn't' in the margin at this point]. This is true, but under present conditions it is practically impossible to do so. There is not a single post in this country of this kind. Only a man with private means could possibly do so and even then he might find difficulties in getting the necessary facilities.[25]

The response of the MRC to Lewis's suggestions was summarized in 1930; Fletcher asked:

Is there a science of experimental medicine for which the actual material for study is the human patient, or is scientific work by the physician or the surgeon limited to the application in his art of scientific results worked out elsewhere in the laboratory and delivered to him for use? The mere fact that these questions can be seriously asked suggests that in the field of clinical medicine there is not yet any stabilised or organised branch of science.[26]

He was quite clear as to the success of the Council's support for Lewis and the Department of Experimental Medicine at UCH. But with regard to the teaching units he wrote that while the teaching had been successful, teaching hindered research:

For teaching purposes the beds must be so filled and kept filled as to illustrate as completely as possible the whole normal range of medical work in all its clinical fields. Research work, on the contrary, requires concentration upon some particular disease or some special aspect of disease. The purposes of clinical education are in this sense not wholly compatible with those of clinical investigation. The heavy demands thus made upon the units in their work of teaching over the whole field of medicine have necessarily limits the volume of spontaneous and successful research work coming from them in aggregate.[27]

He also pointed out that the university and research units had not yet 'produced many men [*sic*] able and willing to devote themselves to a life of clinical research in experimental medicine'. He came to the following conclusions: first, that the experiment of providing a clinical researcher with

[24] MRC 1617: 'List of all assistants passed through the Medical Unit at University College Hospital from January 1920 to July 1929.
[25] MRC 1617: H. MacLean to Fletcher, 14 December 1929.
[26] MRC: *Annual Report 1928–29* (1930), p. 23.
[27] Ibid. p. 27.

proper resources and the right conditions for using them had proved to be an unqualified success; second, that except among the very rare persons combining inclination with good brains and private means there could never be a successful and maintained recruitment of able clinical researchers until there were at least a few stable positions in sight; and third, that the Council wished to recruit in the near future young workers of ability who were prepared to test themselves in this branch of medical research with a view to its becoming their life work. The Council was not only prepared to help these recruits to the utmost of its power in a preliminary period of training and probationary work, but also announced its intention of increasing the number of trained workers in the clinical field from its own permanent staff.[28]

Lewis set out to answer Fletcher's question, 'Is there a science of experimental medicine?' In a long article in the *British Medical Journal (BMJ)* he asserted that 'there is indeed a fertile science that deals primarily with patients and this must be encouraged to a more vigorous growth'. He argued strongly for the creation and training of a group of workers who would devote their lives primarily to research, making disease as this occurred in man the centre point of their studies. He believed that clinical science had reached a stage where it should develop its own training ground for new recruits, and that it should also achieve independence and freedom.[29] The *BMJ* in its leading article, gave enthusiastic support and concluded: 'The report of the Medical Research Council and Sir Thomas Lewis's clear analysis should go far to convince those who have at heart the progress of medicine in Britain that some posts must be created for research physicians.'[30] Lewis did not get his institute, but he had succeeded in persuading the Council of the necessity for training posts in clinical research.

While the *BMJ*'s leading article paid tribute to the MRC, Lewis himself made no reference in his article to his service under the Council, describing himself simply as 'Physician to University College Hospital' and omitting any acknowledgement to the organization which had supported him for 14 years. The year before, Fletcher had asked Lewis why he persisted in describing himself in *Who's who* as: 'attached to the Royal Medical Research Committee'.[31] In a letter to T. R. Elliott which was not in fact sent, Fletcher complained bitterly of Lewis's touchiness, and thought he did not play fair, particularly in failing to acknowledge either his indebtedness to the Council, or Fletcher's generosity in showing him copies of the Council's Annual Report in proof, only to see the material contained within it used by

[28] Ibid. p. 29.
[29] *British Medical Journal* (1930), i, 479–83.
[30] *British Medical Journal* (1930), i, 503–4.
[31] MRC 2011 (2) : Fletcher to Lewis, 20 June 1929.

Lewis before the report's publication.[32] Elliott asked Fletcher not unduly to distress Lewis, in view of his medical history. Fletcher might be forgiven for feeling that Lewis was carrying disloyalty and ingratitude too far, but he was strong enough not to allow such matters to sway his judgement in continuing support for clinical research. At the same time, the University College Hospital Medical School resolved to establish the Department of Clinical Research as an integral part of the institution, with Lewis as physician-in-charge.

In that year, however, there were to be others in the clinical field who were to belabour the Council for a supposed lack of concern with practical medicine. Lord Moynihan, in an address entitled 'the science of medicine' on the occasion of the opening of the Banting Research Institute of the University of Toronto in 1930, attacked the Council (who in his words 'had approximately £500 to spend on research on every working day of the year') , for its concern with mice rather than men, and for its temerity in even asking the question whether there was 'a science of experimental medicine'. To Moynihan the surgical art was a science in itself. He felt his own work in practical surgery deserved scientific recognition and deeply resented not being elected to the Royal Society. In an indirect attack on Fletcher's own research interests, he stated: 'In a standard textbook of physiology as much as a quarter of the text would be taken up with a discussion of the physiology of muscle, when in any textbook of medicine how many pages deal with the injuries or diseases of muscle?'[33] In another address given at Guy's Hospital that same year Moynihan argued that the MRC 'which might exert so magisterial and so incisive an influence upon the progress of medicine, the very purpose for which it was founded, seems too busy with little things, too aloof from the day-to-day practice of medicine'.[34]

Fletcher was clearly irritated by attacks of this sort, but he did continue to encourage the Council's interest in clinical research. In correspondence with H. R. Dean, Professor of Pathology in Cambridge, he reiterated his belief that it was necessary to create research chairs in the clinical field.[35] Other medical schools and universities were also seeking to attract both his interest and MRC support. J. A. Ryle wrote in 1932 to draw his attention to a young clinician at Guy's Hospital, L. J. Witts, of whom he had a high opinion. Fletcher, too, thought highly of Witts, but he had clearly misjudged the person destined to become the first Nuffield Professor of Medicine at Oxford, for he thought he was 'hopelessly booked for busy practice'.[36]

---

[32] MRC PF 136: Fletcher to T. R. Elliott, 17 March 1930 [a line has been drawn through the letter and 'not sent, W. M. F.' written across the top of the page].

[33] *British Medical Journal* (1930), ii, 779–85.

[34] Ibid. pp. 612–4.

[35] MRC 1617: Fletcher, correspondence with H. R. Dean.

[36] MRC 1617: Fletcher, correspondence with J. A. Ryle, August 1932.

It became increasingly clear to Fletcher that the Council, in responding to the demands of clinical research throughout the country, required more formal arrangements to deal with the problem of clinical research. In July 1932, he consulted Wilfred Trotter, the distinguished thyroid surgeon at UCH and then a member of Council, on the need for a Committee 'to aid Council in the problems of clinical research'. The purpose of the Committee was to advise upon applications for research in the clinical field, and to make proposals for the active promotion of medical research by clinical methods.[37] In addition Fletcher thought that the MRC 'might (and I think should) take steps towards some definite co-operation of the Royal College and provision with other bodies for the development of research Studentships'. The Clinical Committee was duly established by Council in October 1932. The initial membership included the clinical members of Council (Lord Dawson, President of the Royal College of Physicians, E. H. Mellanby and Wilfred Trotter), with Lewis as secretary.[38]

That same month, when it became generally known that the Rockefeller Foundation had generously endowed Lewis's own post and given support to his department, the Professor of Physiology in Manchester University, H. S. Raper, enquired in a letter to Fletcher whether the funds released by the Rockefeller endowment might now be available for developments elsewhere.[39] Manchester had established a Clinical Research Department under the direction of the haematologist, J. F. Wilkinson, that year. Fletcher's reply was only moderately enthusiastic. He apologized for his delay in coming to Manchester and promised to visit soon:

There is an urgent need, as we are always preaching, for the proper establishment and equipment of whole-time posts in clinical medicine. Many years ago Manchester led the way in this direction, but bungled the job. They missed Henry Head, and took Murray, who 'sold the pass'. No respectable University ought to have a professor of medicine unless he is competent and equipped for advancing his own subject, as are the professors in other subjects; but we can talk more of all this when I come. It is a matter of the greatest public importance, though this is very little recognised.[40]

He was clearly unhappy about G. R. Murray (the first to treat myxoedema with thyroid extract by injection) who had accepted the Chair at Manchester in 1908, but on a part-time basis only and did little further research until his retirement in 1925. Nevertheless, despite his misgivings Fletcher arranged to visit on 20 December to discuss how the MRC might help the Manchester initiatives.

[37] MRC 1513: Fletcher to W. F. Trotter, 27 July 1932.
[38] MRC 1513: Proceedings of the MRC, 21 October 1932.
[39] MRC 1682: H. S. Raper to Fletcher, 7 October 1932.
[40] MRC 1682: Fletcher to Raper, 11 October 1932.

It was not, however, a particularly propitious time to attempt to interest the Secretary of the MRC in the affairs of a northern University. Lord Dawson had become a member of Council that year. As President of the Royal College of Physicians he, together with Moynihan at the Royal College of Surgeons, represented the most powerful clinical interests in the country at that time. Dawson now saw fit to join Moynihan in attacking the MRC as well as the Royal Society for their supposed lofty attitude to clinical research. Unlike Moynihan's public attack, however, Dawson made his views known in private. In a personal letter to Fletcher in 1932, Dawson wrote, 'For many years there has not been that warmth of feeling in the profession towards the Council which the work of the latter deserves.' Both he and Moynihan believed that the Royal Colleges had as much right to be consulted on matters involving medical research as the Royal Society or the MRC.[41] Fletcher, however, had little sympathy for fashionable practitioners, who to their financial advantage 'hoodwinked' the public with such transient crazes as ultra-violet light treatment, opsonic indices and superstitions such as 'status lymphaticus'. He thought no more highly of College Presidents. The day before he was due to go to Manchester, he replied with seven and a half closely typed foolscap pages, which to this day burn with the suppressed passion with which they were written:

You and Moynihan, the first two medical peers since Lister, have become figureheads of the practising profession, but you have not had the personal footing in the scientific world that Lister had, or that Osler and Allbutt had. Each of you has tended in fact to alienate scientific opinion by your new insistence that headship among successful practitioners is a qualification in itself for leadership in scientific work.[42]

He pointed out that the 'profession' should not be looked upon as represented only by leaders in practice, 'whereas it truly includes all practitioners and hygienists as well as all the investigators in all the numerous fields of curative and preventative medicine and scientific work in genetics, laboratory biology, statistics, sociology and psychology'. And if the Royal College of Physicians wanted to be consulted, what about the British Medical Association, the Royal Society of Medicine and the Scottish Colleges? He pointed out further that the organization of research was not the function of the Royal Colleges, and that where they had been involved, as in cancer research, their record had been 'lamentable'. He also deplored Moynihan's public attacks on the Royal Society and the MRC and his 'ignorant criticisms of British physiology' made in Canada. He concluded with four proposals as to how the Royal College of Physicians, 'whilst maintaining all its present

---

[41] Library of the Royal College of Physicians of London: Lord Dawson of Penn to Fletcher, 15 December 1932.
[42] Library of the Royal College of Physicians of London: Fletcher (unsigned) to Dawson, 9 January 1933.

ceremonial and dignity [might] undertake more actively the task appointed to it'. In particular, as a reflection of his own interests, he thought the Royal College should support a Chair in Medical History at one of the Universities. He concluded:

I am sure you will receive the frankness of this letter in the spirit which you expressed in our talk. It has cleared my own mind at least to set out the picture of our relations as I have been seeing them. These post-war years and the present time in particular are probably among the the most significant in the history of British medicine, . . . Every man of good will must wish to forget any purely personal considerations in giving what help he can to sound progress.[43]

Fletcher's response on this occasion was uncharacteristically vehement. As Sir Harold Himsworth has noted, it was 'hardly the sword play one expects from an experienced public servant'.[44] But in the early months of 1933 it was apparent to many of his colleagues and friends that Sir Walter was losing his customary resilience. He was encouraged in a letter from his old friend and collaborator, Gowland Hopkins, to 'see the whole thing in perspective and let it hurt you no more'. Hopkins maintained,

I think I understand the feelings of 'Distinguished Clinicians' just now. In this country they have been so long in the public eye as infallible augurs that the public think, or has thought, it is they who, standing steeped in wisdom by the bedside, think the great thoughts which advance medicine. But even the Man in the Street is getting better informed and Harley Street is feeling a new and more critical atmosphere. It is feeling chilly.[45]

It was clear, however, that this affair, which occurred shortly before Fletcher's death in 1933, reflected a deeper malaise than was immediately apparent.[46]

When Edward Mellanby succeeded Fletcher as Secretary to the MRC, the Council had become firmly established as an organization of foremost importance in the scientific life of the country. The organization, however, was still relatively small, and no one in 1933 would have foreseen the great expansion of the work of the Council destined to occur during the next two decades. Mellanby, like Fletcher, had been closely involved with Gowland Hopkins in Cambridge, for it had been Hopkins who had stimulated Mellanby's interests in nutrition and metabolism. Mellanby had done pioneer

---

[43] Ibid.

[44] Personal communication to the author: Himsworth, 17 July 1985.

[45] Fletcher, M. (1957). *The bright countenance: a personal biography of Walter Morley Fletcher*, p. 285. Hodder and Stoughton, London.

[46] Fletcher had one great consolation during the last months of his life. His son Charles, reading medicine at his old College in Cambridge, Trinity, had been selected for the Cambridge boat. On the first of April, from an enclosure on Duke's Meadows, he watched the victorious Cambridge crew as they swept to victory. Two days later, he became unwell. Tragically within two months he was dead: Fletcher, *The bright countenance*, p. 288 (see note 45).

work on the discovery of vitamin D and the treatment of rickets. As Professor of Pharmacology in the University of Sheffield, he had held an honorary appointment as Physician to the Sheffield Royal Infirmary, where for thirteen years he had charge of his own beds. Mellanby therefore had a wider knowledge of clinical medicine than Fletcher. He was able to take a broad view of what was needed in medical research. He did not get bogged down in detail and was able to hand over much of the administrative work to the Second Secretary, Landsborough Thomson, who was an outstanding administrator.

During Mellanby's secretaryship there were to be important developments in clinical research, particularly in his own field of nutrition. He himself continued to conduct research with the help of his wife after his move to London. Mellanby was a reserved man, sometimes gruff, and he did not suffer fools gladly. Those who knew him, however, remembered him as 'a wonderful person to work for'.[47] Mellanby continued the correspondence with Manchester where Fletcher had left off, and in 1934 he asked Lewis to review the work of the Clinical Research Department there. It can hardly have helped the Manchester cause when Lewis reported that although there was a great deal of activity, too much was left unfinished.[48] Mellanby arranged to meet Raper, but warned him that 'all my remarks about the Manchester Clinical Research Department would not be of an entirely agreeable nature'.[49] In fact, he threatened that the MRC might withdraw its grants unless the Department was prepared to sever its 'unhealthy links' with commercial interests.

Throughout the 1930s it was undoubtedly the Department of Clinical Research at UCH that was to be the Mecca for all aspiring clinical research workers. G. W. (later Sir George) Pickering, while a student at St Thomas's, had attended one of Lewis's ward rounds in 1928. He described it as 'sparsely attended, as his ward rounds always were. The patients he chose to teach on that day had chronic bronchitis, a theme that few teachers select. He gave a masterly survey of the genesis of physical signs in the chest. I had never heard clinical teaching like it'.[50] Pickering was one of the first of a new generation of clinical research workers to join Lewis's unit, which he did in 1930.[51] Others who were to work in the inspiring atmosphere of Lewis's unit during that memorable decade included E. J. (later Sir Edward) Wayne, E. E. (later Sir Edward) Pochin and J. R. Squire. Lewis also gave great inspiration to those who worked alongside his department in T. R.

[47] Personal communication to the author: R. S. F. Schilling, December 1986.

[48] MRC 1682: Sir Thomas Lewis, notes.

[49] MRC 1682: Mellanby to H. S. Raper, 21 October 1936.

[50] Pickering, G. W. (1955). Thomas Lewis 1881–1945. In *University College Hospital Magazine*, 40, 68.

[51] Clearly, the Council then handled its affairs in a leisurely manner for, although Pickering started work on 1 May 1930, he had still not received a letter of appointment by the 20th of that month: MRC 2011 (2) Lewis to Fletcher, 20 May 1930.

Elliott's medical unit, and who included John McMichael, Harold Himsworth, and Horace Smirk, but there was always a certain rivalry between 'Lewis's boys' and the assistants working on the medical unit under Elliott.

Throughout those years Lewis himself was imbued with all the zeal of a non-conformist preacher in promoting the cause of clinical research. He continued to press the case for what he now termed 'clinical science' in lectures and papers. He strongly supported the views of Sir James Paget, who had written: 'I feel sure that clinical science has as good a claim to the name and rights of self-subsistence of a science as any other department of biology.'[52] In a series of papers and particularly in his Huxley Lecture on 'clinical science within the university' published in 1935, Lewis argued cogently for the recognition of clinical science as a subject in its own right, urging the universities 'to establish that branch of work that studies disease in living people as a science, by removing the obligation to engage in and teach the practical art, and by treating clinical science on precisely the same basis as the allied sciences, physiology and pathology'.[53] In order to encourage the development of clinical science as a distinct entity, Lewis had founded the Medical Research Society in 1930, with the support of a committee that included Francis Fraser, T. R. Elliott, Edward Mellanby and E. B. Verney.[54] He always recognized that his subject also needed a journal. He had himself edited the journal *Heart* since 1907 and in 1932 he changed the name to *Clinical Science* which more closely reflected his own concerns.

By the mid-1930s Lewis was perhaps becoming too successful in his advocacy, for he provoked a powerful response from Sir Frederick Gowland Hopkins, who was at the time President of the Royal Society. Whilst Fletcher had been attacked by the clinical community in his final years, during Mellanby's early years as Secretary the Council was criticized by the scientists for its support of clinical research. In his Address at the Anniversary Meeting of the Royal Society in 1934, Gowland Hopkins specifically referred to Lewis's argument that there was a great need for 'a phalanx of trained clinicians who shall bring clinical science to a new pitch of scientific efficiency and hold it there'. Hopkins expressed his own admiration for the brilliant contributions of Lewis and Mellanby, but he thought that there would be relatively few fields other than cardiology or nutrition that would offer experimental opportunities of equal promise. He went further in stating that if support for clinical science became a national policy, the result might be the transfer to the ward and clinic of much of the financial support that might properly be enjoyed by research in the pure sciences ancillary to medicine.[55]

---

[52] Sir James Paget, cited by Lewis (1935). *British Medical Journal*, **i**, 631.
[53] Lewis (1935). *British Medical Journal*, **i**, 636.
[54] Pochin, E. E. (1981). *Clinical Science*, **61**, 357–60.
[55] Hopkins, F. G. (1934). *Proceedings of the Royal Society Series B.*, **114**; 181–205.

Himsworth has recorded that the only time that he ever saw Sir Thomas Lewis appear depressed was following the delivery of the address.[56]

Lewis continued his proselytizing role as the Council's prophet of clinical research and in October 1933 he invited Mellanby to come and stay with him since he was anxious to go into the whole question of clinical work within the MRC with the new Secretary.[57] Lewis himself continued as secretary to the Clinical Committee and the following month he put forward the proposal that a new Clinical Research Unit should be founded at Guy's Hospital. The new unit would cover a more general field than the Neurological Research Unit at the National Hospital for Nervous Diseases, Queen's Square, set up the same year under the direction of E. A. Carmichael, who had been an assistant in F. R. Fraser's Department at St Bartholomew's Hospital. Lewis proposed that the new unit should be directed by R. T. Grant, who had worked with him during the First World War and had been working on peripheral blood vessels since 1921.[58] Lewis chose Guy's Hospital because it was well known and he hoped that research there would stimulate other teaching hospitals to follow suit. In December, the Dean, T. B. Johnston, outlined the arrangements to be made with the MRC. The Council was to provide the salaries of the director, already chosen by the MRC, a medically-qualified assistant and a technical assistant. Apparatus and research materials were also to be provided by the Council. Guy's for its part, was asked to provide six beds and one laboratory, with the possibility of expanding facilities later. The Dean 'interviewed' Mellanby, who insisted that Grant be appointed 'as an additional Physician to the Hospital' and that the connection between the director and the hospital and medical school be as intimate as possible.[59] The Unit was duly established in 1934 and until the outbreak of war in 1939, Grant continued to study the responses of the blood vessels of the human skin and urticaria, and its relationship to nervous activity. The Guy's Unit was the first to emerge from the inspiring environment of Lewis's Department of Clinical Research at University College Hospital.

The minutes of the Clinical Committee, which continued to meet throughout the 1930s, illustrate how MRC support was now being given to projects undertaken in a number of different medical schools throughout the country. In October 1934, L. J. Witts received support for his work at Guy's on idiopathic hypochromic anaemia, and splenic anaemia.[60] Research into

---

[56] Personal communication to the author: Sir Harold Himsworth, 17 July 1985.

[57] MRC 1513: Lewis to E. H. Mellanby, 29 October 1933.

[58] MRC 1513: Lewis, proposal for a Unit of Clinical Research at Guy's Hospital, 3 November 1933.

[59] MRC 1819: T. B. Johnston, memorandum from the Dean on the suggested formation of a Clinical Research Unit, at Guy's, by the Medical Research Council, December 1933.

[60] MRC 1513: records of the Clinical Committee, 8 October 1934.

liver treatment for pernicious anaemia, a dramatic development stemming from the United States during the previous decade, also received support at Guy's, as well as in Newcastle and Manchester. At the same time, R. G. MacFarlane, working at St Bartholomew's Hospital and supported by the Professor of Pathology, E. H. Kettle, received a grant to work on mechanisms of blood coagulation and on haemophilia. The next year John McMichael, who had returned to the Department of Medicine in Edinburgh after three years at UCH in T. R. Elliott's department, received £100 for developing the 'acetylation method for determination of cardiac output in man'.[61] Other grants were given to W. Melville Arnott in Edinburgh for work on peripheral vascular disease, and to A. H. Hunt and P. R. Allison for research in the surgical field. In 1935, the question of founding a surgical research unit was raised by D. P. D. Wilkie, Professor of Surgery at Edinburgh University and a member of MRC, and in 1938 a Unit for Clinical Research in Surgery was established in Edinburgh under the direction of W. C. Wilson. It was, however, to be short-lived for the Director soon left on his appointment to a professorial chair.

It was clear that Lewis had now become the most powerful figure in clinical research in Britain. He was able to recruit some of the most promising young researchers in the country to his department. He often groomed them as house physicians, taking them on later as full-time assistants. For example, he had recruited E. E. Pochin, 'a man I have had under close supervision for 4 years. Pochin has unusual ability and a strong desire to enter the field of Clinical Science'.[62] At the Clinical Committee, however, Lewis did not always get his way. He did not attend the meeting in November 1937, when an application by G. Bourne of St Bartholomew's Hospital for support in following up 'patients with cardiac pain treated by psychological, medical or surgical methods' was favourably received, despite the fact that Lewis made it known to Mellanby that he would have opposed it had he been present.[63]

The Council continued throughout the 1930s to endorse Fletcher's view that it was vitally necessary to establish full-time positions in academic medicine in the medical schools. It noted with pleasure in 1931 that Aberdeen University was reorganizing its Regius Chairs in order to provide full-time opportunities for teaching and research, and there were other universities that were following suit.[64] If developments in the undergraduate schools were to proceed in a somewhat leisurely fashion at that time there were now to be important initiatives in the postgraduate field both in London and in Oxford which were to lead to a great expansion of the

[61] MRC 1513: records of Clinical Committee, 5 May 1935.
[62] MRC 2011: Lewis to Mellanby, 18 March 1936.
[63] MRC 1513: records of the Clinical Committee, 22 November 1937.
[64] MRC: *Annual report 1931–32* (1933), pp. 10, 11.

opportunities for able men and women to take up full-time academic posts with facilities for clinical research.

In the years after the First World War, the need for effective postgraduate education in medicine had been increasingly recognized and at the same time there was an important body of opinion that considered research to be an essential ingredient of postgraduate study. There had been attempts in London to develop postgraduate education since the later years of the Victorian era, but they had been based solely in the clinic, and as Sir Clifford Allbutt had pointed out: 'Attempts at postgraduate education have failed and must fail, unless they are rooted in the laboratory and the ward.'[65] Osler, at the end of the First World War, played a seminal role in the development of postgraduate education in this country. He considered that Britain could take the place of Vienna in postgraduate education in Europe. Together with Meakins and the future Lord Dawson, he pointed out that doctors returning from war service badly needed educational opportunities and that there was also an increasing flood of postgraduates from all over the old Empire seeking specialist education in London.[66]

In 1921, in response to these initiatives, a Committee was set up under the chairmanship of the Earl of Athlone, which recommended firmly that there should be a school for postgraduate medical education attached to a hospital specifically dedicated for this purpose.[67] In 1925, the teaching hospitals in London were approached by a Committee chaired by Neville Chamberlain for this purpose. All refused, although St Bartholomew's only declined after very careful consideration. Finally it was agreed with the London County Council that the school should be sited at Hammersmith Hospital in west London, where there was thought to be sufficient space for development. The London County Council wanted to encourage a school which might be of importance in raising standards in the municipal hospitals. The new School was formally opened in 1935, nearly a quarter of a century since Osler's evidence to the Haldane Commission. But it was at Hammersmith, to use Osler's own phrase, that there was to be 'the most convincing and active invasion of a hospital by the University in this country'.[68]

The architect of this Flexnerian model, unique in Britain, was Francis Fraser, who came from his Chair at St Bartholomew's to be head of the Department of Medicine, where he had been highly esteemed and had played

[65] Cited by C. E. Newman (1966). *Postgraduate Medical Journal*, **42**, 738–40.
[66] Cushing, *Osler*, Vol. 2, p. 605 (see note 2).
[67] Newman, C. E. (1966). *Postgraduate Medical Journal*, **42**, 738–40.
[68] Booth, C. C. (1985). *British Medical Journal*, **291**, 1771–9.

a crucial role in establishing a Medical Unit.[69] The Postgraduate Medical School was perhaps the only British equivalent to the Johns Hopkins Hospital in the United States, where Osler and his colleagues had had their chance, as noted above, 'to blaze a perfectly new road untrammelled by tradition, vested interest or medical dead wood'. The School was to provide just that vital training in clinical research whose lack in the MRC's clinical units in London had been bewailed by Fletcher.

In 1935 Fraser had tried unsuccessfully to tempt McMichael from Edinburgh to join his department as an assistant. By 1939 he was able to offer him the Readership, which McMichael accepted. McMichael, later to succeed as Professor of Medicine, was to be a key figure in that golden age of Hammersmith, when the 'most advanced and successful school in the British Commonwealth', as it was later described, was in its infancy.[70]

The MRC welcomed the foundation of the school:

The recent opening of the new British Post-Graduate Medical School in London has, among other things, involved the establishment of whole-time professorships in medicine, surgery, and obstetrics. Although these posts are primarily for teaching, they are likely also to give excellent opportunities for research work: furthermore, they are important as additions to the number of senior posts in clinical medicine which offer an alternative to a career in private practice.[71]

At the same time there were to be further important developments in Oxford. It was the distinguished neurosurgeon, Hugh Cairns, then working at the London Hospital, who in the summer of 1935 drew up a memorandum of 'The desirability of establishing a complete school of clinical medicine in Oxford'. The memorandum was sent to Sir Archibald Garrod's successor as Regius Professor of Medicine, Sir Farquhar Buzzard. Buzzard made a powerful plea in his Presidential address to the BMA in July 1936 for the establishment of a new postgraduate school for clinical research, in particular impressing Lord Nuffield who was present. Subsequently Nuffield contributed £2 000 000 to the medical school scheme. It was through this munificence that the University of Oxford was able to establish the Nuffield Chairs in clinical subjects. Hugh Cairns was duly appointed as the first Nuffield Professor of Surgery, and L. J. Witts, after only a brief sojourn as

[69] Sir Ian Wood, the distinguished Australian physician, in his autobiography *Discovery and healing in war and peace* (published by the author: Toorak, Australia, 1984), p. 26, remembered Fraser as a 'splendid teacher' whose weekly ward round was 'the highlight of medical life at Barts'. Fraser's successor at Barts, L. J. Witts, stated in a letter to the MRC, 'During his [Fraser's] tenure of the professorial chair here the Medical Unit has established itself as an integral and much appreciated part of the hospital' (L. J. Witts: MRC 1513: records of the Clinical Committee, 11 March 1935).

[70] F. N. L. Poynter, (1970). Medical education in England since 1600. In *The History of Medical Education*, (ed. C. D. O'Malley) pp. 235–50. University of California Press; Los Angeles.

[71] MRC: *Annual report 1933–34* (1935), p. 12.

Professor of Medicine at St Bartholomew's, became the first Nuffield Professor of Medicine.

The MRC recorded its warm welcome of these proposals since the scheme was 'fully in accord with a policy we have long advocated, particularly in its establishment of senior clinical posts, on a nearly whole-time basis'. It went on to reiterate its declared policy of establishing, 'as opportunities offer and resources permit, positions in our own service for whole-time clinical research. To opportunities of this kind the posts that will now be created at Oxford will form a very important addition. It is to be hoped also that the example will be followed elsewhere'.[72] At the same time, the Council also recorded that a department of clinical research had been established by the University of Cambridge, under the direction of the new Regius Professor of Physic, J. A. (later Sir John) Ryle. A clinical research unit has also been set up at Middlesex Hospital in 1934, supported by a gift of £15 000 from S. A. Courtauld. Landsborough Thomson had written to the Hospital encouragingly: 'Our attitude will be one of benevolence.'[73]

Meanwhile the Council was particularly interested in establishing training posts for work in the clinical field so that there would be researchers available for recruitment to the full-time posts that both the universities and the MRC were seeking to encourage. In 1936, it established six postgraduate studentships for training in methods of research in clinical medicine and experimental pathology. An early applicant for one of these studentships was J. V. (later Professor Sir John) Dacie, who responded to an advertisement in the *Lancet*.[74] A graduate of King's College Medical School, he had been influenced by R. A. McCance whose work there in collaboration with Elsie Widdowson was virtually the only research being conducted at the School at that time. Dacie had been deeply impressed by Janet Vaughan's book on the anaemias and it was she, then working in the Department of Pathology at the newly founded Postgraduate Medical School, who attracted Dacie to the institution where he was later to make his distinguished career in haematology. Another budding clinical scientist who took advantage of the MRC's scheme in that year was D. A. K. (later Sir Douglas) Black, a St Andrews' graduate who was to work in Witts' new Department of Medicine in Oxford.

At the time of the outbreak of the Second World War in 1939, the Council was very much better prepared than its predecessor had been a quarter of a century earlier. Nevertheless, concerned that 'the fruits of some promising research unrelated to war might be frittered away', the Council in 1939, and again in 1940, emphasized the need for continuing its existing programmes of

[72] MRC: *Annual report 1935–36* (1937), p. 11.
[73] MRC 1880: Landsborough Thomson to P. Fildes.
[74] Personal communication to author: Sir John Dacie, 10 November 1986.

work, subject to whatever demands might be made for special investigations into particular problems in the national interest.[75] Wound shock again became a subject of study. The treatment of wound infections had already been markedly influenced by the introduction of the sulphonamides and was to be greatly improved by the introduction of penicillin as a result of the outstanding work that took place in Oxford.

The war provided a fearful blow to Lewis's plans for clinical research. His own department was decimated by the departure of staff to join the war effort. George Pickering had now been appointed to the Chair of Medicine at St Mary's Hospital Medical School. In November 1939 Lewis wrote despairingly to tell Mellanby that his team was 'hopelessly broken'.[76]

By contrast it was the Second World War that was to have a major influence on the development of clinical research at the Postgraduate Medical School. There had been those at Hammersmith who took the view that the function of the postgraduate school was to teach and that research should be the business of the new school in Oxford. At the outbreak of war there were also those who took the gloomy view that the School should be closed down. However, George Gask, Chairman of the School Council, had the courage and imagination to insist that the School should not only continue, but carry out research. In particular, he considered that with its equipment and laboratories the School was in a strong position to carry out research that might be important in a wartime setting. Francis Fraser left to direct the Emergency Medical Services in London, telling his recently appointed Reader as he went: 'Well, McMichael, you just stay here because we have work to do.'[77]

McMichael's own field of research was in cardiovascular physiology. At a time of war, it was clearly important to know more about the effects of haemorrhage, and McMichael's work was effectively supplementing that being undertaken by the MRC's own staff. For the work on blood loss, a method of measuring cardiac output was given priority. At that time McMichael was still using the acetylene method that he had developed in Edinburgh with the Council's support, and he and his colleague Peter Sharpey-Schafer were now stimulated by the paper by Cournand and Ranges, published in the United States in 1941, to use cardiac catheterization to measure cardiac output directly.[78] The new technique enabled them to establish clearly the physiological reaction to blood loss.[79] As McMichael

[75] Landsborough Thomson, A. (1975). *Half a century of medical research*, Vol. II, *The programme of the Medical Research Council (UK)*, p. 293. HMSO, London.

[76] MRC 2011 (5): Lewis to Mellanby, 10 November 1939.

[77] Booth, C. C. (1985). *British Medical Journal*, **291**, 1771–9.

[78] Cournand, A. and Ranges, H. A. (1941). *Proceedings of the Society for Experimental Biology and Medicine*, **46**, 462–6.

[79] Barcroft, H., Edholm, O. G., McMichael, J., and Sharpey-Schafer, E. P. (1944). *Lancet*, **i**, 489–90.

later pointed out, there were no ethical problems with human experimentation of this type since the whole population was anxious to help with the war effort and there was therefore no lack of volunteers, although misgivings were expressed in some quarters, particularly by Lewis himself.[80]

It was the study of crush injuries that was to bring the School and the MRC into fruitful collaboration. At the outbreak of war Hammersmith Hospital became a casualty hospital of 400 beds. When the bombing started in 1940, it was Hammersmith, not being in central London, that received the casualties that were dug out of bombed buildings at a late stage and who often had severe crush injuries. Among these unfortunates were many that developed renal failure, and in 1941 Eric Bywaters published the first of a series of classic papers on what appeared to be a new syndrome, crush injury with subsequent renal failure.[81] With the support of the Council and the collaboration of Sir James Walton, consultant surgeon at the London Hospital, Bywaters formed an MRC team to visit every major bombing in the home counties, and sometimes as far afield as York, Norfolk, and Bristol. He intended not only to document the early stages of this apparently new type of kidney damage, but also wanted to learn how to prevent it. The team consisted of Sir James Walton, Bywaters, and a driver who had to cope with the blackout and no signposts, which had been removed to confuse possible enemy invaders. Much of the work was unfruitful, but a full study was completed of cases of crush syndrome following a compression tragedy among a crowd at Bethnal Green underground station.[82]

Meanwhile, R. T. Grant, with the help of E. B. Reeve, had been studying shock in air raid casualties in the Clinical Research Unit at Guy's Hospital. After the building was seriously damaged by enemy action, the Unit was transferred to the Royal Victoria Infirmary, Newcastle-on-Tyne, where Erasmus Barlow joined Reeve and Grant. Ludwig Wittgenstein, the renowned Cambridge philosopher, worked as a war-time technician in the Unit. Towards the end of 1943 the Council's Shock Committee concluded that more detailed observations were required to elucidate how serious injuries caused shock. Furthermore it concluded that sufficient clinical material could only be found on the battlefield. The Council and the War Office therefore decided to send a 'British Traumatic Shock Team' to Italy in early 1944 and this was led by R. T. Grant, seconded from the Council's service to the RAMC as a Lieutenant-Colonel. It is said that Grant chose the Italian field of war as being less liable to disastrous retreats that might lead to the loss of his records. Bywaters now became the second director of the Newcastle Unit. There, with Barlow and with the help of Bernard Shaw,

[80] McMichael, J. (1962). Foreword. In *Cardiac catheterisation and angiocardiology* (eds. D. Veral and R. G. Grainger).. Churchill Livingston, Edinburgh.
[81] E. G. L. Bywaters and D. Beall (1941). *British Medical Journal*, i, 427–32.
[82] Personal communication to the author: E. G. L. Bywaters, 16 January 1987.

Professor of Pathology in the University of Newcastle, he studied serious industrial injuries, many of which ended in renal failure following fracture, muscle disruption, and from myoglobinuria. By 1945, with the resumption of enemy bombing using V1 and V2s, Bywaters returned to Hammersmith, where, after the end of hostilities, he was to receive the first Kolf Dialysis machine from Holland. The earliest renal dialyses in this country were therefore undertaken at Hammersmith under the auspices of the MRC.[83]

Lewis had meanwhile continued to teach and to carry out his own research. J. R. Squire had joined his department in 1939 and was to stay until 1942 when he joined the RAMC. During the winter of 1940–1, and in order to avoid interruption from the continuous night bombing of that period, Lewis and the clinical students were evacuated to Cardiff. Not much was gained from this move for the enemy switched their bombing attacks to port towns almost as soon as the move was completed. N. B. Myant's clearest memories of that period as a UCH student at Cardiff are not of listening to Lewis's lectures or ward teaching, but of spending many nights in cold and flimsy air raid shelters.[84] After about a year the clinical students were moved back to Stanborough's Hospital, between Watford and Rickmansworth and near to Lewis's home at Loudwater. Harold Himsworth, who had succeeded Elliott as Professor of Medicine in 1939, was working on nutritional liver disease in the rat, and for a while, Himsworth's rodents were also housed at Stanborough's Hospital.

Although Lewis did not allow the war to disturb his vision of the future, it is clear that he found these later years profoundly frustrating. In June 1942, he prepared another memorandum on the position of clinical research following the war, which he sent to the MRC from Stanborough's Hospital with a covering letter.[85] He pointed out that at the outbreak of war there had been 'the most promising group of young clinical research workers that this country has ever seen'. The group was organized with its own society (the Medical Research Society) and journal (*Clinical Science*). He believed that it was important that these workers should receive ample facilities for their work following the war. There had been by the outbreak of the war a growing tendency among some of the ablest young students to prefer full-time research to consultant work, resulting in a sufficiently large pool of highly trained researchers available for 'an independent and self-sufficient team in Clinical Science'. Another development before the war had been a growing tendency for the London hospitals to recruit more practising staff without appropriate training or aptitude for research. Yet the control of facilities for research in the hospitals remained chiefly in the latter's hands. This was

[83] Ibid.
[84] Personal communication to the author: N. B. Myant, 22 December 1986.
[85] MRC 445: Lewis to Mellanby, with a memorandum to the MRC (the position of clinical research when the war ends), 11 June 1942.

becoming more problematic as the difference in outlook between the members of the honorary staff and research workers grew. There was also the problem that hospitals were increasingly under the control of local government with little knowledge and understanding of the need for research into the 'ground work of progressive medicine'. The university research units were important but they also bore the brunt of routine technical teaching. Lewis believed that the nucleus for a further and permanent system lay in the MRC-controlled units for clinical research in the London teaching hospitals, and advocated greater centralization. A central organization for clinical science was, in his opinion, imperative.

At that time, with the war at its height, it was clear that nothing effective could be done, and the Council deferred further consideration. Lewis's proposal, however, was to be given practical expression by the Council's foundation of its Clinical Research Centre in the post-war era (see below).

Throughout the war, Lewis, with the help of Mellanby, pulled all the strings that he knew to ensure that his young researchers were able to continue investigative work despite the exigencies of war. In the letter that accompanied his memorandum to Mellanby in June 1942, when Squire joined the RAMC, Lewis had expressed his confidence 'that you will do everything you can to make his work go smoothly'.[86] Myant was conscripted into the RAMC at the end of 1943. Lewis tried unsuccessfully to have him posted to a virology unit then being formed by Charles Stuart-Harris. He was due to go to France three days after the Normandy invasion, but a broken arm prevented his participation. At the end of 1944, he was mysteriously sent by flying-boat to Bombay, then on to Delhi and to Dehra Dun, where he was met by Major J. R. Squire. He was to work with Squire in a tented unit called the User Trials Establishment.[87] The extent to which the activities of Squire and his colleagues contributed to the war effort in South East Asia is uncertain, but, as Lewis recognized, it was important for future clinical research workers that the circumstances of war should not be allowed to atrophy their critical faculties.

By now Lewis's health was causing concern. He had had his third coronary occlusion and early in 1945 it was rumoured that he had contracted pneumonia.[88] On 16 March, he wrote his last letter to Mellanby. He was deeply concerned about the future of the young researchers he had trained and who were still languishing in the armed services. Pochin had visited him that same day. Lewis was also depressed about the future of his own unit after his retirement. He wrote:

[86] Ibid.

[87] Personal communication to the author: N. B. Myant, 22 December 1986.

[88] Howarth, S. (Lady McMichael) Sir Thomas Lewis: personal recollections. Typescript in the author's possession.

I cannot help feeling that there is something radically wrong, with all the lip service that is being given to the immediate future of Clinical Research and higher teaching if the men required for this rebuilding are to be robbed of any opportunity of re-training for it. I think that there is a strong case for the present release of a limited number of such men and that the MRC is the proper body to emphasise the imperative need of this release. What are you waiting for? The German surrender? The Japanese defeat? What is the plan? Am I right in thinking there is no plan?[89]

The following day Lewis died suddenly from his fourth and last coronary attack. The letter was typed by his secretary and sent to Council on Lady Lewis's instructions. In an appropriate tribute to the architect of clinical research in the modern era, virtually all the staff of the Department of Medicine at Hammersmith attended Lewis's Memorial Service. He was buried in the small churchyard in Llangorst in Breconshire. There, in that lovely part of Wales, an upright stone faces the nearby lake. Upon the stone there is a bronze medallion from which, as Sheila Howarth has written, 'the eyes of Lewis fix you with unwinking stare'.[90]

Lewis's contribution to clinical research under the auspices of the MRC was immeasurable. It was he who virtually alone convinced the Council in its early days of the need to 'forward the science of experimental medicine and its study of the bedside' and he inspired a whole generation of clinical research workers whose work was to be the foundation of the expansion in academic medicine that followed the Second World War. It was not his fault that some of his pupils, and later others, carried on the purely physiological approach to clinical research for too long, at a time when biochemistry, immunology, and cell biology were becoming more important. There were, however, those who considered that his championing of clinical science as a subject in its own right had caused a rift to develop between clinical research and the basic sciences at University College. Sir Charles Lovett-Evans, Professor of Physiology, thought that Lewis had created an entirely artificial subject called 'clinical science', which was simply human physiology applied to the problems of clinical medicine.[91]

At Hammersmith, where McMichael had succeeded Fraser as Professor of Medicine and Ian Aird came to the Chair of Surgery, there now began a period of expansion which lasted for the next twenty years. This was associated with a flowering of the research effort which had been so effectively established during the school's first decade. The MRC made a particular contribution through the establishment there of the Cyclotron Unit, where the production of short-lived radioactive isotopes was to be particularly exploited by respiratory physiologists such as Philip Hugh Jones and J. B. West. It would be heartening to be able to relate that there was a

---

[89] MRC 2011 (6): Lewis to Mellanby, 16 March 1945.
[90] Howarth, personal recollections (see note 88).
[91] Ibid.

similar enthusiasm for clinical research in all the London undergraduate schools during those early years after the war. At UCH, the Department of Medicine carried on distinguished work under Himsworth's leadership. Sharpey-Schafer became Professor of Medicine at St Thomas's and there built up an outstanding staff. But in other schools that then had academic departments there was friction between full-time academics and part-time staff in consultant practice. Clinical investigators were still not accepted by many physicians at that time and there was a general resistance to the introduction of invasive techniques of investigation, for example cardiac catheterization and liver biopsy, which had been developed by McMichael and Sheila Sherlock at Hammersmith. There were also those who questioned the ethics of such human investigation.[92] Medical schools in London were frankly critical of Hammersmith's approach and often warned their young alumni not to go to work there. At one London School, when the first full-time professor was appointed, a distinguished part-time physician commented: 'Good God, doesn't he sample blood from his patient's brachial arteries?'[93] In retrospect, it appears that ethical standards that had been appropriate in the context of global war were increasingly inappropriate in times of peace. Nevertheless, it must be questioned whether the great achievements of those years would have been possible if the strict ethical standards of today had been applied.

There was only a gradual increase in academic units in the London schools during those early post-war years. The Middlesex Hospital Medical School appointed its first Professor of Medicine in 1946. St George's Hospital Medical School did not follow suit until 1958. The Royal Free Hospital appointed Sheila (later Dame Sheila) Sherlock to the Chair of Medicine in 1959, and the Westminster Hospital took M. D. Milne, who had worked in Manchester with Platt and D. A. K. Black, from Hammersmith in 1960. The last London undergraduate school to establish an academic Department of Medicine was King's College Hospital Medical School and that was not until 1965. In 1968, Peart pointed out that academic medicine was still a young discipline in Britain, particularly in comparison with the United States.[94]

It is against this background that the MRC's commitment to clinical research in the post-war period must be considered. A number of new units in the clinical field had been created during the war, for example, the Burns Research Unit in Birmingham under the direction of Leonard Colebrook. In 1941, the Radiotherapeutic Research Unit, directed by Constance Wood, was set up at Hammersmith where in the 1950s it was to develop into the Cyclotron Unit, as noted above. This was the first of a series of MRC Units

---

[92] Pappworth, M. H. (1967). *Human guinea pigs: experimentation on man.* Routledge and Kegan Paul; London.
[93] Personal communication to the author: Sir John Butterfield, 6 February 1987.
[94] Peart, W. S. (1967). *British Medical Journal,* ii, 616.

that were to benefit from the stimulating environment of the Postgraduate Medical School, where the majority of the staff worked full time. In 1946, the MRC set up a Blood Transfusion Research Unit there, under the direction of P. L. Mollison. Several other important Units were to be founded within the next two years. The Council established the Common Cold Unit at Salisbury under the direction of C. H. (later Sir Christopher) Andrewes in 1946.

After the death of Lewis, the Council together with University College Hospital had invited E. E. (later Sir Edward) Pochin to become the new Director of the Department of Clinical Research, which he accepted.[95] Pochin, who as an undergraduate in Cambridge in 1932 had played tennis with Sir Walter Fletcher, had worked with Lewis before the war on the abnormalities of the eye in thyrotoxicosis. In 1941, Mellanby sent him to the tank gunnery school at Lulworth in Dorset where he carried out valuable work on the problems of tank crews working in confined spaces. At the end of the war Mellanby arranged for him to attend as a British observer at the Bikini Atoll atomic bomb tests.[96] He soon became involved in the use of radioisotopes in medicine, and the Department under his leadership was to undertake pioneering work in this field. He began to build up his team in 1946 when Erasmus Barlow and E. A. G. Goldie were recruited. The following year N. B. Myant, after a period of rehabilitation as a house physician with McMichael at Hammersmith following his demobilization, formally joined the Department. Pochin had already begun work, the first to be carried out in Britain, on the application of radioisotopes to the study of thyrotoxicosis and he later extended his work to include the treatment of thyroid cancer.[97]

The Department, however, continued Lewis's tradition of maintaining a general rather than a limited specialist interest. D. A. W. Edwards, who came to the Unit in 1948, and E. N. Rowlands who joined the next year, became important contributors to gastroenterology.

It was a reflection of the importance of new scientific developments to clinical investigation that Myant, recognizing that for the future he needed more experience in biochemistry, spent a year with I. M. London at Columbia University in New York in 1952–3. On his return he went to see G. J. Popjak who had just moved from the National Institute for Medical Research

[95] S. C. Shanks to Pochin, 3 December 1945 (in possession of Sir Edward Pochin).

[96] Personal communication to the author: Sir Edward Pochin, 1 April 1987.

[97] Myant remembers that: 'the work was very challenging and we had to teach ourselves how to interpret experiments *in vivo* with radioactive tracers and how to measure the ^{131}I content of the thyroid gland. All this would be very elementary now but in the 1940s there were no books or review articles to help us. Pochin's analytical prowess and mathematical fluency were invaluable, and so was the electronics expertise of E. A. G. Goldie, who died of lung cancer before we published our first paper in 1949. This comparatively brief period, when we were applying a whole new technology, was very exciting and I have never experienced anything quite like it since. In a small way it was analogous to the early years of molecular biology': Personal communication to the author: N. B. Myant, 22 December 1986.

(NIMR) to Hammersmith to direct the newly established Experimental Radiopathology Research Unit. Popjak had no interest in radiopathology but he had already embarked on his distinguished studies of cholesterol biosynthesis and metabolism and Myant now joined his unit. He started the studies of lipid metabolism which later, after Popjak's departure to work for Shell Research at Sittingbourne in Kent, led to his being appointed to head his own Lipid Research Unit at Hammersmith.[98]

The Pneumokoniosis Unit, set up in 1945 under the direction of C. M. Fletcher, the son of Sir Walter (see Chapter 7), was to have a major impact on certain areas of clinical research during the early post-war years. The Unit was involved in pulmonary physiology and it was necessary to develop methods of measuring pulmonary function. J. C. Gilson and Philip Hugh Jones were deeply involved in the development of simple tests for assessing maximum breathing capacity, and the forced expiratory volume (FEV) was later found to be the most useful. Those who worked in the Unit included Martin Wright, who invented the peak respiratory flow meter which bears his name, and both W. A. Briscoe and J. B. West, who were later to distinguish themselves as pulmonary physiologists in the United States, worked in the Unit during their formative years.

The Unit was also to be the first to recognize the importance of observer variation in clinical research. At that time the existence of such variation was unrecognized except as a measure of unsatisfactory training in medical students and young doctors. Fletcher and his colleagues encountered it first in their radiological studies. In collaboration with R. V. Christie's Unit at St Bartholomew's Hospital, they went on to show that there were grave errors in eliciting the physical signs reputed to detect emphysema and that such signs were not only inaccurate, but to a large extent irrelevant. These studies upset senior members of the practising profession who at that time, when so much of medicine depended upon authority, were often reluctant to admit their inadequacies. When Fletcher left to take up a post as senior lecturer in McMichael's department at Hammersmith in 1952, he was succeeded by J. C. Gilson, who was to prove an equally inspiring leader. As Schilling has recalled, the success of the MRC's larger units to a great extent depended upon their leaders and the Pneumokoniosis Unit was well served during those years.[99]

In 1949, Himsworth succeeded Mellanby as Secretary to the Council. As a practising clinician, he was clearly concerned to stimulate and encourage clinical research. He had also played a significant role, during his tenure of the Chair of Medicine at UCH, in extending Lewis's physiological approach by encouraging a biochemical approach to clinical

[98] Landsborough Thomson, *Medical research*, Vol. II, p. 368 (see note 75).
[99] Personal communication to the author: R. S. F. Schilling, December 1986.

research. It was Himsworth who was responsible for the appointment of C. E. Dent to the staff of the medical school. Dent was a distinguished clinical investigator who exploited the techniques of biochemistry and of paper chromatography in the investigation of genetic and metabolic disorders.

Himsworth was to serve as Secretary during the years that followed the implementation of the National Health Service (NHS) Act of 1946. The Act was to have important consequences for clinical research. It gave Ministers powers not only to conduct research but also to assist others to do so. A joint committee comprising representatives from the Health Departments and the MRC was set up under the Chairmanship of Sir Henry (Later Lord) Cohen in 1952. Their recommendations included the founding of a central organization for the promotion of clinical research, to be called the Clinical Research Board, as part of the MRC, with extra funding to be allocated at a later stage. At the same time, facilities for decentralized research were to be provided by Regional Hospital Boards, Boards of Governors and Hospital Management Committees.[100]

The appointment of the Clinical Research Board was announced in October 1953.[101] It was proposed that Sir Geoffrey Jefferson, the distinguished Manchester neurosurgeon, should be appointed Chairman. There were to be ten members, five proposed from a panel of names prepared by the Health Departments and five from the MRC. The latter had already agreed that its representatives should be its clinical members. At that time these were Sir James Learmonth, Sir James Spence, Aubrey Lewis and Robert Platt. The Health Department nominees were Sir Henry Cohen, Sir James Patterson Ross, E. C. Dodds, Bryan Windeyer, and Dugald Baird. The Chief Medical Officer of the Health Department was also to be there as an assessor, and Himsworth, as Secretary of the MRC, was also invited to attend. Himsworth made it clear that he had every intention of taking an active part.[102]

From 1950 to 1970 there was to be a great expansion in the activities of the MRC throughout the country. The budget of the Council increased every year and this, together with the progressive increase in the number of clinical academic departments and full-time staff in the expanding university sector, provided a base for research development that was vital to the exploitation of the new biological sciences in the study of human disease. In that period, the Council founded 82 new Research Units. The Unit for Research on the Molecular Structure of Biological Systems had already been set up in Cambridge in 1947 and was later to develop into the Molecular Biology Research Unit. In 1968, it became the MRC's highly distinguished

[100] Landsborough Thomson, *Medical Research*, Vol. II, p. 24 (see note 75).
[101] MRC A41/1: Parliamentary debates, 14 July 1953; ibid. Appointment of Clinical Research Board: memorandum to MRC, 8 October 1953.
[102] MRC A41/1: Himsworth, interview with Sir John Charles, 6 August 1953.

Laboratory of Molecular Biology. Other units which continued to carry out important work in the basic sciences emerged, but of the 82 newly formed units, as many as 46 were in the clinical field. Many of these units were set up in university departments and directed by university professors. Examples were the Body Temperature Research Unit directed by Sir George Pickering, first at St Mary's Hospital Medical School then at Oxford, the Obstetric Medicine Research Unit under the honorary direction of Sir Dugald Baird in Aberdeen, the Research Unit on Metabolic Disturbances in Surgery under L. M. Pirah in Leeds, and the Abnormal Haemoglobin Research Unit under H. Lehmann at St Bartholomew's Hospital.

These developments might suggest that the MRC had developed a highly satisfactory relationship with the medical schools at that time. In general that was true, but there were still medical schools in London whose commitment to clinical research under the Council was less than whole-hearted. Furthermore, it appeared to clinical members of the Council that there were still insufficient researchers of high quality available to undertake the work required by the Council. In 1955 the Council was concerned about the future of R. T. Grant's Clinical Research Unit at Guy's Hospital with the director due to retire in 1957. Robert Platt wrote to Himsworth from Manchester in October, recommending for the Council's consideration Douglas Black and Bill Stanbury, for both of whom he had a high opinion.[103] Neither candidate was acceptable to the Dean of Guy's, however. A year later, the Council was still seeking a successor to Grant, which apparently depressed Platt. Platt pointed out that none of the applicants for a vacant Chair in Medicine at St Bartholomew's and St Mary's had been considered suitable ('except Peart, who is entirely unknown except as a pharmacologist'), and now it seemed that there was 'nobody suitable even to take charge of a research department'.[104] The problem of recruiting suitable heads for important clinical Units was a recurring theme throughout the Council's history.

It became increasingly clear that Guy's Hospital Medical School was less interested in continuing the MRC's Unit than in creating a new Chair of Experimental Medicine with the help of the University Grants Committee.[105] The MRC also seemed to consider this a satisfactory alternative. A committee of the MRC, set up to consider the matter, recommended: 'The Unit should not be maintained but [that] if an approach was received from Professor G. Payling Wright and Professor R. H. S. Thompson, consideration should be given to including clinical studies in their programme of work on demyelinating diseases at Guy's Hospital supported by the Council.'[106]

[103] MRC D28/32: R. Platt to Himsworth, 7 October 1955.
[104] MRC D28/32: R. Platt to Himsworth, 9 July 1956.
[105] MRC D28/32: E. R. Boland to Himsworth, 12 October 1956.
[106] MRC D28/32: Minutes of MRC, 12 April 1957.

Himsworth had a remarkable capacity, invaluable for an MRC Secretary, to recognize talent and ability. In 1956, W. M. Court-Brown, who had worked at Hammersmith and collaborated with Richard Doll on radiation-induced leukaemia, developed a Group for Research on the General Effects of Radiation at the Western General Hospital in Edinburgh, which later became the MRC Clinical and Population Cytogenetics Unit. There, with P. A. Jacobs and their colleagues, he carried out distinguished work on the relationship between chromosomal abnormalities and human disease and behaviour.[107] Sadly Court-Brown himself died prematurely of coronary heart disease in 1968. The Blood Coagulation Research Unit was established in Oxford at the Churchill Hospital in 1959 under the direction of R. G. MacFarlane, who had worked at both St Bartholomew's Hospital and the newly established Postgraduate Medical School before going to Oxford during the war. His close associate, Rosemary Biggs, recalled his statement during the 1950s: 'If we can see how Factor VIII works, we can measure it; if we can measure it we can make it; if we can make it, we can treat patients.' This reckoning led to the work of the next two decades that introduced effective treatment for haemophilia in the modern era.[108]

Other research, such as into environmental problems, was also undertaken by the MRC. The Air Pollution Research Unit, set up at St Bartholomew's Hospital in 1955 under the direction of P. J. Lawther, was a response to the disastrous London smog of November 1952, when so many died of pulmonary infection. The Unit was to play a major role in ridding London of the traditional winter gloom so beloved of Hollywood. The Atheroma Research Unit was deprived by the premature death of its director in 1965, but the Unit was reconstituted in Glasgow as the Blood Pressure Research Unit, an equally important subject for research. The Rheumatism Research Unit, established in 1958, was an example of a clinical unit which was set up in a non-teaching environment. E. G. L. Bywaters, who returned to work in the Department of Medicine at Hammersmith after the war, moved from renal work to his original research interest, rheumatology. With the assistance of Paul Wood, Tom Cotton, and Sir John Parkinson, he started a Unit for Childhood Rheumatism at the Canadian Red Cross Memorial Hospital at Taplow within the grounds of Cliveden, which he had visited early in the war to give a seminar to the Canadians on Crush Syndrome. The Hospital had been built on the Astor Estate in 1940 for the 5th Canadian Army, and the Canadian Government had left it to the British nation in 1945 for the purpose of research in childhood rheumatism. Rheumatic fever was then a major problem, not only demanding long hospitalization, but also leading to long-

---

[107] MRC *SRS* 305: Court Brown, W. M., *et al.* (1964). *Abnormalities of the sex chromosome complement in man*. HMSO, London.
[108] Biggs, R. (1987). Obituary of R. G. MacFarlane. *Lancet*, i, 932.

standing residual heart disease. The Unit was run from 1947 by a governing body including representatives of the Royal College of Physicians, the Ministry of Health and the University of London. They enlisted help from the Helen Hay Witney Foundation for new laboratories with a promise from the Ministry of Health to provide an equal matching grant, which it ultimately did. The Unit was finally so well established that the MRC agreed to take it over in 1958. So it was that Bywaters again became Director of an MRC Unit. It was successful in establishing an international reputation for work on rheumatic disease in childhood, to which Barbara Ansell made an important contribution. Bywaters also continued to have links with the Postgraduate Medical School, for he had a part-time appointment in the Department of Medicine as Professor of Rheumatology.[109]

During this period other units were created in NHS hospitals. A Social Science Research Unit had been established at the Central Middlesex Hospital under the direction of J. N. Morris in 1948, but the Gastro-enterology Research Unit, established in 1961, was a particularly good example of a unit set up in the environment of a district general hospital. The Central Middlesex Hospital, with support from the MRC, was to play a major role in the encouragement of gastroenterology as a specialty in the post-war era. Francis (later Sir Francis) Avery-Jones had worked on the treatment of haematemesis and melaena with L. J. Witts at St Bartholomew's Hospital before the outbreak of war.[110] During the war, now at Central Middlesex Hospital, he had studied dyspepsia in the staff of local industrial concerns such as the tinned food business Heinz. After the war he decided to investigate the incidence and occupational hazard of peptic ulcer and he obtained an MRC grant for carrying out this work. The MRC suggested that Richard Doll should be his research assistant. Together they produced a detailed report which was published in the MRC Special Report Series.[111]

Following the publication of Doll and Avery-Jones's report in 1951, Himsworth invited Avery-Jones to speak at one of the Council's noon sessions. There Avery-Jones developed the idea that a physiological approach to gastroenterological problems might be appropriate in a centre where there was an abundance of clinical work. The Nuffield Foundation

[109] Personal communication to the author: E. G. L. Bywaters, 16 January 1987.

[110] Witts, L. J. (1937). *British Medical Journal*, i, 847–52.

[111] MRC *SRS* 276: Doll, R. and Avery-Jones, F. (1951). *Occupational factors in the aetiology of gastric and duodenal ulcers with an estimate of their incidence in the general population.* HMSO, London. This was the beginning of a fruitful association, for after Doll joined Bradford Hill's Department of Statistics at the London School of Hygiene and Tropical Medicine in 1947, Avery-Jones gave him responsibility for four beds in his department for the investigation of the methods of treatment of peptic ulcer. Doll established, with the help of detailed and accurate statistical methods, that only bed rest, stopping smoking or the drug carbenoxolone were at that time effective methods of treatment. Their association lasted until Doll was appointed Regius Professor of Medicine at Oxford in succession to Sir George Pickering in 1969: Personal commuication to author: Sir Francis Avery-Jones, November 1986.

had already built a department for gastroenterological investigation for Avery-Jones and the establishment of the MRC Unit in 1961 at the Central Middlesex Hospital took place in the space provided by this development.[112]
E. N. Rowlands, whilst working in Pochin's Unit at UCH, had already created an important working relationship with the gastroenterology department and he was now appointed director. D. A. W. Edwards of Pochin's Unit was also closely involved with this venture.

The initiative for creating a centralized organization for clinical research, as envisaged by Lewis, came from Himsworth himself. As a close colleague of Sir Thomas Lewis, he knew of the 1929 letter to Fletcher but had been unaware of Lewis's 1942 memorandum to Mellanby (see above). Himsworth had been convinced by his own research experience that, with the increasing development of techniques for investigating human disease, a new era was opening for clinical research and that it would make an increasing contribution, not only to the work with the care of patients but also to biomedical science in general. At the end of the Second World War, when still Professor of Medicine at UCH, he had learned with dismay of the decision of the MRC to move its National Institute from Hampstead to a site in Mill Hill surrounded by fields and totally isolated from direct contact with research in the clinical and para-clinical fields. He had at that time urged Mellanby and the then Chief Medical Officer of the Department of Health, Sir Wilson Jameson, both of whom he knew well from wartime work, to transfer the still unopened building at Mill Hill to the Agricultural Research Council, which was then needing a central institute, and instead to rebuild the NIMR alongside a good non-teaching hospital such as the Central Middlesex. Both Mellanby and Jameson were against the idea. Even if it had at that time been desirable, the building industry was at full stretch repairing bomb damage. Materials such as steel were in short supply and finance was difficult, so that by 1949, when Himsworth became the MRC's Secretary, he had abandoned any hope for a central institute for clinical research and he looked to individual Research Units to cover the Council's needs in the clinical field. By the mid-1950s, however, experience with the working of MRC Units was beginning to raise increasing doubts in his mind whether these, although admirable for many purposes, would in themselves enable the Council to respond sufficiently to the developing situation in the clinical and para-clinical fields. Clinical research was multidisciplinary, but being guests in other people's houses limited the MRC's freedom. Furthermore, a Unit concerned with rheumatic disease, for example, was having to make do with a newly qualified PhD to meet its need for major biochemistry. In theory, such a Unit should be able to obtain ancillary support from the academic departments of the host institution, but unlike the Heads of Departments in an Institute, as for example at NIMR, the heads of University Units were under no obligation to provide this. Moreover, although the Council was always careful when setting up a Unit to site it at a place where relevant work was in progress in the surrounding departments, the Heads of these might change and their successors might well have quite different research interests.[113]

So the idea of a clinical research institute began to be reconsidered by Himsworth and he was supported by the views of the Chairman of the Clinical Research Board, Sir Geoffrey Jefferson. A Committee composed of clinical and para-clinical members of the Council was set up to review the MRC's provision for research in the clinical field and to make recommendations. At the outset, the Committee doubted whether any change in the existing arrangements was required, but it took exhaustive evidence from Unit directors and finally recommended unanimously that there were compelling reasons for setting up an institute in which an adequate concentration of clinical and para-clinical research groups was brought together on one site, in association with a district general hospital. It was this report that formed the basis of the Council's submission to the Government in 1959.[114] With the warm support of Lord Hailsham, Minister for Science, the concurrence of the Minister of Health, and the provisional support of the Secretary of State for Scotland (who expressed the view, routinely expected of all Scottish Ministers, that any further institute of this kind should be set up north of the border), the plan was approved in principle.

The decision that the proposed centre should be associated with a non-teaching rather than a teaching hospital was made on the grounds that it would be difficult to have two bodies deciding research policy and competing for beds on one site. In the early days of the NHS, the teaching hospitals still sheltered behind powerful Boards of Governors and were effectively administered separately from the remainder of the Health Service. The decision by the MRC, then thought by some to be too much oriented to basic science, to link its clinical research centre with the work of a district hospital comprehensively serving a defined community, was particularly welcomed by the Department of Health.

At first, thought was given to siting the projected centre at Chase Farm or at the Central Middlesex Hospital, but Sir John Charles, Chief Medical Officer at the Department of Health, pointed out that the North West Metropolitan Regional Hospital Board, as it then was, was intending to build a new district hospital at Northwick Park near Harrow, since there were no effective hospital services in that area of outer London. The opportunity was

[113] Booth, C. C. (1986). *Quarterly Journal of Medicine*, **59**, 435–47.
[114] MRC 59/245: Clinical Research Centre Archives, 'Organisation of medical research: proposed new Clinical Research Centre'.

therefore seized to build the new Clinical Research Centre at the same time as the district hospital and both the architectural design and the organization of the Northwick Park site were to integrate the hospital and the centre as a single unit.

John Squire, pupil of Sir Thomas Lewis and well known to Himsworth and the MRC as a Unit Director, was appointed the first Director of the projected Centre. Squire differed from his mentor, Lewis, in that his interest lay primarily in long-term planning, organization and administration, and unlike Lewis, he was numerate, liking to 'turn in a page or two of integral calculus in his reports' and with a love for gadgets.[115] Squire applied himself with enthusiasm and dynamic energy to the problems of recruiting staff and designing the research centre, integrating its laboratories and wards effectively with the planning phases of the district general hospital. It was a herculean task carried out whilst he continued his departmental work in the University of Birmingham. However, in January 1966, during a visit to London, Squire, a heavy smoker, developed angina, and tragically died shortly after the age of 52.[116] No single person with Squire's leadership qualities could be found to replace him, and the Council decided to appoint a director and deputy director jointly as successors. G. M. (later Sir Graham) Bull was appointed as director, and Richard Doll, who was to have directed an Epidemiology and Health Care Unit at Northwick Park, was appointed as his deputy. Bull had spent the early years of his research career at Hammersmith where he had succeeded Bywaters in studies of acute renal failure. With Joekes and Lowe, he had developed the conservative method of treatment associated with his name. Later he had been Professor of Medicine in Belfast. Until Doll's appointment as Regius Professor of Medicine in Oxford, they worked on planning and recruitment together.

It was clear from the start that Northwick Park Hospital was to be entirely different from Hammersmith and other teaching centres in London. Whereas Hammersmith had built up an excellent reputation as a tertiary referral centre through the years and was providing first-class training at postgraduate level, as were many of the London teaching hospitals, the work of the Clinical Research Centre was to be oriented to the study of those diseases which formed the bulk of the work of a district general hospital. At the same time it was to develop a national role in the encouragement of clinical research. Sir Thomas Lewis, in his 1929 memorandum to the MRC, had stated that the research workers in his projected institute should be 'free from the distractions presented by the petty and mainly diagnostic problems of disease in obscure cases and in which they can settle down to a more profound and uninterrupted study of the natural history of selected

---

[115] Personal communication to the author: N. B. Myant, 22 December 1986.
[116] Obituary, *Lancet* (1966), i, 157.

diseases'.[117] The Northwick Park model, with its district hospital providing an excellent service to the community and with 160 extra beds provided by the Health Authorities for research, was to give the research staff precisely that opportunity.

Sir Harold Himsworth retired from the secretaryship in 1968 at a time of great optimism for the future of clinical research in this country. The Clinical Research Centre was formally opened in 1970 by Her Majesty the Queen, in the presence of Sir Harold and the then Secretary of State for Education and Science, Margaret Thatcher. The Bishop of Willesden gave spiritual support. The Postgraduate Medical School had by now become Royal and was described by the historian Noel Poynter as 'an example of what can be achieved when the restrictions imposed by tradition and vested interest are loosened. This institution with its brilliant record has been of tremendous value in radically changing the attitudes of British doctors to medical education and the way it should be organised'.[118] In the universities throughout the country there were well-found departments in the clinical field staffed by men and women with a full-time commitment to teaching and research. The old rivalries between full-time academics and part-time staff had largely disappeared and in the best schools part-time staff were developing their own laboratories and research programmes. It was a reflection of the amount of money available in those heady days that the MRC had been able to set up a series of research groups in the universities, the resources being provided by the MRC for an initial five year period with a guarantee by the University Grants Committee to provide funds for complete takeover of the Group at the end of that time. In the half century since Lewis had established his pioneering research department at UCH, and the universities had begun to create full-time chairs in medicine and surgery, so much had been achieved. The credit for a great deal of that achievement is due to the MRC.

Acknowledgements

I am grateful to many friends and colleagues who have responded to my enquiries about the Medical Research Council's endeavours in the field of clinical research. I owe a particular debt to the following: Sir Christopher Andrewes, Sir Melville Arnott, Dr Rosemary Biggs, Dr E. G. L. Bywaters, Sir Richard Doll, Sir John Butterfield, Dr C. M. Fletcher, Dr R. T. Grant, Sir Charles Stuart Harris, Dr Sheila Howarth (Lady McMichael), Sir Francis

---

[117] MRC 2011 (2): Lewis to Fletcher, 31 May 1929.
[118] Poynter, F. N. L. (1970). Medical education in England since 1600. In *The history of medical education* (ed. C. D. O'Malley), pp. 235–50. University of California Press, Los Angeles. pp. 235–50.

Avery Jones, Professor J. N. Morris, Dr N. B. Myant, Sir Edward Pochin, Dr E. N. Rowlands, and Professor R. S. F. Schilling. I also thank Miss Mary Nicholas for her guidance through the labyrinth of the archives of the Medical Research Council. Some of the data included in this chapter was included in a paper on Clinical Research and the MRC, previously published in the *Quarterly Journal of Medicine* (1986, **59**, 435–47) and I am grateful to the Editor for permission to use this material. As I acknowledged in that paper, I am also particularly indebted to Sir Harold Himsworth for his account of the considerations that weighed with the Council in the decision to set up the Clinical Research Centre.

Index

Errors

cf. Bond (206) .   p. 59

? 46 ?

p 53 — Dunn School, 1915 ?

Steve Sturdy

Wellcome Unit for the
History of Medicine

Manchester University

April 1990.

Dryden — of his Life — what is going on over
    version & Heteronymia?

Author — job of excessively unobtrusive view of
    'pure' & 'applied' distinction — though generally
    useful — but how idiosyncratic & slobbly?

A & B — survey & review — little analysis.